INTERFERON

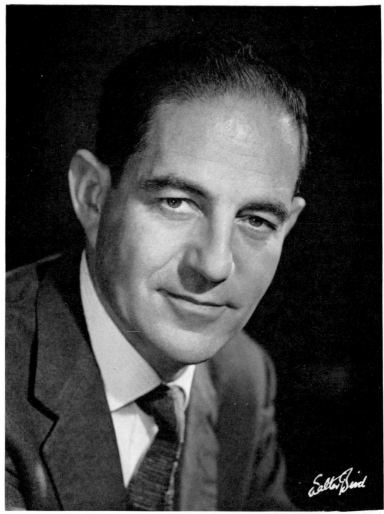

ALICK ISAACS, 1921–1967

INTERFERON

Ciba Foundation Symposium
Dedicated to Alick Isaacs, F.R.S.

Edited by
G. E. W. WOLSTENHOLME
and
MAEVE O'CONNOR

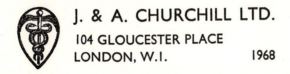

J. & A. CHURCHILL LTD.
104 GLOUCESTER PLACE
LONDON, W.I.   1968

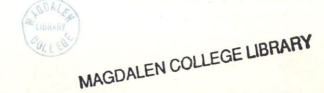

First published 1967

Containing 54 illustrations

Standard Book Number 7000 1339 3

The Ciba Foundation

The Ciba Foundation was opened in 1949 to promote international co-operation in medical and chemical research among scientists from all parts of the world. Its house at 41 Portland Place, London, has become a meeting place well known to workers in many fields of science. Every year the Foundation organizes from six to ten three-day symposia and three or four one-day study groups, all of which are published in book form. Many other informal meetings are held in the house, organized either by the Foundation or by other scientific groups needing a place to meet. In addition, bedrooms are available for scientists visiting London, whether or not they are attending a meeting in the building.

The Ciba Foundation owes its existence to the generosity of CIBA Ltd, Basle, who, realising the disruption of scientific communication caused by the war and by problems of distance, decided to set up a philanthropic institution whose aim would be to overcome such barriers. London was chosen as its site for reasons dictated by the special advantages of English charitable trust law (ensuring the independence of its actions), as well as those of language and geography.

The Foundation's many activities are controlled by a small group of distinguished trustees. Within the general framework of biological science, interpreted in its broadest sense, these activities are well summed up by the Ciba Foundation's motto, *Consocient Gentes*—let the nations come together.

Contents

CONTENTS

Membership

1*

E. Mécs Institute of Microbiology, Medical University, Szeged

T. C. Merigan Division of Infectious Diseases, Stanford University School of Medicine, Palo Alto, California

H. G. Pereira WHO World Influenza Centre, National Institute for Medical Research, London

Z. Rotem Scientific Counsellor, Embassy of Israel; and National Institute for Medical Research, London

J. A. Sonnabend National Institute for Medical Research, London

M. G. P. Stoker Institute of Virology, University of Glasgow

D. A. J. Tyrrell Common Cold Research Unit, Harvard Hospital, Salisbury

R. R. Wagner The University of Virginia, Charlottesville, Virginia

Preface

IN his opening remarks here, Michael Stoker speaks of the remarkable way in which Alick Isaacs, in his short and brilliant life, was responsible for so much of the research and inspiration which formed the background to this meeting. It had earlier been a disappointment to us at the Ciba Foundation when Alick Isaacs had been too ill to take part in a conference on Myxoviruses in 1964; when his health improved and he suggested a symposium on Interferon, we seized the chance of marking the tenth anniversary of its discovery, when we could pay tribute to work of such importance done almost on our doorstep, at a time when the development of interferon seemed full of fresh promise.

Alick joined enthusiastically in the detailed organization of the symposium, but sadly it soon became obvious that he would not be fit to play a full leading role in it, and his death came just when the preparations were complete.

This symposium is therefore a gesture of thankfulness to Alick Isaacs both for his work and his friendship. The tribute to him will be all the more meaningful if these papers and discussions awaken in even one reader ideas for further development in this field of research.

We are most grateful to all who have contributed to this occasion, in particular to Michael Stoker for his appropriately friendly chairmanship, and to Joseph Sonnabend for his generous and expert help in editing the discussions.

CHAIRMAN'S OPENING REMARKS

M. G. P. STOKER

We are here to discuss interferon, and the one person who is missing is the person who is most responsible for bringing us together. We would not be here if Dr. Alick Isaacs and Dr. Lindenmann had not discovered interferon. We would not be here if Dr. Isaacs, with Dr. Wolstenholme and the Executive Council of the Ciba Foundation, had not initiated this particular symposium. Alick Isaacs died early this year, and the shock was particularly great to those of us who are here. It is appropriate, and certainly our wish, that the symposium and the book should be dedicated to him.

Dr. Isaacs' career and contribution to science have been, and are still being, reviewed by others much more competent than I am. In particular, Sir Christopher Andrewes is preparing an authoritative obituary which will be published by the Royal Society. I am certainly not going to review the history of interferon in detail before a company of acknowledged experts in this field—and I include amongst the acknowledged experts Dr. Sue Isaacs. Although pre-eminent in her own field, she must know more about interferon than a great many virologists. We are very happy that she is with us on this occasion at the beginning of the meeting, and that she will also be with us on some subsequent occasions during the next few days.

Even if interferon had never been discovered, Dr. Isaacs would still be remembered as a very eminent virologist: his work, which he continued for over twenty years with the utmost vigour, gave him a very considerable reputation. This particularly applies to his studies on influenza virus in all its aspects, from epidemiology to virus structure. But the supreme event in his scientific life was the publication of two papers, one with Dr. J. Lindenmann (1957. *Proc. R. Soc. B*, **147**, 258) and the other with Dr. Lindenmann and Dr. R. C. Valentine (1957. *Proc. R. Soc. B*, **147**, 268). It falls to very few of us to make a single outstanding contribution which has such a tremendous repercussion over many years and which leads to innumerable meetings, books, and not least to a Ciba Foundation symposium ten years later.

I first heard about interferon in a pub near University College which I am sure is familiar to many of us—it ought to be called "The Grapevine":

I

Dr. Isaacs and I went there as usual after a meeting; he was obviously excited and out came the idea of interferon. A lot of very interesting scientific gossip may be heard in that particular pub, but I suppose this was the most important thing I ever heard there.

After the original discovery and publication, he threw himself with typical and enormous energy into both the practical and theoretical aspects of the subject, and did indeed lay much of the ground work for what was to follow. The idea of interferon immediately had great appeal, not only amongst medical people, who saw it as a possible therapeutic weapon, but also amongst virologists who were concerned with basic aspects of virus-cell interaction; despite this appeal, however, it was not taken up experimentally in many other laboratories outside Mill Hill for several years. In fact there were centres where the whole idea was criticized and regarded rather cynically. Many of us will remember the word "misinterpreton" which was circulating. It is true, of course, that some of Dr. Isaacs' theories and ideas have subsequently turned out to be wrong, as happens to all of us. We know now that some of his observations were due to impurities in early preparations, and now it is much easier to interpret things. But the basic idea was not wrong: it was not "misinterpreton". He had enormous faith in interferon, and his enthusiasm and faith kept it going in the two or three, perhaps rather lonely, years when it was being criticized and not taken up very widely. Eventually, of course others entered the game with equal enthusiasm. This has led in the last few years to the second phase of interest in interferon, with tentative interpretation of its production and action in the context of modern molecular biology. If Alick Isaacs had not kept the project going during the early period, however, there might have been a very long delay before this second expansion of investigation took place, and I feel that he should be remembered for this as well as the original observation.

You will perhaps wonder why I am here as chairman. There are two kinds of chairman. One is the authoritative figure who knows the contents of every paper in advance, who knows who is going to ask what question in the discussion and what the answer is going to be; this is the paternalistic type of chairman. I am the other sort: indeed I must be one of the few virologists who has never published a paper on interferon. In fact I did once do some work on interferon, and was about to post an article to a journal, but on re-reading it I decided that the subject was much to difficult and complicated. So I tore it up—it is the only paper I have destroyed at that stage.

Dr. Isaacs is responsible for my being chairman, and I suspect he knew in his kindly way that amongst his colleagues and friends, I was the one who most needed educating. He was absolutely right, and I am going to enjoy being educated by you all during the coming three days.

Finally, may I remind you of Alick Isaacs' main characteristic—his joyful and bubbling enthusiasm, described very movingly by Dr. John Humphrey at the memorial ceremony. If this meeting is to be dedicated to Alick Isaacs it would be no service to him if we made it a funereal and mournful occasion. On the contrary we should proceed with the light-hearted enthusiasm which he himself would have shown.

CELLULAR EVENTS PRECEDING INTERFERON FORMATION

D. C. BURKE, J. J. SKEHEL, A. J. HAY AND SHAN WALTERS

Department of Biological Chemistry, Marischal College,
University of Aberdeen

VIRUS-INDUCED interferon formation may be represented as follows (Fig. 1). The virus, which may be either infective or inactivated, invades

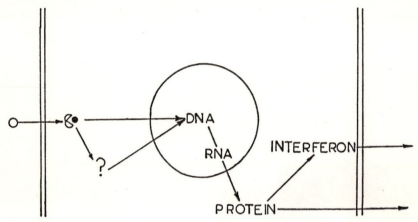

FIG. 1. A hypothetical scheme for interferon production.

the cell and presumably uncoats, although we do not know whether uncoating is necessary or not. Then some virus component, or some product of the virus-cell interaction, proceeds to the nucleus and there initiates, by a process similar to derepression, the formation of an interferon messenger RNA. This RNA then codes for the protein interferon, or possibly for a precursor of interferon. This scheme is no more than a working hypothesis, but it does accommodate all the available evidence, and provides a framework for the interpretation of results.

THE NATURE OF THE INTERFERON INDUCER

What component of the virus is responsible for the induction of interferon formation—the virus protein, virus nucleic acid, or some other component or combination of components? The inducer is more stable to heat and ultraviolet irradiation than virus infectivity, since non–infective viruses which can still induce interferon formation can readily be prepared. However the ability of several myxoviruses to produce interferon is destroyed by increased ultraviolet irradiation; therefore it is likely that the inducer absorbs ultraviolet light, and is probably protein or nucleic acid. The production of low titres of inhibitory material by treatment of cells with nucleic acids led Isaacs (1963) to the concept of "foreign nucleic acid" as the inducer for interferon formation. However the inhibitory material was never fully characterized, and other workers have found it difficult to repeat these observations. It is possible that this inhibitory material is similar to the preformed material released after treatment of animals with bacterial endotoxin.

We have made two attempts to identify the nature of the interferon inducer. The first approach was to see whether isolated virus nucleic acid

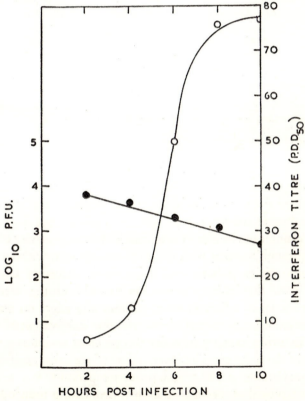

FIG. 2. The production of virus (—●—●—) and interferon (—○—○—) when chick cells were incubated at 42° after infection with SFV for 1 hr. at 37°.

would induce interferon formation. In order to obtain an unequivocal answer it was necessary to use a biological system in which interferon but not virus protein was formed. Infection of chick embryo cells with Semliki Forest virus (SFV) at 37° C, followed by incubation at 42°, was satisfactory for this purpose, since at 42° interferon but not virus was formed (Fig. 2), and we have been unable to detect any virus-induced protein synthesis at 42° (see below). SFV readily yielded an infective nucleic acid (Cheng, 1958) and it was thus possible to obtain an undegraded nucleic acid from a virus capable of inducing interferon formation. However a high virus multiplicity was necessary in order to obtain maximum interferon yields (Table I), and this meant that very large amounts of

TABLE I

EFFECT OF VIRUS MULTIPLICITY ON VIRUS AND INTERFERON YIELD

Multiplicity of exposure (p.f.u. SFV/cell)	Virus yield per culture ($\log_{10}$/p.f.u.)	Interferon yield per culture (PDD_{50})
$3 \cdot 6 \times 10^2$	8·88	84
$1 \cdot 2 \times 10^2$	8·55	98
$4 \cdot 0 \times 10^1$	8·66	40
$1 \cdot 3 \times 10^1$	8·38	30
4·5	8·50	12
1·5	8·50	4

Chick cells (7×10^6) were infected with varying multiplicities of partially purified SFV for 1 hour at 37°. Virus was harvested after 8 hours at 37°, and interferon after 12 hours at 42°.
p.f.u.: plaque-forming units.
PDD_{50}: plaque-depressing doses.

infective virus nucleic acid would have to be prepared. In addition, the high molarity salt treatment, needed to force virus nucleic acid into the cells, depressed the virus-induced interferon response, and it was decided to attempt another approach.

Hydroxylamine has been shown to inactivate the infectivity of a number of viruses through reaction with the virus nucleic acid, without any effect on viral antigenicity (Schafer and Rott, 1962). Recently Grossgebauer (1966) has found that hydroxylamine inactivated both the infectivity and interfering ability of influenza virus without any effect on antigenicity. We have examined the effect of hydroxylamine inactivation of SFV on its interferon-inducing capacity in order to obtain more information about the nature of the inducer. The inactivation of partially purified SFV by 0·2 M-hydroxylamine at pH 7 and room temperature was a first-order reaction, in a typical experiment, the virus titre falling four $\log_{10}$ units in five hours (Fig. 3). Samples of virus were removed after inactivation for varying times, and after dialysis they were examined for their ability to

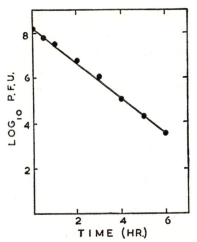

FIG. 3. Inactivation of SFV by 0·2M-
hydroxylamine.

produce infectious virus, virus haemagglutinin, virus-induced RNA
synthesis (Taylor, 1965) and virus-induced RNA polymerase (Martin and
Sonnabend, 1967). There was no effect of hydroxylamine inactivation
until the multiplicity of infection fell below one, when all these virus-
induced properties were inactivated with first-order kinetics (Fig. 4).

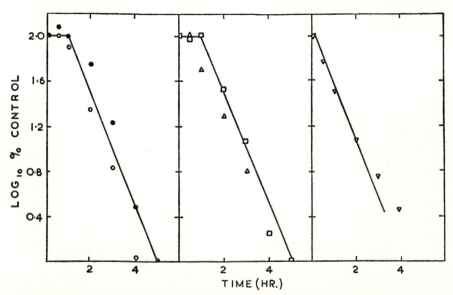

FIG. 4. The production of infectious virus (—●—●—), virus haemagglutinin (—○—○—),
virus-induced RNA synthesis (—□—□—), virus-induced RNA polymerase (—△—△—),
and interferon (—▽—▽—) by SFV inactivated for different times with 0·2M-hydroxylamine.

The inactivated virus samples were also examined for their interferon-inducing capacity by incubation of cells at 42° after infection at 37°. The interferon-producing capacity was inactivated by hydroxylamine at the same rate as that of the other virus-induced properties, suggesting that complete virus nucleic acid is essential for induction of interferon production by this virus.

EARLY STAGES IN INTERFERON FORMATION

In a number of systems virus multiplication and interferon production proceed concomitantly, although either one may be selectively inhibited in various ways. If both processes depend on intact virus nucleic acid for initiation, how much do the two processes have in common? Are some of the early stages of virus multiplication also necessary for interferon formation, and if so, which stages? We have looked for evidence of involvement of the early stages of virus multiplication in interferon production by SFV at 42°.

Viral nucleic acid synthesis is readily detected by treating the cells with actinomycin and pulsing with radioactive uridine (Taylor, 1965), and we have used this method to look for viral nucleic acid synthesis early in interferon production. The treatment with actinomycin inhibited subsequent interferon formation, but it was assumed that any necessary viral nucleic acid synthesis occurred before the actinomycin-sensitive step

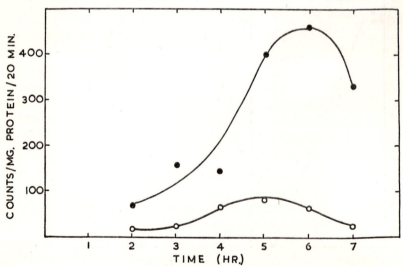

FIG. 5. Production of virus-induced RNA polymerase when chick cells were incubated at 37° (—●—●—) or 42° (—○—○—) after infection with SFV for 1 hr. at 37°. The enzyme was assayed at 37° essentially as described by Martin and Sonnabend (1967).

in interferon production. No viral nucleic acid synthesis could be detected and it was concluded that viral nucleic acid synthesis was unnecessary for interferon production (Burke, Skehel and Low, 1967).

A stage prior to viral nucleic acid formation is the formation of the virus-induced RNA polymerase. This protein appears to be the first virus-coded property to be expressed. We therefore looked for virus-induced RNA polymerase in SFV-infected cells at 37° and at 42°. Fig 5 shows that polymerase was detectable when the cells were incubated at 37° but not at 42°, and therefore this polymerase is not necessary for interferon formation. The failure to find polymerase at 42° could be due to inhibition of either its formation or its action by incubation at the increased temperature, since polymerase formation is autocatalytic. However, the polymerase formed at 37° was active when assayed at 42°, suggesting that the enzyme is not *formed* at 42°. The product formed by this enzyme is predominantly double-stranded RNA (Martin and Sonnabend, 1967), and if two polymerases are involved in virus RNA replication, it is probably the first to be formed. Thus the pathways that lead to virus multiplication and interferon production part very early after infection—at least before formation of the polymerase.

It was possible that other virus-coded proteins were formed as an early stage of interferon formation, and a search was made for these, using radioisotopes. No stimulation of the rate of protein synthesis could be detected after infection of chick cells with SFV at 37° and only a small stimulation was detectable when actinomycin-treated cells were used (the inhibitor was added to depress host-cell protein synthesis). This was presumably because viral protein synthesis represented only a small portion of the total protein synthesis. However the synthesis of virus-induced proteins could be detected by fractionation of the proteins by polyacryl-amide gel electrophoresis (Summers, Maizel and Darnell, 1965). SFV-infected cells were pulse-labelled with [^{3}H]valine and control cells with [^{14}C]valine at intervals after infection. The harvested cells were mixed and fractionated by polyacrylamide gel electrophoresis. Measurement of the [^{3}H]/[^{14}C] ratio revealed the presence of several virus-coded proteins, two of which have been identified as components of the virus coat protein (Fig. 6). In this system, mobility is governed largely by molecular size, and the fast-moving components around fraction 60 are probably incomplete polypeptide chains. The other components have not yet been identified. When cells were incubated at 42° after infection, none of these proteins could be detected and we concluded that the formation of virus-coded proteins was not essential for interferon production.

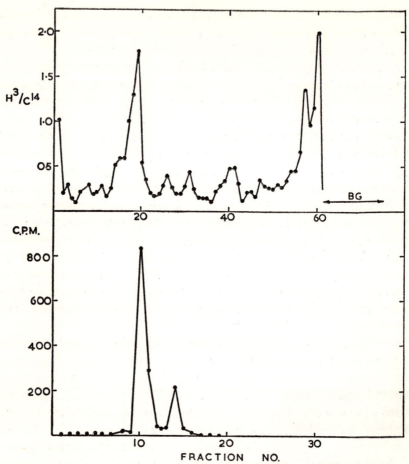

Fig. 6. (a) Production of virus-induced proteins in SFV-infected cells. Chick cells were treated for 4 hr. at 37° with 0·5 μg./ml. of actinomycin, infected with SFV for 1 hr. at 37°, and then incubated at 37°. Isotope was added at hourly intervals for 8 hr.; the figure shows the result obtained when it was present from 6 to 7 hr. after infection (BG=background counting rate).
(b) Proteins from SFV. The virus was grown in actinomycin-treated cells in the presence of [³H]valine, purified as described by Cheng (1961), and the proteins extracted and fractionated as in (a).

SYNTHESIS OF THE INTERFERON MESSENGER RNA

The inhibition of interferon production by actinomycin (Heller, 1963) suggests that the formation of the messenger RNA for interferon synthesis is directed by cellular DNA rather than by the virus nucleic acid. This interpretation accounts for the frequent observations of the species specificity of interferon (Lockart, 1966), and the induction of an apparently identical interferon by either a DNA or an RNA virus (Lampson *et al.*,

1965), but it assumes that actinomycin inhibits interferon production by acting solely as an inhibitor of DNA-dependent RNA synthesis. Actinomycin, however, exerts a number of other effects, including inhibition of DNA synthesis (Baserga *et al.*, 1965), inhibition of RNA transfer from the nucleus to the cytoplasm (Levy, 1963), and inhibition of protein synthesis by a process reversible by glucose (Honig and Rabinowitz, 1966). It has been claimed to cause breakdown of messenger RNA (Wiesner *et al.*, 1965), although the interpretation of the results which led to this conclusion has been challenged (Chantrenne, 1965). It seemed important to establish that actinomycin inhibited interferon formation because of its primary effect rather than because of some secondary effect, and we therefore investigated the effect of actinomycin and of two other inhibitors of RNA synthesis on interferon production initiated by three different viruses.

The other inhibitors were 4,5,6-trichloro-1β-D-ribofuranosyl benzimidazole (TRB) and 2-mercapto-1-(β-4-pyridethyl) benzimidazole (MPB). Both compounds exerted their primary effect on RNA synthesis, although there was also some depression of DNA and of protein synthesis (Walters, Burke and Skehel, 1967). In addition, MPB caused an immediate and competitive inhibition of nucleoside phosphorylation, probably due to inhibition of the nucleoside kinase (Skehel *et al.*, 1967). Viruses which are sensitive to actinomycin (fowl plague and influenza viruses) were more sensitive to the effect of both MPB and TRB than were viruses insensitive to actinomycin (Newcastle disease, parainfluenza 1 and Semliki Forest viruses). The similarity of the antiviral spectrum to that of actinomycin suggested that MPB and TRB were possibly acting as preferential inhibitors of DNA-directed RNA synthesis. However it is unlikely that the substituted benzimidazoles were acting in exactly the same way as actinomycin, since their structures are so different. Results obtained with cell-free systems support this suggestion since DNA-directed RNA synthesis was much more sensitive to MPB than was DNA-directed DNA synthesis or RNA-directed RNA synthesis (Keir and Burke, unpublished; Martin, unpublished).

Actinomycin, TRB and MPB inhibited interferon production induced by Chikungunya virus, ultraviolet-irradiated Newcastle disease virus (u.v.-NDV) or ultraviolet-irradiated influenza virus (u.v.-MEL) at doses where their principal effect was on RNA synthesis. The structures of these compounds are so different that they are unlikely to inhibit interferon production by a common secondary process, and we concluded that DNA-directed RNA synthesis is essential for interferon production.

Several workers (Wagner, 1964; Wagner and Huang, 1966; Levy, Axelrod and Baron, 1965; Ho and Breinig, 1965) have added actinomycin during the course of interferon formation in order to obtain data about the time of formation and the stability of the interferon messenger RNA. Interpretation assumes that the production of interferon messenger RNA is the rate-limiting process for interferon synthesis, and that actinomycin has no effect on the stability of the messenger RNA. Their results indicated that synthesis of a stable messenger RNA was complete shortly after infection. Addition of actinomycin or MPB to the Chikungunya virus-induced system gave similar results (Table II), addition one hour after infection

TABLE II

EFFECT OF ADDITION OF ACTINOMYCIN AND MPB ON INTERFERON PRODUCTION BY CHIKUNGUNYA VIRUS

Time of addition of inhibitor (hr.)	Titre at time of addition (PDD_{50})	Interferon yield between time of addition and 9 hr. after addition (PDD_{50})		
		Control	Actinomycin (0·5 µg./ml.)	MPB (50 µg./ml.)
0	0	113	<2	22
1	2	75	14	25
3	25	54	52	53
4	37	56	55	57
5	58	48	50	44
7	81	40	39	32

causing substantial inhibition of interferon production but addition three hours after infection having no effect. However when u.v.-NDV was used as an inducer, interferon formation did not become insensitive to the effects of actinomycin and MPB until 12 to 15 hours after infection (Table III). In both cases the inhibitors ceased to be effective shortly after the end

TABLE III

EFFECT OF ADDITION OF ACTINOMYCIN AND MPB ON INTERFERON PRODUCTION INDUCED BY u.v.-NDV

Time of addition of inhibitor (hr.)	Titre at time of addition (PDD_{50})	Interferon yield between time of addition and 48 hr. post-infection (PDD_{50})		
		Control	Actinomycin (0·5 µg./ml.)	MPB (50 µg./ml.)
0	0	130	3	4
8	12	81	10	12
12	25	63	25	32
16	90	52	50	50
20	103	44	44	38

of the lag period, indicating that formation of the interferon messenger RNA was the last stage in the lag period, whatever its length. In both cases the messenger RNA was stable for at least six hours. However, in the ultraviolet-irradiated influenza-virus-induced system, interferon production remained sensitive to the effects of actinomycin and TRB throughout the period of production, the messenger RNA having a half-life of about two to four hours (Table IV). The reason for this difference is not known;

TABLE IV

EFFECT OF ADDITION OF ACTINOMYCIN AND TRB DURING INTERFERON FORMATION INDUCED BY U.V.-MEL

		Interferon yield between time of addition and 47 hr. after infection (PDD_{50})			
			Actinomycin		
Time of addition of inhibitor (hr.)	Titre at time of addition (PDD_{50})	Control	(0·5 µg./ml.)	(0·06 µg./ml.)	TRB (10 mM)
0	0	210	<2	<2	16
18	76	140	34	34	60
22	104	84	26	26	48
26	128	56	26	26	30
30	152	37	18	21	23
35	181	26	21	18	30

it may be significant that influenza is the only actinomycin-sensitive virus that has been used for interferon production, and it is possible that the stability of the interferon messenger RNA may be dependent in some way on an early stage of virus infection, which in this case is actinomycin-sensitive.

An attempt to demonstrate the formation of the interferon messenger RNA was made, using the Chikungunya virus-induced system at 42° (Burke and Walters, 1966). Interferon-producing cells were labelled for 40 minutes with [^{3}H]uridine at hourly intervals for five hours after infection, while control cells received [^{14}C]uridine under similar conditions. The cells were mixed and successively extracted with phenol at 2°, and with phenol plus 0·5 per cent sodium dodecyl sulphate at 50°. The former extracted mainly cytoplasmic RNA (Fenwick, 1964), while the latter extract consisted mainly of rapidly labelled ribosomal RNA precursor found in the nucleus (Scherrer, Latham and Darnell, 1963). The extracts were centrifuged at 20,000 rev./min. for 16 hours on gradients of 5 to 25 per cent sucrose. Appearance of a new RNA in the interferon-producing cells would have increased the ratio of [^{3}H]/[^{14}C], but no rise could be detected. However we do not know how sensitive this method is, and it is very likely that the amount of interferon messenger RNA is below the limit of detection. A similar attempt to detect new protein formation in interferon-producing cells was made by labelling interferon-producing cells with [^{3}H]valine and control cells with [^{14}C]valine. The cells were mixed and the extracted proteins fractionated by a polyacrylamide gel electrophoresis. Again no increase in [^{3}H]/[^{14}C] could be detected. These failures are not too surprising in view of the very high biological activity of interferon, which is at least 10^6 units/mg. protein (Fantes, 1967). The cells were producing about 45 units of interferon per hour or only about 0·05 μg. of interferon per hour. However it was possible that other proteins, as well as interferon, were produced after treatment with virus. If this was so, we were unable to detect them.

SUMMARY

Results obtained by use of Semliki Forest virus partially inactivated with hydroxylamine suggest that the complete virus nucleic acid is essential for induction of interferon formation. The pathways leading to virus production and interferon formation appear to part shortly after infection since neither virus-directed protein nor nucleic acid synthesis are necessary for interferon formation. Three inhibitors of DNA-directed RNA synthesis inhibited interferon production, showing that such synthesis was a necessary stage in interferon formation. The interferon messenger RNA was stable in two virus-induced systems but not in a third. An attempt to detect the formation of the interferon messenger RNA directly was not successful.

REFERENCES

BASERGA, R., ESTENSEN, R. D., PETERSON, R. O., and LAYDE, J. P. (1965). *Proc. natn. Acad. Sci. U.S.A.*, **54**, 745–751.

BURKE, D. C., SKEHEL, J. J., and LOW, M. (1967). *J. gen. Virol.*, **1**, 235–237.

BURKE, D. C., and WALTERS, S. (1966). *Biochem. J.*, **101**, 25–26 P.

CHANTRENNE, H. (1965). *Biochim. biophys. Acta*, **95**, 351–353.

CHENG, P. Y. (1958). *Nature, Lond.*, **181**, 1800.

CHENG, P. Y. (1961). *Virology*, **14**, 124–131.

FANTES, K. H. (1967). *J. gen. Virol.*, **1**, 257–267.

FENWICK, M. L. (1964). *Biochim. biophys. Acta*, **87**, 388–396.

GROSSGEBAUER, K. (1966). *Z. Naturf.*, **21b**, 1063–1072.

HELLER, E. (1963). *Virology*, **21**, 652–656.

HO, M., and BREINIG, M. (1965). *Virology*, **25**, 331–339.

HONIG, G. R., and RABINOWITZ, M. (1966). *J. biol. Chem.*, **241**, 1681–1687.

ISAACS, A. (1963). *Nature, Lond.*, **197**, 564–566.

LAMPSON, G. P., TYTELL, A. A., NEMES, M. M., and HILLEMAN, M. R. (1965). *Proc. Soc. exp. Biol. Med.*, **118**, 441–448.

LEVY, H. B. (1963). *Proc. Soc. exp. Biol. Med.*, **113**, 886–889.

LEVY, H. B., AXELROD, D., and BARON, S. (1965). *Proc. Soc. exp. Biol. Med.*, **118**, 384–385.

LOCKART, R. Z. (1966). In *Interferons*, pp. 1–20, ed. Finter, N. B. Amsterdam: North-Holland Publishing Co.

MARTIN, E. M., and SONNABEND, J. A. (1967). *J. gen. Virol.*, **1**, 97–109.

SCHAFER, W., and ROTT, R. (1962). *Z. Hyg. InfektKrankh.*, **148**, 256–269.

SCHERRER, K., LATHAM, H., and DARNELL, J. E. (1963). *Proc. natn. Acad. Sci. U.S.A.*, **49**, 240–248.

SKEHEL, J. J., HAY, A. J., BURKE, D. C., and CARTWRIGHT, L. N. (1967). *Biochim. biophys. Acta*, **142**, 430–439.

Summers, D. F., Maizel, J. V., Jr., and Darnell, J. E., Jr. (1965). *Proc. natn. Acad. Sci. U.S.A.*, **54,** 505–513.

Taylor, J. (1965). *Virology*, **25**, 340–349.

Wagner, R. R. (1964). *Nature, Lond.*, **204**, 49–51.

Wagner, R. R., and Huang, A. S. (1966). *Virology*, **28**, 1–10.

Walters, S., Burke, D. C., and Skehel, J. J. (1967). *J. gen. Virol.*, **1**, 349–362.

Wiesner, R., Acs, G., Reich, E., and Shafiq, A. (1965). *J. Cell Biol.*, **27**, 47–52.

DISCUSSION

De Maeyer: The ratio of virus particles to plaque-forming units in your Semliki Forest preparations with hydroxylamine might explain the apparent initial lack of effect; if the curve in Fig. 4 is extrapolated the ratio would be 10:1.

Burke: We don't know the ratio, but we do know that our preparations contain particles which will haemagglutinate but are not infective. Nothing is yet known about the role of non-infective virus particles in interferon production. The extrapolation to 10 in Fig. 4 reflects the original high multiplicity of infection, and no effect of hydroxylamine was detectable until the number of infective particles per cell fell below one.

Levy: The harmful effect of a high salt concentration has kept many people from doing these experiments with viral RNA. Has anyone used something like polyornithine to aid absorption? In a system which gave rapid production of interferon before new virus production, one could possibly see whether the viral RNA really is the effective agent. The polyornithine system gives titres of 10^6 infectious doses/ml. of viral RNA solution (Dianzani, Buckler and Baron, in preparation).

Ho: Dr. Burke, when you used viruses inactivated by u.v. irradiation the nucleic acid had been damaged and this presumably prevented viral subunit replication. What is the general significance of these results? With many other types of inactivated virus the ability to replicate viral subunits is not necessary for the induction of interferon.

Burke: We expected that interferon-producing ability might be inactivated more slowly than the other properties measured. The myxoviruses might be atypical. Isn't there some evidence that the RNA in them is a little unusual and might be polyploid? C. Scholtissek and R. Rott (1964. *Virology*, **22**, 169) obtained some interesting results when they showed that fowl plague virus, inactivated with Bayer 139, still initiated some virus-induced functions, but the Newcastle disease virus was different from this. Certainly with fowl plague virus it looks as if one doesn't need the whole nucleic acid to initiate some viral-induced functions. It is just possible, in some of the myxoviruses anyway, that part of the nucleic acid is sufficient to induce interferon formation. At the moment, we can't explain why interferon-producing viruses can be produced by heat inactivation; there may be another mechanism here.

Ho: Is it possible that hydroxylamine is acting quite differently, perhaps by specifically inactivating the interferon-inducing sequences, if there are such?

Burke: You may be quite right about hydroxylamine. We have checked its effect only on the haemagglutination ability of the virus we are inactivating. On long treatments with hydroxylamine the haemagglutination titres drop, but not under the conditions we have used here. The effect on infectivity is very much faster than the effect on the haemagglutination activity.

Crick: You said that you need intact viral RNA in your experiment, but what does "intact" mean?

Burke: When virus particles are treated with hydroxylamine the ability to produce interferon is inactivated as fast as all other virus-induced properties. Maybe these properties are controlled by cytosine-rich stretches but we generally assume that they need the whole nucleic acid—all the genetic information. The inactivation slopes are the same, but with different target sizes there might be different slopes.

Joklik: There are two factors which control the half-life of any particular messenger RNA. The first is that in the same cell and in the same milieu one particular messenger RNA may be more stable than another, that is, the "intrinsic" stability. The second concerns the conditions in the cell—for instance early vaccinia messenger RNA has a different stability in two different cell systems (L cells and HeLa cells). It is not inconceivable, therefore, that in some cell systems lysosomal breakdown or something like that occurs first and alters the intracellular milieu. So a difference in the half-lives can be readily understood.

Burke: All these experiments were done under the same conditions.

Joklik: But they were done with different viruses, and that is the point. Why did you do the experiments with infectious nucleic acid? The problem is to find out whether interferon would still be produced in the absence of nucleic acid or if nucleic acid were inactivated.

Burke: We are planning to do that. The nucleic acid work was done last year and we moved from there to hydroxylamine. We can separate Semliki Forest virus into two components, both of which haemagglutinate and the heavier of which contains the RNA, and now we want to look at these as inducers of interferon.

Joklik: It is rather difficult to believe that infectious nucleic acid is in fact essential for interferon production.

Burke: Have you an alternative suggestion?

Joklik: It is some disruptive reaction—something which is not a property of an infectious nucleic acid molecule but rather of some protein getting into a cell, as a result of which a chain of reactions is set up which leads to some sort of derepression.

Wagner: Of course, one can split off some protein products which retain haemagglutinating activity and test their capacity to induce interferon synthesis. Is this worth an experiment?

Burke: Haemagglutination of Semliki Forest virus can be inactivated with pronase, and this would be one way of looking at it.

Wagner: With myxovirus systems one could get a haemagglutinating particle relatively free of nucleic acid and see if this would act as an inducer.

Chany: Trypsin treatment of NDV does not prevent viral multiplication in the cell. In some of our experiments trypsin destroyed the interferon-inducing ability of the virus.

Burke: The trouble is that the virus has been broken up and if the results are negative one never knows whether the products are getting into the cells.

Chany: The virus is not broken up in these experiments because it is fully infectious after trypsin treatment.

Ho: Some old experiments seem to corroborate your hypothesis that it may be the nucleic acid of a virus which induces interference and interferon. K. Paucker and W. Henle (1958. *Virology*, **6**, 198–214) showed before the days of interferon that the interfering activity of influenza virus was associated with the ribonucleoprotein subunit or complement-fixing antigens of influenza virus. They also showed that the haemagglutinin had no interfering ability. W. Schäfer purified the haemagglutinin from fowl plague virus. He (and T. Tokumaru [1958]. *Z. Naturf.*, **13b**, 704–713) demonstrated that this did not induce interference, and Schäfer also showed, in unpublished work, that it did not induce interferon.

Burke: But the point there is that no haemagglutinin activity got into the cells.

Ho: The haemagglutinin, which is a surface antigen, and which in Paucker and Henle's work possessed receptor-destroying enzyme activity, would be expected to adsorb to cells.

Gresser: We should perhaps distinguish between interferon induction *in vitro* and *in vivo*. Dr. Chany mentioned that treating NDV with trypsin reduced the ability of the virus to induce interferon *in vitro*. In contrast, however, trypsin-treated NDV induces as high titres of interferon in the mouse as does untreated NDV (Gresser, unpublished observations). The infectivity of Sendai virus is diminished by trypsin (Gresser, I., and Enders, J. F. [1961]. *Virology*, **13**, 420). When trypsin-treated Sendai virus is inoculated into an animal, only a slight decrease in interferon production occurs compared to that in controls, although there has been more than 99·99 per cent decrease in infectivity.

Chany: Much may also depend on the cell. In many instances u.v.-inactivated virus can produce interferon in one cell but absolutely none in another cell. There are probably several mechanisms by which the virus can trigger interferon production in the cell.

Burke: The 42° system does not work in mouse cells; SFV does not produce interferon in mouse cells, though it does in chick cells, but I don't know why.

Baron: Do you think the small production of polymerase in the SFV system at 42° was significant and truly viral in origin?

Burke: I think it may be truly viral. It came up at the right time under standard conditions. When one is looking at very low levels of incorporation, one has to rely on a small count. I am tempted to think that it is not significant for interferon production. What I don't understand is why we were unable to pick up virus

RNA synthesis when we could pick up polymerase, because the first should be easier. Polymerase was still partially active at 42° when we assayed it *in vitro*, but it appears to be fairly labile in the cells. If cells are moved from 37° to 42° then the polymerase decayed after about one hour. Other people have found this too, but we do not have sufficient evidence to decide finally whether it is the production or the action of polymerase which is inhibited at 42°.

Martin: With reference to Dr. Baron's question, we have come across a similar situation in looking at the effect of interferon on the development of the Semliki Forest viral RNA polymerase. With the interferon-treated cells we have seen an increase during infection in the ability of cell extracts to incorporate GTP into RNA. However, the incorporation is not dependent on the addition of all four nucleoside triphosphates. When we extracted the RNA and looked at the product, we found that most of it was low molecular weight material which was obviously not viral RNA (see Sonnabend, Martin and Mécs, this volume, pp. 143–156). The increased polymerase activity in the interferon-treated cells as compared with that in the uninfected controls was of the same order as Dr. Burke saw in his infected cells incubated at the higher temperature. Perhaps the cell responds by producing a defective polymerase—or unmasking a cellular one—which just adds labelled precursors to the ends of pre-existing RNA.

Burke: This is possible, but we used as a control in all cases exactly the same incubation mixture, though without the three 5′-triphosphates. The increase was still seen, but of course the incorporation levels are low.

THE SYSTEMIC INDUCTION OF INTERFERON

Monto Ho, Bosko Postic and Yang H. Ke

Department of Epidemiology and Microbiology, Graduate School of Public Health,
University of Pittsburgh, Pittsburgh, Pennsylvania

We would like to summarize some of our studies on what might be called "systemic" induction of interferon in one experimental animal, the rabbit. Systemic induction originated with the demonstration by Baron and Buckler (1963) that high titres of circulating interferon could be obtained in intact mice after an intravenous inoculation of a non-replicating virus. Before 1963, induction of interferon in animals was mostly "local" and "infectious", that is, interferon was produced in a local lesion infected with a virus (see Finter, 1966). The systemic method has been particularly useful for discovering various non-viral inducers of interferon. The list of such agents has accumulated largely in the last few years (Table I). Many

TABLE I

INDUCERS OF INTERFERON

Micro-organisms
(1) Viruses: both DNA, RNA cytocidal and oncogenic viruses; active and inactivated.
(2) Trachoma-inclusion conjunctivitis (TRIC) agent.
(3) Rickettsia.
(4) Bacteria (especially Gram-negative ones), living and killed.
(5) Mycoplasma.
(6) Protozoa (*Toxoplasma gondii*).

Products of Micro-organisms
(1) Bacterial products (bacterial endotoxins).
(2) Fungal products (statolon, helenine).

Others
(1) Nucleic acids (animal and plant).
(2) Phytohaemagglutinin.
(3) Pyran copolymer.
(4) Cycloheximide.

of them are only effective systemically. They have to be inoculated intravenously or intraperitoneally, usually in fairly substantial doses, so that they gain ready access via the blood stream to the interferon-forming tissues.

A complete comparative study of the mechanism of induction of interferon by these various agents is not yet available. Perhaps because bacterial endotoxin was the first non-viral inducer used in our laboratory (Ho,

1964*a*), we have concentrated on a comparison between viruses and bacterial endotoxin. As events have borne out, these two classes of inducers represent two distinct mechanisms between which most of the others may lie.

A great deal is known about the induction of interferon by viruses. Most of the data have been obtained from cell cultures, which yield in general better data than experimental animals (see Ho, 1964*b*; Finter, 1966). Following the work of Heller (1963) and Wagner (1963), who showed that actinomycin D inhibited the production of interferon without affecting the replication of the RNA virus inducer of interferon, it has been generally assumed that the synthesis of interferon requires the synthesis of DNA-dependent RNA, or cell messenger RNA. This is still the best evidence that interferon is a cell and not a viral protein. We further ascertained in the u.v.-irradiated Newcastle disease virus–chick fibroblast system that the synthesis of messenger RNA for interferon is completed about four hours after inoculation of the inducer, and that no messenger synthesis takes place thereafter. It functions for 12 to 24 hours (Ho, 1964*b*). Similar results with some variation have been obtained in other interferon-forming systems in cell cultures (see Finter, 1966). It was further found that interferon synthesis was inhibited by puromycin, indicating that new protein synthesis was necessary (Ho and Breinig, 1965; Burke, 1966). This result is of course consistent with the interpretation of the actinomycin data. One might keep in mind, however, that there is still no direct proof that the interferon molecule is actually synthesized *de novo*. It might still be argued that interferon exists in a precursor state in all cells, and the demonstrated requirement for messenger RNA and protein synthesis is for an intermediate enzyme or protein which activates the precursor molecule.

COMPARATIVE STUDIES OF THE INDUCTION OF VIRUS–INDUCED INTERFERON AND ENDOTOXIN–INDUCED INTERFERON

After it had been found that a small intravenous dose of endotoxin ($\geqslant 2\,\mu\text{g.}$) would induce circulating interferon in rabbits, it became important to ascertain whether the induction of endotoxin-induced interferon (EII) was similar to that of virus-induced interferon (VII) (Ho, 1964*a*). We noted that EII differed from VII in several aspects. It was more labile at pH 2 and $56°$ C. These differences were reinforced by the finding of Hallum, Youngner and Stinebring (1965) that EII in the mouse is of larger molecular weight than VII. We confirmed this for rabbit EII, but found in addition that both EII and VII were heterogeneous in molecular size (Ke, Ho and Merigan, 1966).

With respect to the induction of EII, we first attempted to find out if it was inhibited by actinomycin and puromycin (Ho and Kono, 1965a; Ke et al., 1966). To do this, we first ascertained that in the rabbit, as well as in the earlier cell culture studies, both actinomycin and puromycin inhibited the formation of Sindbis-virus-induced interferon (Tables II and III). In

TABLE II

EFFECT OF ACTINOMYCIN D ON THE INDUCTION OF VIRUS- AND ENDOTOXIN-
INDUCED INTERFERON IN RABBITS

(1) *Sindbis-virus-induced interferon*

	No actinomycin		Actinomycin-treated	
Hours	No. samples	Mean titre	No. samples	Mean titre
1·5–2	10	37	4	0
4	12	1,587	5	18
7	14	2,723	5	91

(2) *Endotoxin-induced interferon*

0	17	<2	ND	ND
2	24	43	11	46
4	19	23	7	20
7	15	9	3	<2

Amounts inoculated per kilogram were: Actinomycin—1·0 to 2·0 mg.; Sindbis virus—about 10^{10} p.f.u.; *E. coli* endotoxin (Boivin)—usually 20 µg. ND=Not done.

TABLE III

EFFECT OF PUROMYCIN ON THE INDUCTION OF VIRUS- AND
ENDOTOXIN-INDUCED INTERFERON

(1) *Sindbis-virus-induced interferon*

	No actinomycin		Actinomycin-treated	
Hours	No. samples	Mean titre	No. samples	Mean titre
4	4	404	4	4
7	4	1,312	4	17

(2) *Endotoxin-induced interferon*

2	4	19	4	11
4	4	52	4	58

Small (0·3–0·5 kg.) rabbits were inoculated with 40 mg. puromycin/100 g. body weight in divided doses which inhibited [^{14}C]leucine uptake in liver protein by 96–100 per cent. The animals received either 10^9 p.f.u. Sindbis virus or 5 µg. endotoxin.

sharp contrast to this, these two antimetabolites had no effect on the production of EII. This was important evidence that the mechanism of formation of EII is quite different. Apparently no detectable protein synthetic activity is necessary, but what metabolic determinants are necessary for the release of the EII is not yet known (Ho, 1967).

After obtaining the above results, and considering what we know about the physiology of endotoxin (Atkins, 1960; Landy and Braun, 1964), we next decided to compare the effect of alteration of the physiological *milieu intérieur* on the induction of EII and VII. In almost every physiological or pharmacological alteration we have studied, a marked difference in the response of EII and VII production was found.

In Table IV, our data regarding the effect of body temperature are

TABLE IV

EFFECT OF BODY TEMPERATURE ON VII AND EII FORMATION

Environmental condition	Mean body temp.	Peak VII titre	Peak EII titre
35° not shorn	41°	831	24
25° not shorn	40°	776	16
25° shorn	39·2°	200	69
4° shorn	38·1°	30	30

Rabbits weighing 1 kg. received 3×10^9 p.f.u. NDV or 10 µg. endotoxin. Each titre is the geometric mean of four or more titrations.

summarized (Postic *et al.*, 1966). The body temperature of the rabbit may be easily altered, within limits, by changing the ambient temperature and by shearing. The normal body temperature is about 40°. VII was enhanced at 41°, as would be expected from work in cell cultures (see Finter, 1966). Such an elevation had no effect on EII production, but paradoxically a lowering of body temperature by shearing exerted an accentuating effect. This result has been consistently confirmed in our laboratory.

Adrenal corticosteroids also affected EII and VII production in markedly different ways (Postic *et al.*, 1967). Although it is well known that cortisol depresses interferon formation both *in vivo* and *in vitro* (see Finter, 1966), this effect is much more dramatic with respect to EII production. This point was best brought out by adrenalectomy, a process which eliminates the physiological source of corticosteroids. We were unable to affect VII production after ablation of the adrenal glands, but EII production was increased about tenfold (Table V).

TABLE V

THE EFFECT OF ADRENALECTOMY ON ENDOTOXIN-INDUCED INTERFERON

Adrenalectomy	Cortisol postoperatively	No. samples	Serum interferon*
Yes	None	7	388
Yes	25 mg. daily	3	6
No	None	7	28

* Geometric mean titres of samples obtained on the seventh postoperative day and 2 hours after 10 µg. of endotoxin i.v.

The data on temperature and steroid effects are not yet interpretable in cellular, biochemical or metabolic terms. But they are important in providing methods for altering EII production. It is remarkable that although such lethal metabolic poisons as actinomycin and puromycin do not affect EII production, an alteration of body temperature or hormonal status does. It is an indication that EII production is perhaps a host response somewhat analogous to the secretion of hormones which is subject to physiological controls not entirely analysable on a cellular basis. One point in favour of this outlook is the fact that we have been unable to induce EII in cultures of embryo, renal, spleen, peripheral and peritoneal white cells *in vitro* (see Ho *et al.*, 1966, and Ho, unpublished data). For this reason the recent reports of Nagano and co-workers (1966) and Wagner and Smith (1968) that such *in vitro* studies may be possible deserve close attention.

FATE OF INOCULATED AND INDUCED INTERFERON

There have not been many studies in animal hosts on the physiology of interferon. Recently we performed some on the rate of disappearance of interferon, its distribution in tissues, and its renal excretion.

Interferon disappears very rapidly after it is inoculated in the blood stream. Therefore, large amounts must be administered initially in order to study the kinetics of its disappearance. We found that the half-time of virus-induced interferon in the homologous (rabbit) host was only 11 minutes (Ho and Postic, 1967a). This agrees well with calculations based on the data of Baron and co-workers (1966), and Gresser and co-workers (1967) for the mouse. Where does the interferon go to? Some of it is excreted, but proportionately not very much (see below). Subrahmanyan and Mims (1966) studied the distribution of interferon in mice after an intravenous inoculation of 340 units. Only very small amounts were detected in the blood, liver, kidney and lungs 5 to 13 minutes after inoculation. The disappearance of interferon was too rapid for the relatively small amount inoculated to be followed with any precision.

Recently, we inoculated a large dose of interferon into a pregnant rabbit.

TABLE VI

DISTRIBUTION OF VII INOCULATED IN THE PREGNANT RABBIT

Minutes post-injection	Tissue assayed	Interferon titre	% Amount injected
1	Maternal serum	205	29·5
5	Maternal serum	66	9·5
30	Maternal serum	24	3·4
30	Maternal liver	150	13·4
30	Maternal spleen	300	0·4
30	Embryo blood	4	<0·1
30	Amniotic fluid	2	<0·1

A 4·5 kg. rabbit received 6·5 ml. VII with a titre of 24,000 units/ml. Serum volume assumed to be 5 per cent of body weight; liver=140 g.; spleen=2·5 g.; embryo blood=10 ml.

Thirty minutes after inoculation, only 3·4 per cent was recoverable in the serum, but about 14 per cent could be found in the liver and spleen (Table VI; Postic and Ho, unpublished data). There seems to be a definite barrier for transplacental migration of interferon. Whether this may be partly due to placental accumulation of interferon is not known (see below and Table VII). The accumulation of interferon in the reticuloendothelial

TABLE VII

DISTRIBUTION OF SINDBIS VIRUS AND INDUCED INTERFERON IN THE PREGNANT RABBIT

Hours after virus inoculation

Tissue	2 Virus*	2 Interferon†	4 Virus	4 Interferon	7 Virus	7 Interferon
Mother						
Serum	2·92	512	0·70	512	3·48	2,048
Liver	5·92	40	3·17	40	1·17	160
Spleen	5·11	320	3·00	160	0·70	640
Kidney	3·11	160	1·00	80	3·55	160
Urine	N.F.	64	N.F.	64	N.F.	2,048
Placenta	3·40	20	0·70	80	3·00	640
Embryo						
Amniotic fluid	N.F.	4	N.F.	<5	N.F.	45
Blood	0·85	6	0·23	4	N.F.	64
Viscera	N.F.	<5	N.F.	<5	N.F.	10
Skin, muscle	N.F.	<5	N.F.	<5	N.F.	<5

* Log p.f.u. per 0·1 ml. or 0·1 g.
† 1/dilution per 0·3 ml. or 0·3 g.
N.F.=none found.

system and its rapid clearance from the circulation suggest the hypothesis that although interferon is a cell protein which resembles serum proteins physicochemically, it is handled very much differently from serum proteins. It behaves much more like a foreign substance against which the body has already had an immune experience. The theoretical and practical implications of this hypothesis are far-reaching. But more data are desirable at this time.

An important question concerning the induction of interferon is the amount induced. We thought that one simple method of measuring how much interferon is induced is to measure how much is excreted. To do this accurately, we must first determine what proportion of a renal load of interferon is excreted. After inoculating a dose of interferon intravenously, we found by measuring total urine interferon over a 24-hour period that only about 0·2 to 2 per cent was recovered, a relatively small proportion of the amount administered. But in separate animals, large amounts (100,000 to 300,000 units) of interferon were recovered in the urine after inoculation of 10^9 p.f.u. Newcastle disease virus (NDV) to induce interferon. If we assume that the recovered amount represented 0·2 to 2 per cent of the total renal load, the latter calculated out to be 5×10^6 to 150×10 units of interferon. This should approximate the total amount of interferon induced in a rabbit weighing 1 kg. It is clear that induction of interferon is a much more effective way of getting large amounts of interferon in the animal than the injection of exogenous interferon (Ho and Postic, 1967*a*).

The efficiency of renal excretion of VII and EII was also studied (Ho and Postic, 1967*b*). Since detectable plasma levels of interferon are maintained for two to ten hours after induction with either bacterial endotoxin or with viruses, and quantitative collection of urine in the rabbit was feasible with an in-dwelling Foley catheter, renal clearances of both virus- and endotoxin-induced interferon could be determined from the familiar renal plasma clearance formula UV/Pt (U = urine interferon concentration, $V =$ volume of urine collected over a time period t, and $P =$ mean plasma interferon concentration during t). We found in the 1 kg. rabbit, which has a plasma volume of about 45 ml.:

(1) Renal clearance of virus-induced interferon (VII) averaged 30·6 ml. of plasma cleared per hour;

(2) Comparable value for endotoxin-induced interferon (EII) was 1·2 ml. of plasma cleared per hour;

(3) For comparison, creatinine clearance, a good indicator of glomerular filtration, was 136 ml. plasma per hour. The injection of endotoxin or virus *per se* had no significant effect on such clearance. These results indicated that the two types of interferon were cleared quite differently. EII was cleared poorly by the kidney, perhaps because it contained somewhat more of the larger molecule species (Ke, Ho and Merigan, 1966). In contrast, the renal clearance of VII was quite substantial. How much of this may have been due to the kidney producing VII is as yet unexplored. It appears that one reason why a relatively small proportion of either VII or EII is actually excreted is that interferon diffuses rapidly in the tissue spaces; it is perhaps trapped in the reticuloendothelial system, and becomes unavailable for excretion.

THE ORIGIN OF SYSTEMICALLY INDUCED INTERFERON

Earlier, we had postulated that the reticuloendothelial system (RES) is the important system for the formation of interferon after an intravenous inoculation (Kono and Ho, 1965). This view has been fairly generally accepted, although when studied closely it is a difficult proposition to prove rigorously. Our hypothesis is based on the following three considerations:

The *first* is that tissues of the reticuloendothelial system form interferon better than other tissues. We found that cell suspensions obtained from liver and spleen made interferon faster and in greater amounts than cells from, for example, the kidney. This would account for the rapid as well as high interferon titres obtained after an intravenous inoculation. It is a clear indication that although interferon formation, unlike antibody formation, is not the function of specialized cells, there do appear to be cells which produce it better than others. This viewpoint has recently been strengthened by Kono's work (1967) in which he compares interferon production in bovine leucocytes and other bovine tissues. He found that bovine leucocytes produced, per cell, more interferon faster than renal cells. Furthermore, with continued cultivation for 12 days the amount of interferon produced by leucocytes increased. The conclusion seems warranted that the common denominator of the reticuloendothelial system, i.e. the phagocyte, may be either the most important interferon former, or a mediator of its formation in systemic induction. One might explain Kono's results by assuming that the number of phagocytizing cells, i.e. macrophages, increased with the prolonged cultivation of white cells.

The *second* consideration is exemplified by results obtained by Dr. Kono while he was in our laboratory (Kono and Ho, 1965; and unpublished data). We determined interferon levels in various tissues 60 to 90 minutes after inoculation of the virus, before the serum levels had reached their peak levels. The tissues with the highest levels were tissues of the reticuloendothelial system, i.e. spleen, liver, white cells and bone marrow. The amount of virus in these tissues was also measured. Generally speaking, there was a good correlation between the amount of virus absorbed by a tissue and the amount of interferon formed. Clearly one reason why the RES plays a role in interferon formation may be that this system traps the inducer, whether it be a virus, bacterium or endotoxin. Perfusion of the tissues did not correlate well with interferon formation. The kidney and brain, for example, though freely perfused by large quantities of blood during life, did not contain large amounts of interferon. On the other hand, the portion of the reticuloendothelial system that was not perfused at all, such as the lymph nodes, did not and would not be expected to produce interferon.

In a more recent experiment, we measured the distribution of virus and VII at two, four, and seven hours after 10^{10} p.f.u. Sindbis virus in pregnant rabbits weighing 4 to 5 kg. (Table VII; Postic and Ho, unpublished data). Of the various organs, the spleen contained the highest concentration of interferon. Less was found in the liver, which is consistent with the results of Subrahmanyan and Mims (1966), and may be due to a catabolic effect of this tissue on interferon. There was remarkably little interferon in foetal tissues, due no doubt to the inability of both the inducer and interferon to permeate the placental barrier freely. Comparable amounts were found in the liver and kidney. This may represent the amount filtered through the renal glomeruli. A relatively high interferon concentration was found in the urine seven hours after virus inoculation. Alternatively it may be postulated that the kidney produces some VII (see above), perhaps of the later-appearing type.

The *third* basis for identifying the reticuloendothelial system as the system responsible for the formation of interferon is that interferon formation is reduced after the RES has been blocked. Previously, we reported that rabbits whose RES had been "blocked" by 5–10 ml. of 25 per cent thorium dioxide (Thorotrast) per kilogram produced less interferon in response to Sindbis virus (Kono and Ho, 1965). The three-hour titres were uniformly decreased although the peak titres were not. Our recent experience is recorded in Table VIII. Different patterns appeared to emerge, depending

TABLE VIII

EFFECT OF THOROTRAST ON SERUM VIRUS- AND ENDOTOXIN-INDUCED INTERFERON

		Interferon (hours after inducer)†			
Thorotrast*	Inducer	2	3	4	7
−18	Sindbis		3		39
−2	Sindbis		6		<2
None	Sindbis		83		135
−18	NDV	64		45	89
−2	NDV	64		128	89
None	NDV	1,190		3,470	710
−18	Endotoxin	72		2	
−2	Endotoxin	27			
None	Endotoxin	61		13	

* Inoculated 18 or 2 hours before the inducer.
† Geometric mean titre from two to four rabbits.

on the time of pretreatment with Thorotrast and the type of inducer used. With Sindbis virus as the inducer there was a reduction in the three-hour interferon titre when Thorotrast was given 18 hours before the virus. The seven-hour titre was more convincingly reduced if Thorotrast was given two hours before virus. With NDV as an inducer, there was a general decrease in the interferon titres three, four and seven hours after inoculation, irrespective of whether Thorotrast was given 18 or two hours before the inducer. When endotoxin was used as an inducer, there was certainly no evidence that Thorotrast inoculated 18 hours earlier decreased EII levels. However, when Thorotrast was given two hours before the inducer, there was an indication of reduced response.

Generally speaking, Thorotrast inoculated two hours before the inducer seems to be more effective than Thorotrast inoculated 18 hours before. There may be a gradation of effect depending on the type of inducer. This may be due to variations in the uptake of the inducer substance by the reticuloendothelial system.

What is the precise role of the phagocytic function of the RES in interferon formation? There are still insufficient data on this point, but perhaps the simplest formulation is that, analogous to the trapping of antigens by macrophages in antibody-forming organs to facilitate the production of antibody (Nossal, Ada and Austin, 1964), the reticuloendothelial system traps and concentrates the inducer and makes it available to the interferon-producing cells. If there were no phagocytosis of the inducer, then the only way to induce interferon would be for cells to absorb the inducer, probably an inefficient process short of actual infection. For example, the brain or kidney tissue may not form interferon after an intravenous inoculation since it does not fix viruses in sufficient quantities. However, should an infection of the brain or an encephalitis ensue, interferon may readily be found in the brain (Finter, 1966).

Parenthetically, this may be the reason why certain inducers such as endotoxin have not been found to act *in vitro*. They may not be taken up by the usual primary or secondary cells in culture. It is, therefore, not surprising that it is the macrophage that has been reported to produce EII (Nagano *et al.*, 1966).

If the phagocytes are important in the formation of interferon, one may logically ask what type is involved? One way to study the role of phagocytes is to try to prepare an animal free of them. This is of course difficult if not impossible to do. One type may be reduced, if not entirely eliminated, namely the polymorphonuclear leucocytes (PMN): the common nitrogen mustard, mechlorethamine (Mustargen), can be used to reduce the peripheral white count by about 75 per cent (as calculated from data presented in Table IX) four days after the first inoculation. At this time, most of the PMN's have disappeared from the peripheral smear, the remaining cells being mononuclear cells, mostly lymphocytes. If these animals are induced with either endotoxin or NDV, their response is nearly normal. There is no evidence of reduced induction of interferon. From this, we assume that the PMN is not the essential source for systemic interferon production. This is further indirect evidence for the role of the

TABLE IX

EFFECT OF MECHLORETHAMINE (MUSTARGEN) ON INTERFERON PRODUCTION

Dose of Mustargen (mg.)			White cell count		% PMN	Inducer	Serum interferon at hours		
Day 0	Day 1	Day 2	Day 0	Day 4	Day 4	Day 4	2	4	7
2	1	1	5,600	1,640	8	Endotoxin	256	Died	—
2	1	1	8,600	2,920	0	Endotoxin	16	Died	—
2	0	0	8,200	1,000	0	Endotoxin	64	45	21
2	0	0	6,800	880	4	Endotoxin	128	64	6
0	0	0	—	—	—	Endotoxin	44	23	9
2	0	0	6,600	1,280	4	NDV	512	2,048	256
2	0	0	6,800	2,800	0	NDV	256	1,024	128
0	0	0	—	—	—	NDV	512	708	256

PMN = polymorphonuclear leucocytes.
Each row of figures represents data from a separate animal; 10 µg. endotoxin or $10^{9.6}$ p.f.u. NDV inoculated.

macrophage as the essential phagocytizing cell leading to interferon formation.

RELATIONSHIP OF THE RES TO TOLERANCE

Any theory of interferon formation must also explain the phenomenon of tolerance to reinduction. It is now clearly established that after the inoculation of either virus or bacterial endotoxin, the animal becomes refractory or tolerant to a second inoculation for about six days after the first inoculation (Ho and Kono, 1965b; Youngner and Stinebring, 1965). There is "crossed tolerance" in that one inoculation of endotoxin will also render the rabbit or mouse tolerant to induction of interferon by a virus. Similarly, an inoculation of virus will also render the mouse and the rat hyporeactive to endotoxin (Youngner and Stinebring, 1965; De Somer and Billiau, 1966), although the latter sequence of inoculations did not result in tolerance in the rabbit (Ho, Kono and Breinig, 1965).

The explanation for this interesting phenomenon is unknown, but several theories may be considered. It is possible that multiple mechanisms may be involved, as is the case with tolerance to pyrogens and endotoxins (Landy and Braun, 1964). It is instructive to recall briefly the history of tolerance to the pyrogenicity of endotoxin. In classic experiments, Beeson (1947) suggested that tolerance was based upon increased phagocytosis or clearance of endotoxin by the RES of the tolerant animal. Evidence obtained by Farr and co-workers (1954) for a serum humoral mediator of tolerance was largely ignored until recently. It is now apparent that Beeson's explanation by itself is no longer sufficient. Humoral factors, whether they be immunological, opsonic (Freedman and Sultzer, 1964) or enzymic (Rutenburg et al., 1965) in character, appear to play at least a

2*

supporting role in tolerance to the pyrogenic and toxic effects of endotoxin. It appears prudent, therefore, to consider all these possibilities in tolerance to interferon induction.

The *first* and perhaps simplest theory is that tolerance in the animal host is mediated by a diffusible humoral factor. It is well-known that interferon production in cell culture is a "one-shot" affair, as the continued presence of the inducer in cell culture does not result in continuous interferon production. This characteristic hall-mark of interferon production has been

TABLE X

INDUCTION OF INTERFERON BY NDV IN LEUCOCYTES FROM TOLERANT RABBITS

Treatment of rabbits	Leucocytes per ml.	Inducer	Interferon titre
Endotoxin	10^7	NDV	128, 128, 128
Endotoxin	10^6	NDV	64, 32, 32
Pertussis vaccine	10^7	NDV	256, 512, 512
Pertussis vaccine	10^6	NDV	64, 128, 128
None	10^7	NDV	128, 256
None	10^6	NDV	64, 64
None	10^8	None	<2, <2

Rabbits (1 kg.) were made tolerant after receiving 10 µg. endotoxin or 2·0 ml. pertussis vaccine (10^{11} cells) 24 and 72 hours before collection of leucocytes by bleeding. Leucocytes were incubated at 37° after inoculation of NDV at input multiplicity of 10; and assayed after 24 hours for interferon production. Each number represents a titre from a separate sample.

convincingly shown by Paucker and Boxaca (1967) to be due to a responsiveness-suppressing factor closely associated with interferon. They assume that whenever interferon is induced, this factor is also produced and provides for the negative feedback and cellular refractoriness.

Some of the difficulties in extending this mechanism to the intact animal have been mentioned (Ho and Postic, 1967a). No general transmissible humoral factor has been identified in the tolerant animal. The alternative would be that the humoral factor is rapidly fixed by the cells, and is not easily detected. In this case, one would expect cells of a tolerant animal to be more resistant to interferon induction. However, we found that white blood cells from animals made tolerant either by bacterial endotoxin or pertussis vaccine could still be induced to produce as much interferon as did cells from normal animals (Table X; Ho and Postic, unpublished data and 1967a). Recently we have tested liver, lung and spleen cells from animals made tolerant with endotoxin, and these cells could also be induced to produce as much interferon after inoculation of NDV as comparable cells from normal animals.

Although there is little evidence to support a general humoral theory to explain tolerance, in the limited case of tolerance produced by endotoxin against the interferon-inducing effect of endotoxin, a humoral factor which correlates well with the state of tolerance has been described (Ho, Kono and Breinig, 1965). It turns out that this is similar to the endotoxin-inactivating factor found in normal serum (Ho and Kass, 1958; Skarnes *et al.*, 1958), subsequently assumed to be enzymic in character. What is new is that with a perhaps more sensitive measurement of endotoxin activity, i.e. induction

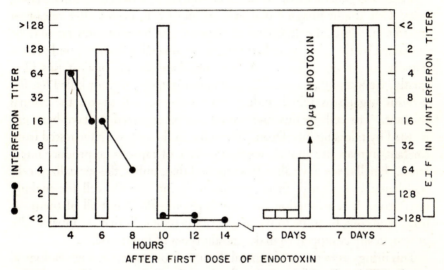

FIG. 1. Development of tolerance and endotoxin-inactivating factor (EIF) after an inoculation of endotoxin.

Interferon titres in four rabbits weighing 1 kg. each are represented by lines connecting two dots. The animals all received the first 10 µg. dose of endotoxin at time 0, and a second dose at 4, 6, 10, and 12 hours respectively. Serum was titrated for EIF (Ho, Kono and Breinig, 1965) as follows: a 1 ml. sample was incubated with 10 µg. endotoxin for 1 hour at 37°; this mixture was then inoculated into a fresh rabbit, and its serum was titrated for interferon two hours later. An interferon titre less than 1:16 signified the presence of endotoxin-inactivating activity. Normal serum incubated with this dose of endotoxin showed no inactivating effect.

of interferon, we have shown that this factor is increased in the state of tolerance (Ho, Kono and Breinig, 1965).

Fig. 1 illustrates the time of onset of tolerance, and the concomitant development of the endotoxin-inactivating factor (EIF). Endotoxin inoculated four or six hours after the first dose had no effect on the exponential decline in serum interferon titres resulting from the first inoculation. It appears that tolerance had already developed four hours after an inoculation of endotoxin, and certainly by ten hours. By ten hours, serum interferon from the first dose had largely disappeared and a second dose of endotoxin at this time produced no detectable interferon levels. EIF was detectable four

hours after the initial dose of endotoxin. It remained elevated until about
the sixth day, when tolerance had largely disappeared. If another dose of
endotoxin was given at this time, tolerance was re-established and the EIF
rose again, as shown by levels 24 hours later. In a pluralistic view of the
mechanism of tolerance, EIF is definitely a candidate for a role in tolerance
to endotoxin.

The *second* general theory to account for tolerance is that it is mediated by
cells. One might imagine that exhaustion of cells occurs after release of
interferon. Thus, the difference in responses to different inducers may be
explained by the selective exhaustion of certain cells which respond prefer-
entially to certain inducers. A few considerations are against this idea.
Firstly, we found that a small dose of endotoxin (0·1 µg.) or killed *Bacillus
pertussis* organisms which induce no interferon still makes the animal
tolerant. The cells in this case would not be expected to have been ex-
hausted by releasing interferon. Secondly, in the cells we have tested from
tolerant animals (see above), we find no lack of capacity to produce interferon. Finally, we have already suggested that, unlike the specialized cells
which make antibody, there appears to be no specific cell for making
interferon. It is a function of many types of cells if not all of them. It
may, therefore, be futile to try to identify certain cells that are intrinsically
or genetically equipped to make certain types of interferon.

This brings us to the *third* general theory of tolerance, i.e. a physiological
theory. This is based on an analysis of the tissues that are producing
interferon, and on ascribing tolerance to a functional alteration of such
tissues or systems, Since we have postulated that the reticuloendothelial
system is the system producing interferon, it follows that tolerance may
represent a functional alteration of such a system. The following considerations support this theory:

(1) *The non-specificity of tolerance:* The inoculation of particular inducers
will affect the RES to a varying extent in different animals. For example,
in the rabbit endotoxin produces a greater alteration than viruses; consequently, it produces a tolerance that extends to virus inducers, although the
reverse does not occur.

(2) *The graded tolerance response:* Tolerance is not an "all-or-none"
phenomenon. It is "graded" with respect to the type of inducer and to the
duration. For example, rabbits preinoculated with pertussis vaccine
produced tolerance to endotoxin and NDV, but not to Sindbis virus
(Table XI; Ho and Postic, 1967a). The duration of tolerance to endotoxin
induction was 7 to 12 days, but it was even longer with respect to NDV.
Possibly these two viruses are handled differently by the RES. Sindbis virus

persists longer in the blood stream. Recent evidence by De Maeyer (1967) that X-irradiation affects the interferon-inducing capacity of these two viruses differently is consistent with this idea.

(3) *Alterations of RE function:* We have already mentioned that non-specific alteration of the RES can affect interferon formation. Thus, blockade of the RES by Thorotrast reduces interferon formation. Pre-treatment of mice with *Mycobacterium tuberculosis* enhanced interferon induction by endotoxin (Youngner and Stinebring, 1965). This is associated with increased phagocytic capacity of the RES (Lurie, 1960).

TABLE XI

TOLERANCE TO INDUCTION OF INTERFERON AFTER PERTUSSIS VACCINE

Day vaccine given before inducer	Type of inducer given	Interferon titre
None	Endotoxin	52
1	Endotoxin	3
7	Endotoxin	2
12	Endotoxin	25
None	NDV	723
1	NDV	2
2	NDV	6
12	NDV	84
None	Sindbis	111
2	Sindbis	256

Pertussis vaccine (about 12 antigenic units or 10^{11} cells) was administered intravenously before 10 μg. endotoxin or about 10^9 p.f.u. of virus. "None" signifies that no vaccine was given. Each titre represents the mean obtained from two to six animals bled two hours after endotoxin or four hours after virus.

On the other hand, pretreatment of mice with cytomegalovirus reduced interferon induction by Newcastle disease virus (Osborn and Medearis, 1967). It has been shown by Wagner, Iio and Hornick (1963) that systemic virus infections such as sandfly fever and dengue, unlike many bacterial infections, are associated with decreased RE function as measured by the clearance of radioactively labelled aggregated albumin.

Nevertheless, it must be admitted that much more work is required before the precise alteration of the RES in association with tolerance is understood. It may be predicted on *a priori* grounds that the one easily measurable function of RES, i.e. its non-specific phagocytic function, will not be perfectly correlated with the development of tolerance. We know, for example, that after an inoculation of endotoxin the non-specific phagocytic function of the RES, as measured by the clearance of colloidal substances, undergoes a biphasic response. An initial depression shortly after such an inoculation is followed by an enhancement of the phagocytic response which is sustained for a week or so (Biozzi, Benacerraf and

Halpern, 1955). Hence both depression and elevation of non-specific RES clearance is associated with resistance to induction.

It would, therefore, be important to study non-specific as well as specific clearance values of the RES in the tolerant state. Another important parameter to bear in mind is the clearance of interferon itself. Is it possible that tolerance represents an accelerated elimination and phagocytosis of *interferon* by the reticuloendothelial system with or without the benefit of opsonins?

SUMMARY

Systemic induction of interferon involves maximum exposure of the interferon-forming tissues to a viral or non-viral inducer of interferon. The mechanism by which viruses induce interferon is quite different from that by which endotoxin induces it. The production of virus-induced interferon is inhibited by actinomycin and puromycin, while that of endotoxin-induced interferon is not. The two mechanisms may also be differentiated by their temperature requirement and sensitivity to corticosteroids.

Interferon disappears rapidly from the circulation. There is some evidence that it may be concentrated in the reticuloendothelial system. The disappearance is not accounted for by renal excretion. The renal clearance of virus-induced interferon is very much higher than that of endotoxin-induced interferon.

It is assumed that interferon is produced by the reticuloendothelial system. Thorotrast blockade of this system reduces interferon production.

Tolerance or refractoriness to interferon induction recurs after one injection of inducer. No theory yet put forward accounts for all aspects of this interesting phenomenon.

Acknowledgement

Work reported from the authors' laboratory was supported by Grant AI-02953 from the National Institutes of Health (U.S. Public Health Service).

REFERENCES

ATKINS, E. (1960). *Physiol. Rev.*, **40**, 580–646.
BARON, S., and BUCKLER, C. E. (1963). *Science*, **141**, 1061–1063.
BARON, S., BUCKLER, C. E., McCLOSKEY, R. V., and KIRSCHSTEIN, R. L. (1966). *J. Immun.*, **96**, 12–16.
BEESON, P. B. (1947). *J. exp. Med.*, **86**, 29–38.
BIOZZI, G., BENACERRAF, B., and HALPERN, B. N. (1955). *Br. J. exp. Path.*, **36**, 226–235.
BURKE, D. C. (1966). In *Interferons*, pp. 55–86, ed. Finter, N. B. Amsterdam: North-Holland Publishing Co.

DE MAEYER, E. (1967). *Arch. ges. Virusforsch.*, in press.
DE SOMER, P., and BILLIAU, A. (1966). *Arch. ges Virusforsch.*, **19**, 143–154.
FARR, R. S., CLARK, S. L., JR., PROFFITT, J. E., and CAMPBELL, D. H. (1954). *Am. J. Physiol.*, **177**, 269–278.
FINTER, N. B. (ed.) (1966). *Interferons.* Amsterdam: North-Holland Publishing Co.
FREEDMAN, H. H., and SULTZER, M. (1964). In *Bacterial Endotoxins*, pp. 537–545, ed. Landy, M., and Braun, W. Rahway, N.J.: Quinn & Boden Co.
GRESSER, I., COPPEY, J., FALCOFF, E., and FONTAINE, D. (1967). *Proc. Soc. exp. Biol. Med.*, **124**, 84–91.
HALLUM, J. V., YOUNGNER, J. S., and STINEBRING, W. R. (1965). *Virology*, **27**, 429–431.
HELLER, E. (1963). *Virology*, **21**, 652–656.
HO, M. (1964a). *Science*, **146**, 1472–1474.
HO, M. (1964b). *Bact. Rev.*, **28**, 367–381.
HO, M. (1967). *Jap. J. exp. Med.*, in press.
HO, M., and BREINIG, M. K. (1965). *Virology*, **25**, 331–339.
HO, M., FANTES, K. H., BURKE, D. C., and FINTER, N. B. (1966). In *Interferons*, pp. 181–201, ed. Finter, N. B. Amsterdam: North-Holland Publishing Co.
HO, M., and KASS, E. H. (1958). *J. Lab. clin. Med.*, **51**, 297–311.
HO, M., and KONO, Y. (1965a). *Proc. natn. Acad. Sci. U.S.A.*, **53**, 220–224.
HO, M., and KONO, Y. (1965b). *J. clin. Invest.*, **44**, 1059.
HO, M., KONO, Y., and BREINIG, M. K. (1965). *Proc. Soc. exp. Biol. Med.*, **119**, 1227–1232.
HO, M., and POSTIC, B. (1967a). In *First International Conference on Vaccines against Viral and Rickettsial Diseases of Man*, pp. 632–649. Washington, D.C.: PAHO/WHO Scientific Publication 147.
HO, M., and POSTIC, B. (1967b). *Nature, Lond.*, **214**, 1230–1231.
KE, Y. H., HO, M., and MERIGAN, T. C. (1966). *Nature, Lond.*, **211**, 541–542.
KE, Y. H., SINGER, S. H., POSTIC, B., and HO, M. (1966). *Proc. Soc. exp. Biol. Med.*, **121**, 181–183.
KONO, Y. (1967). *Proc. Soc. exp. Biol. Med.*, **124**, 155–160.
KONO, Y., and HO, M. (1965). *Virology*, **25**, 162–166.
LANDY, M., and BRAUN, W. (eds.) (1964). *Bacterial Endotoxins.* Rahway, N.J.: Quinn & Boden Co.
LURIE, M. B. (1960). *Ann. N.Y. Acad. Sci.*, **88**, 83–98.
NAGANO, Y., KOJIMA, Y., ARAKAWA, J., and KANASHIRO, R. S. (1966). *Jap. J. exp. Med.*, **36**, 481–487.
NOSSAL, G. J. V., ADA, G. L., and AUSTIN, C. M. (1964). *Aust. J. exp. Biol. med. Sci.*, **42**, 311–330.
OSBORN, J., and MEDEARIS, D. N. (1967). *Proc. Soc. exp. Biol. Med.*, **124**, 347–352.
PAUCKER, K., and BOXACA, M. (1967). *Bact. Rev.*, **31**, 145–156.
POSTIC, B., DE ANGELIS, C., BREINIG, M. K., and HO, M. (1966). *J. Bact.*, **91**, 1277–1281.
POSTIC, B., DE ANGELIS, C., BREINIG, M. K., and HO, M. (1967). *Proc. Soc. exp. Biol. Med.*, **125**, 89–92.
RUTENBURG, S. H., RUTENBURG, A. M., SMITH, E. E., and FINE, J. (1965). *Proc. Soc. exp. Biol. Med.*, **118**, 620–623.
SKARNES, R. C., ROSEN, F. S., SHEAR, M. J., and LANDY, M. (1958). *J. exp. Med.*, **108**, 685–699.
SUBRAHMANYAN, T. P., and MIMS, C. A. (1966). *Br. J. exp. Path.*, **47**, 168–176.
WAGNER, H. N., IIO, M., and HORNICK, R. B. (1963). *J. clin. Invest.*, **42**, 990.
WAGNER, R. R. (1963). *Trans. Ass. Am. Physns*, **76**, 92–101.
WAGNER, R. R., and SMITH, T. J. (1968). This volume, pp. 95–106.
YOUNGNER, J. S., and STINEBRING, W. R. (1965). *Nature, Lond.*, **208**, 456–458.

DISCUSSION

De Maeyer: In collaboration with Dr. R. Fauve, from the Pasteur Institute in Paris, we observed the "spontaneous" release of a substance with the characteristics of interferon in cultures of mouse peritoneal macrophages (unpublished results). Dr. Wagner indicates, in his abstract, that he made a similar observation with rabbit macrophages, which would support the theory that some kind of preformed interferon exists.

Secondly, I agree, but with reservations, to the role assigned to the reticuloendothelial system in interferon induction. In eight-week-old C3H mice we found induction of interferon to be very sensitive to total body X-irradiation. A small dose of 125 r. is sufficient to decrease by 80 per cent the normal amounts of circulating interferon obtained four days after irradiation, while after a dose of 250 r. interferon levels are reduced to 1 per cent of those of non-irradiated animals. With Sindbis virus, on the other hand, we find that the amounts of induced interferon come down significantly only after 1,000 r. It is well established that the reticuloendothelial system is resistant to small doses of irradiation, which almost excludes the possibility that macrophages play a prominent role in the induction of circulating interferon with NDV in the mouse. The experiments with Sindbis virus however suggest that macrophages play a role in the induction of interferon with this virus.

Ho: I think these results tend to confirm the role of the reticuloendothelial system. We believe that the RES has a different avidity for and response to these two viruses. First, the differences you observe with NDV and Sindbis virus agree very nicely with the other differences we have seen with these two viruses. They respond differently to tolerance and the interferons they induce have different times of peak appearance. Secondly, B. N. Jaroslow and G. J. V. Nossal (1966. *Aust. J. exp. Biol. med. Sci.*, **44**, 609–628) and others, working on irradiation and antibody formation, find that it is practically impossible to eliminate completely all parameters of the phagocytic activity for an antigen with extremely high irradiation doses. It is therefore very difficult to eliminate the phagocytic function of the RES by irradiation. In addition, post-irradiation stimulation makes precise interpretation even more difficult. The dose as well as the time parameter must be carefully considered.

De Maeyer: It is certainly risky to use just one parameter, but in talking about interferon induction *in vivo*, we should always say which virus was used.

Gresser: Dr. Ho, can homologous interferon be considered a foreign substance if the animal synthesizes interferon as a natural response to viral infection?

The figures we obtained for interferon excretion in mouse urine were very similar to yours in the rabbit, i.e. 0·1 to 0·5 per cent of the total amount administered.

We were unable to recover interferon from the amniotic fluid of the mouse, even when we inoculated interferon preparations titering 1:100,000. Have you attempted to recover interferon from the amniotic fluid?

The time intervals that you demonstrated make me wonder whether phagocytes act indirectly by transmitting a factor to other cells.

Lastly, is it possible that the reduced amounts of interferon that you find after a second or third challenge of virus are being masked by the presence of a factor in the serum or tissue tested that counteracts interferon? In other words the same amount of interferon may be produced after a third challenge but another factor, or factors, may also be liberated which prevents the detection of interferon in your assay system.

Ho: The interferon used was homologous (rabbit) serum interferon. Incubation of tolerant serum with the inducer, except when endotoxin was used, does not inactivate the inducer. No transmissible inactivating factor has been shown—in fact it has not been possible to transmit tolerance. So I don't believe that there is a factor which prevents the detection of interferon. A tentative theory struck us recently which could explain at least the non-specificity of tolerance and why different inducers produce the same phenomenon. That is that tolerance represents an immunological response to interferon. In the state of tolerance, opsonins are produced which facilitate the rapid clearing of any interferon produced. The idea is that clearing of interferon itself is accentuated in the tolerant state. This has the merit of explaining why the most varied inducers produce tolerance. There are, of course, lots of difficulties with this theory also. Why does tolerance only last for a few days, for example? The only answer I can give is that perhaps the opsonin involved is a particularly short-lived one.

Tyrrell: Does the high rate of clearance really indicate that the interferon is a foreign protein? Several physiological proteins—insulin, for example—under appropriate circumstances disappear quite rapidly from the circulation, although they are certainly not foreign in any way.

Secondly, you gave exact figures for renal clearance rates, but these are very difficult to calculate when the concentration is declining rapidly; they are most satisfactorily calculated when there is a dynamic equilibrium, with a constant level in the blood and a constant rate of excretion in the urine. Did you take this into account, first from the point of view of calculating the mean concentration, and then from the point of view of timing when the urine had to be collected in relation to the blood level? It takes some time for what is filtered to get from the glomerulus to the bladder.

Ho: We are quite satisfied with the virus-induced interferon because high levels of interferon are sustained for some hours. It is true that we have to wait an hour or two for its appearance in urine, but it is difficult to work with less than the amount of urine which can be collected in an hour or two hours. I am less satisfied with our data on endotoxin-induced interferon, although I think they definitely indicate a lower clearance. The amount of interferon induced is less, but still we can get measurable serum and urine levels for about four hours. It is of course important in renal clearance work to measure the actual interferon concentration in the serum at the same time as the urine is collected. We did this by measuring serum levels at intervals and got the mean titre, which is an accepted procedure, although it may not be as good as a constant intravenous infusion of interferon to maintain a constant serum level.

The alternative to the foreign protein idea would be to say that interferon is taken up by tissues and cells, as happens with insulin.

Levy: The question of clearance is a little more complicated than has been indicated. Unfortunately a biological test has to be used for interferon and when we talk about finding 1 per cent in the urine, we mean we find 1 per cent of the biological activity in the urine. That may represent 95 per cent of the interferon molecules, most of which have been inactivated. Until a book-keeping system can be used whereby one can recover all the interferon put into the body, one can't really say how much is going into the urine. The different rates of clearance of endotoxin-induced and virus-induced interferon might just be due to different rates of inactivation.

Ho: Yes, I think you are right. In this respect, all we have done is to show that urine *per se* does not directly inactivate the interferon in question, but this of course does not eliminate what happens in the glomerular epithelium. It is not yet possible to eliminate all the possibilities you mention.

Chany: The refractory state you described, Professor Ho, can be obtained not only in the whole animal but also *in vitro*, in the amniotic membrane, as I shall show in my paper. This is obtained with the u.v.-irradiated virus. In this *in vitro* system of course antibody plays no part. Therefore one would think that the refractory state can be due to interferon itself or maybe to some other factor which is antagonistic to the interferon.

Ho: It has been known for a long time that the induction of interferon *in vitro* is not continuous but is a one-shot affair. There is also good evidence, as you said, that the refractoriness to repeated induction is transmitted by a soluble factor—in other words by something that is interferon or associated with interferon. But there is much less evidence *in vivo*.

Stoker: In dealing with whole animals, and especially when thinking about pre-formed interferon, one must always remember that animals already contain a large number of latent viruses.

STATOLON, AS AN INDUCER OF INTERFERON

W. J. Kleinschmidt and L. F. Ellis

Lilly Research Laboratories, Indianapolis

POTENTIATION OF STATOLON ACTIVITY

THE properties of statolon, its low solubility, sedimentability, and tendency to aggregate have continuously accented its macromolecular,

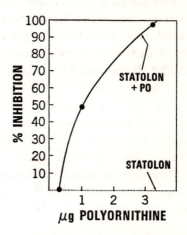

Fig. 1. Potentiation of statolon activity by poly-L-ornithine (PO).

possibly even particulate, nature. Basic polyamino acids are known to increase phagocytosis of particulate materials in leucocytes (De Vries *et al.*, 1955). We asked the question: could a stimulator of phagocytosis such as a basic polyamino acid possibly affect the uptake of statolon by cells?

It was reasoned that an increased uptake of statolon should increase its interferon-inducing capacity and result in greater protection of cells against virus infection. When poly-L-ornithine was applied to cells along with statolon, a potentiation of antiviral activity was evident. Fig. 1 shows the results of such an experiment. Statolon, diluted to a point just below its effective concentration, was applied to monolayers of mouse L cells. To other monolayers were added the same solutions of statolon supplemented with poly-L-ornithine. (Poly-L-ornithine HBr, mol. wt. 100,000 was purchased from Pilot Chemicals, Watertown, Massachusetts, and

39

poly-L-ornithine HBr, mol. wt. 60,000, was obtained from Calbiochem, Los Angeles, California.) After 24 hours at 37° C the fluids were removed, the cells were washed and then infected with vesicular stomatitis virus (VSV) to test for viral inhibitory activity. It can be seen that poly-L-ornithine potentiates the antiviral activity of statolon. An enhancement of inhibition is seen with increased concentration of the polyamino acid. Poly-L-ornithine itself possesses no viral inhibitory activity at the concentrations employed. We explain the potentiation of statolon activity by poly-L-ornithine as resulting from an increased uptake of statolon which in turn brings about a stimulation of interferon production.

POTENTIATION OF INTERFERON ACTIVITY

There has been considerable discussion recently on whether interferon penetrates cells or attaches only to the surface of the cells and acts from the outside. Both positive and negative results have been obtained in adsorption of interferon in serial transfer experiments by several investigators (Buckler, Baron and Levy, 1966; Burke, 1966; Ke, Armstrong and Ho, 1966; Wagner, 1966). Poly-L-ornithine increases not only the penetration of particulate materials into cells, but also that of smaller molecules. Ryser and Hancock (1965) have recently shown that poly-L-ornithine increases the uptake by cells of labelled serum albumin. The use of poly-L-ornithine then permitted another approach to the problem of the site of interferon action, extracellular or intracellular.

Interferon was diluted 10^{-3} to produce about 35 per cent virus inhibition when in contact with cells for three hours. Interferon, alone and together

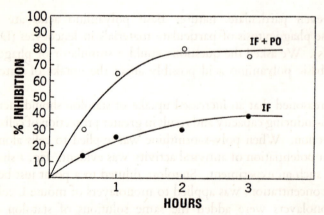

Fig. 2. Potentiation of interferon (IF) activity by poly-L-ornithine (PO). Poly-L-ornithine was applied at a concentration of 3 µg./ml.; the volume was 2·5 ml.

with poly-L-ornithine, was added to L-cell monolayers. After 30 minutes, and after one, two, and three hours, the fluids were removed, the cells were washed and then infected with VSV. The results (Fig. 2) show that poly-L-ornithine also potentiates the activity of interferon. The activity was found to be elevated at each hour, being proportionately higher at the beginning and coming to a plateau at two and three hours.

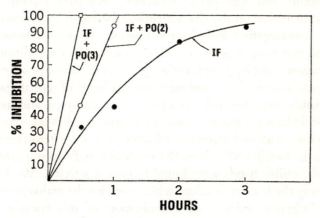

FIG. 3. Potentiation of interferon (IF) activity by poly-L-ornithine (PO). The figures in parentheses indicate the concentration of poly-L-ornithine (μg./ml.) employed.

The experiment was repeated with a slightly higher concentration of interferon ($10^{-2.75}$ dilution). The potentiation is again observed (Fig. 3), and is seen to increase with concentration of the poly-L-ornithine. An experiment has been conducted to determine the actual potentiation in interferon activity produced by poly-L-ornithine. With 3 and 4·5 μg. poly-L-ornithine/ml. the increase in activity over interferon alone was sixfold and 10·7-fold, respectively, in three hours. Poly-L-ornithine at concentrations 0 to 4·5 μg./ml. had no effect on the cells or on plaque formation. At 6 μg./ml. and above an increase in the number of plaques was observed, no doubt due to a greater uptake of virus stimulated by poly-L-ornithine; at 7·5 μg./ml. the number increased to two to three times that in controls. At 10 μg./ml. toxicity to the cells is manifest. The results in these experiments again concur with the interpretation that an increased uptake of interferon is mediated by the poly-L-ornithine.

FURTHER PURIFICATION OF STATOLON

The procedure for isolating statolon from the fermentation filtrate has consisted essentially of precipitation with a water-miscible organic solvent. In early attempts to identify the active molecule of such statolon preparations, our evidence indicated that the antiviral activity was associated with a polysaccharide fraction (Kleinschmidt and Probst, 1962). Statolon, however, admittedly was not pure and because of this there was, of course, uncertainty as to its identity. But further attempts to refine statolon always led to failure, primarily because of its properties of low solubility and aggregative tendency. We have recently obtained further information on the characteristics of statolon by means of sucrose gradient centrifugation and electron microscopic studies, from which it was found that its aggregation could be prevented by the addition of NaCl to the gradients and by maintaining a pH near 9. Statolon solutions were placed on sucrose gradients and after 16 to 24 hours of centrifugation, two visible bands were formed. Fractions were collected and assayed for interferon-inducing capacity with the mouse L-cell-VSV system or by injecting mice with such fractions and determining interferon levels of their sera with the L-cell-VSV system (Kleinschmidt and Murphy, 1965, 1967).

Both the visible bands were found to possess activity. We have so far studied only the heavier fraction, which contains the major portion of the activity. Electron microscope examination of this fraction disclosed numerous particles possessing the typical morphology of viruses. Higher magnification of negatively stained preparations revealed that the particles were hexagonal and approximately 30 mμ in diameter (Fig. 4).

The evidence that interferon-inducing activity is associated with these particles is based on the following observations. Interferon-stimulating activity was found to correlate with the number of particles distributed in the fractions. The band containing the most particles showed a higher interferon-inducing capacity both in tissue culture and in animals. Fractions adjacent to this band demonstrated less activity and correspondingly fewer particles. No particles were seen in inactive fractions.

Evidence indicates that the mould *Penicillium stoloniferum* is the source of the particles. Uninoculated media incubated for the same length of time as is employed for normal statolon fermentation (five to seven days) showed neither interferon-inducing activity nor the presence of particles. Neither activity nor particles were detected in inoculated media until after four days of incubation had ensued. Another primary piece of evidence that the particles are derived from the mould is the demonstration, with the electron microscope, of particles within thin sections of mycelia which possess the morphology of those obtained by gradient centrifugation (Fig. 5).

We refer to the particles as virus-like because we have not been able as yet to demonstrate the property of infectivity, nor have we satisfactorily shown

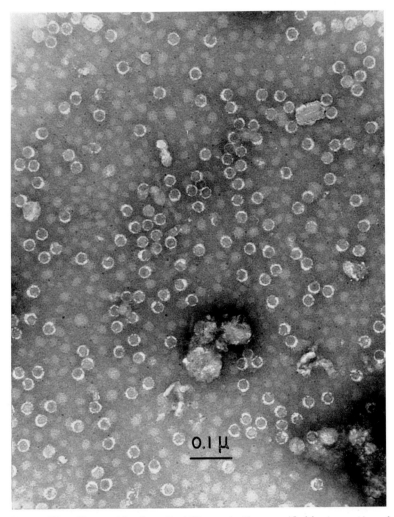

Fig. 4. Virus-like particles from *Penicillium stoloniferum* purified by isopycnic and rate zonal density gradient centrifugation. Negative stain with phosphotungstic acid.

[*To face page 42*

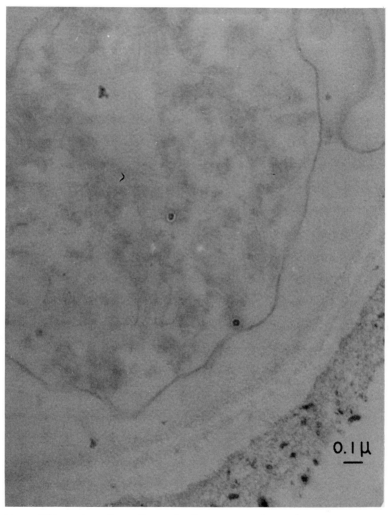

Fig. 5. Thin section of *Penicillium stoloniferum* fixed with glutaraldehyde and post-fixed with osmium tetroxide. Section was stained with uranyl acetate.

nucleic acid to be associated with the particle *per se*. We have failed to detect infectivity by cellular lysis, but since cell destruction during replication is not a characteristic of all viruses, it may be that replication of this particle may also occur without lysis. The particles possess a density of approximately 1·20. This density is relatively low for viruses and means that the particles contain little nucleic acid, perhaps insufficient for coding the necessary proteins for replication. The particle may be an incomplete virus. Elucidation of the problem of the nucleic acid content is imperative and it is at present being pursued, as is the question of infectivity.

To our knowledge this is the first report of particles with viral morphology associated with the class Fungi Imperfecti. It is possible that two known disease abnormalities of Fungi Imperfecti are caused by viruses, but in neither of these instances has the infective agent been identified (Lindberg, 1959; Jinks, 1959; Grogan and Campbell, 1966). Hollings (1962) and Hollings, Gandy and Last (1963) have clearly identified the virus that causes dieback disease of cultivated mushrooms (Homobasidiomycetes). Lindegren and Bang (1961) and Lindegren, Bang and Hirano (1962) have reported evidence that a phage occurs in a yeast, but micrographs of particles identified as the phage reveal structures lacking the uniformity normally associated with viruses.

We are aware that hexagonal intracellular crystalline inclusions of ergosterol have been observed in the mould *Neurospora crassa* by Tsuda and Tatum (1961). Some ergosterol is found associated with the heavier statolon band of the sucrose gradient. Exhaustive extraction of statolon solutions with chloroform or ether, however, removes all the ergosterol without a significant loss in activity or particles.

Particles are not detectable by electron microscopy in the lighter band (35 per cent sucrose), which contains a minor portion of the total interferon-inducing activity. Further study is needed to show whether the activity of this fraction is mould-derived or virus-derived.

Interferon studies have played an important role in detecting these particles with virus morphology in a mould of the Fungi Imperfecti class. Viruses of fungi may not be as rare as was once thought (Luria, 1953; Smith and Williams, 1958), but their detectability is made difficult by the presence of other cellular components. Interferon determinations combined with density gradient centrifugation and electron microscope studies may be helpful in uncovering the existence of other viruses of fungi.

Eventual conclusive identification of statolon as a virus would mean that a non-mammalian virus is capable of stimulating the production of interferon. A recognition mechanism that is stimulated into operation in cells on infection by a mammalian virus as a means of defence against that virus is apparently also triggered into action by the virus-like statolon particles. Not only has the finding of these particles with virus morphology added to the interferon story, but should these particles prove to be viruses, new studies with moulds, such as the introduction of genetic material via transduction, may also have been made feasible.

PROTECTION AGAINST YABA VIRUS IN MONKEYS

We have recently attempted to develop an assay for the testing of statolon or other interferon-inducing substances in primates in order to aid the determination of the clinical possibilities of these substances. A non-lethal virus was considered to be necessary, and Yaba virus was chosen. Protection against this virus could be determined by observing the prevention of tumour formation or by measuring the size of tumours when they did develop. (The Yaba virus was obtained from Dr. Julian L. Ambrus, Roswell Park Memorial Institute, Springville Laboratories, Springville, N.Y.)

Statolon was injected into three cynomolgus monkeys subcutaneously in the abdominal area at a dose of 19·3 mg./kg. (statolon weight based on non-dialysable solids). Other monkeys, serving as controls, were injected with equivalent quantities of 1 per cent $NaHCO_3$. Twenty-four hours later all were infected subcutaneously with four dilutions of Yaba virus (10^{-3} to 10^{-6}) at four different sites on their backs (Ambrus et al., 1963). Six days after the initial statolon injection another dose was administered to bolster interferon levels while avoiding the period of tolerance to further stimulation, as seen in the mouse (Kleinschmidt and Murphy, 1967). Monkeys were bled about 20 hours after each injection of statolon. Unfortunately the interferon response, assayed on BSC1 green monkey cells (Kleinschmidt and Murphy, 1967) was minimal, very likely because of lack of sensitivity of these cells to cynomolgus monkey interferon. So correlation of interferon levels to protection could not be made.

Nevertheless, protection was observed. Delayed tumour development was seen in one of the monkeys treated with statolon. At 25 days after infection all the control monkeys, but only one of the treated animals, had tumours at the sites at which Yaba virus dilutions of 10^{-3} and 10^{-4} had been given. At 35 days, tumours had developed as shown in Table I. One of the treated monkeys was still completely protected; another developed a tumour only at the site of highest virus concentration. The protection exerted by statolon is shown by the mean tumour diameters, calculated by dividing the sum of the tumour diameters by the number of monkeys included in the test. The test as applied to the cynomolgus monkeys was based on information obtained from the mouse and the African green monkey. Refinement of the assay by determination of optimum

TABLE I

PROTECTION AFFORDED BY STATOLON AGAINST VARIOUS DILUTIONS OF YABA VIRUS INJECTED INTO MONKEYS

Dimensions of tumours (mm.)

Monkey no.		Dilution of Yaba virus			
		10^{-3}	10^{-4}	10^{-5}	10^{-6}
		Statolon-treated			
127		17·5	0	0	0
129		0	0	0	0
131		21·5	19·5	11	0
	Mean diameter	13	6·5	3·7	0
		Not treated			
128		29	26	15	0
130		23·5	18·5	0	0
132		23	14	0	0
	Mean diameter	25·1	19·5	5	0

conditions, e.g. statolon injection and virus infection schedules, for the cynomolgus monkey should result in a satisfactory test procedure with the Yaba virus.

SUMMARY

We have observed a potentiation of antiviral activity of both statolon and interferon by poly-L-ornithine. The potentiated activity increases with the concentration of poly-L-ornithine, which itself possesses no viral inhibitory activity at the concentration employed. Since poly-L-ornithine increases the penetration of substances into cells, our results can be explained by an increase in uptake of statolon and interferon by the cells. This observation supports the concept that interferon penetrates into mammalian cells and acts intracellularly rather than from outside the cell.

Density gradient centrifugation and electron microscopic studies have enabled us to obtain further information on the physical characteristics of statolon. Particles possessing the morphology of viruses are found in an isopycnic band after centrifugation of statolon preparations on a sucrose gradient. These particles, hexagonal in shape and 30 mµ in diameter, are associated with interferon-inducing activity. Electron microscopic examination of thin sections of mycelia of *Penicillium stoloniferum* have also revealed the presence of particles with the same characteristics as those obtained by gradient centrifugation.

An attempt has been made to develop a method for testing statolon and other interferon-inducing substances in primates to aid determination of their clinical potentialities. Cynomolgus monkeys, treated with statolon and untreated controls, were infected with Yaba virus. A degree of protection is observed in animals receiving statolon.

ACKNOWLEDGEMENTS

We thank E. L. Hayes, M. M. Hoehn, E. B. Murphy, R. Schlegel, V. C. Spurling, R. M. VanFrank, and F. Streightoff and his group for assistance in these studies.

REFERENCES

AMBRUS, J. L., FELTZ, E. T., GRACE, J. T., JR., and OWEN, G. (1963). *Natn. Cancer Inst. Monogr.*, **10**, pp. 447–458.

BUCKLER, C. E., BARON, S., and LEVY, H. B. (1966). *Science*, **152**, 80–82.

BURKE, D. C. (1966). Personal communication. IEG No. 6, Memo 173.

DE VRIES, A., SALGO, J., MATOTH, Y., NEVO, A., and KATCHALSKI, E. (1955). *Archs int. Pharmacodyn. Thér.*, **104**, 1–10.

GROGAN, R. G., and CAMPBELL, R. N. (1966). *A. Rev. Phytopathol.*, **4**, 29–52.

HOLLINGS, M. (1962). *Nature, Lond.*, **196**, 962–965.

HOLLINGS, M., GANDY, D. G., and LAST, F. T. (1963). *Endeavour*, **22**, 112–117.

JINKS, J. L. (1959). *J. gen. Microbiol.*, **21**, 397–409.

KE, Y., ARMSTRONG, J., and HO, M. (1966). Personal communication. IEG No. 6, Memo 235.

KLEINSCHMIDT, W. J., and MURPHY, E. B. (1965). *Virology*, **27**, 484–489.

KLEINSCHMIDT, W. J., and MURPHY, E. B. (1967). *Bact. Rev.*, **31**, 132–137.

KLEINSCHMIDT, W. J., and PROBST, G. W. (1962). *Antibiotics Chemother.*, **12**, 298–309.

LINDBERG, G. D. (1959). *Phytopathology*, **49**, 29–32.

LINDEGREN, C. C., and BANG, Y. N. (1961). *Antonie van Leeuwenhoek*, **27**, 1–18.

LINDEGREN, C. C., BANG, Y. N., and HIRANO, T. (1962). *Trans. N.Y. Acad. Sci.*, **24**, 540–566.

LURIA, S. E. (1953). In *General Virology*, p. 15. New York: John Wiley and Sons.

RYSER, H. J. P., and HANCOCK, R. (1965). *Science*, **150**, 501–503.

SMITH, K. M., and WILLIAMS, R. C. (1958). *Endeavour*, **17**, 12–21.

TSUDA, S., and TATUM, E. L. (1961). *J. biophys. biochem. Cytol.*, **11**, 171–177.

WAGNER, R. R. (1966). Personal communication. IEG No. 6, Memo 154.

DISCUSSION

Baron: If poly-L-ornithine increases the activity of interferon by sixfold to ten-fold it would suggest that without poly-L-ornithine most of the applied interferon is at an ineffective extracellular site, with only a small amount of applied interferon reaching the active site. If poly-L-ornithine actually increases cellular uptake of interferon then it would help the large portion of interferon to reach the active site.

Has statolon been shown to be antigenic?

Kleinschmidt: We have not shown this yet, but the rabbits should be producing antibodies right now.

These experiments were of course just run for three hours. If we ran an experiment to determine the potentiation activity for 24 hours this might help to elucidate your first point. It may be that the activity is just speeded up, that is the uptake is increased, and one sees this in three hours but not in 24 hours.

Wagner: Don't you have to measure the disappearance of interferon from the medium in contact with the cells before you can say that it is taken up?

Kleinschmidt: To do that we would have had to eliminate the poly-L-ornithine and in the process interferon would also be lost.

Chain: Crude statolon contains protein, but the more we purify it and remove the protein, the less active it seems to become.

Kleinschmidt: We have not determined this. The polysaccharide fraction contains a lot of amino sugars, which would account for plenty of nitrogen, and I know extraneous proteins are present.

Joklik: What percentage of the weight of crude statolon is accounted for by the particles which you see?

Kleinschmidt: We think it is between $0 \cdot 1$ and $0 \cdot 5$ per cent, so really there is not very much there. We have also calculated that it takes about 10^{10} particles to protect a mouse. We have not been able to estimate how many are needed to protect one cell.

Chain: Is the view that these particles resemble viruses only based on their morphological appearance as crystalloids of regular form, as is revealed by the electron microscope? Many polysaccharides may assume crystalline form under appropriate conditions. For instance, starch can readily be converted into Schardinger dextrins; the α-form crystallizes in hexagonal plates.

Kleinschmidt: We may be just imagining this, but the points of light at the ends indicate capsomeres. Tsuda and Tatum's finding (1961, *loc. cit.*) of ergosterol crystals in *Neurospora* was exciting, but these again were not of uniform size. One similarity is that only one or two of these crystals are found in a small area of mycelia too.

Burke: Statolon appears to be the only non-viral agent which will produce interferon in tissue culture. We haven't been able to produce interferon with the material you sent us, Dr. Kleinschmidt, though we can get interference. We did look at production of antibody against statolon because we are interested in assaying interferon in the presence of statolon. We found we could do this by adding the statolon/interferon mixture to cells and then challenging after three or four hours, when interferon but not statolon is active. We also looked at the antigenic properties of the statolon you sent us. We raised antibody which gave precipitin lines on Ouchterlony plates and which after agar gel electrophoresis gave three separate bands, but this antiserum had no effect on the interfering ability of the statolon preparation.

Levy: If these particles are virus particles would you expect to need pH 9 to solubilize the antiviral action, Dr. Kleinschmidt? In other words why do you have to dissolve statolon in sodium bicarbonate to get it active?

Kleinschmidt: What the pH 9 and the salt do here is to solubilize all the contaminating material of the statolon, permitting the virus to be released.

Levy: It would be worth testing. If you brought it down to pH 7 again and precipitated out the active principle, would this be consistent with it being a virus?

Kleinschmidt: We could test this but there is probably still enough contaminating material to permit aggregation.

Tyrrell: Your finding of a density of 1·2 for the particles doesn't seem to tie up with Dr. Burke's suggestion that nucleic acid might be the inducer of interferon production. This density would suggest that these were incomplete particles which had lost their nucleic acid. They also look like hollow shell-like particles which wouldn't contain nucleic acid. The other difficulty is that your Fig. 4 shows many other particles which are much less clearly defined and have a great range of sizes, which I presume you ignore when you count the uniform particles with a hexagonal outline. Are the other particles distributed in the same bands as the virus-like particles, or uniformly through the whole of the gradient? It is possible that the effects are produced by the things which don't look like virus particles.

Kleinschmidt: We consistently find a correlation between the number of particles and the activity of the preparations. Of course there is a lot of background material that is not virus-like, but it is difficult to get at it. When we use velocity sedimentation instead of equilibrium sedimentation the activity still correlates with the number of particles.

Tyrrell: Have you ever found fractions which are inactive and contain these small irregular-sized particles in large numbers but have none of the regular-sized virus-like particles?

Kleinschmidt: We wanted to wait until we had more pure material before we ran chemical studies on the other fraction. The background "particles" that you are referring to in Fig. 4 are ascribed to phosphotungstate salt.

Chany: The statolon particles look very much like Kilham's rat virus, which we know has 32 capsomeres. Do they haemagglutinate?

Kleinschmidt: We have not tested for haemagglutination.

Andrewes: A lot of the particles with shiny outlines in Fig. 4 are very thick on one side and have a signet-ring appearance. What virus are they like?

Pereira: An adenovirus that is breaking up looks very much like that. Some of the capsomeres accumulate at the margin and break into these groups of nine which in profile look fairly similar to those in Fig. 4. They look more like incomplete viruses or viruses that are breaking than like full particles.

Crick: Is there any phosphorus? Is there a small amount of nucleic acid, or any lipid? I think most of these questions will be answered when statolon is purified.

Chain: There is very little phosphorus in our purified statolon preparations.

Crick: You wouldn't get very much if there was a small amount of nucleic acid. Is your nitrogen compatible with it being mainly protein?

Chain: It is the protein content we measure; some of our purified preparations contain about 2 per cent protein.

Kleinschmidt: Do your fractions give positive tests for polysaccharide?

Chain: Yes, it is a heparin-like substance.

Crick: The particles in your Fig. 4 look much more like aggregates of protein molecules than like polysaccharide, Dr. Kleinschmidt.

INTERFERON INDUCTION IN MOUSE AND MAN WITH VIRAL AND NON-VIRAL STIMULI

Thomas C. Merigan

Division of Infectious Diseases, Department of Medicine, Stanford University School of Medicine, Palo Alto, California

GREAT hope has existed for the clinical potential of interferon since its discovery in 1957. We have been interested in evaluating various inducers of interferon production with an eye towards their possible application in clinical medicine, either in prophylaxis or therapy of virus infections. Animal models have been useful for such studies, and in particular the mouse model has been instructive to us. I would like first to discuss results obtained, in our laboratory and elsewhere, by employing viruses for the systemic induction of human interferon, before going on to results obtained in the mouse and man with a new class of non-viral inducers.

VIRAL INDUCERS IN MAN

The induction of interferon in man by many viral stimuli has been described; our work has focused on myxovirus inducers. First, it was found that, during infection with an attenuated strain (Edmonston) of measles virus, circulating interferon was present 7 to 11 days after vaccination of non-immune children (Petralli, Merigan and Wilbur, 1965*a*). More recently, naturally occurring mumps virus infection proved to have comparable levels of interferon in the serum for an apparently similar duration of time (Waddell, Merigan and Wilbur, 1967). In both, the interferon was present during the symptoms of the infection: fever and, rarely, rash with the Edmonston vaccine, and parotitis or other symptoms during the mumps infection. These results with myxoviruses *in vivo*, and the known potency of Newcastle disease virus (NDV) in inducing interferon in human cells in tissue culture, made it reasonable to study the effects of NDV in man in some detail.

We obtained a highly attenuated strain of NDV (73-T) which has been subjected to multiple passages in tissue culture in another laboratory and had already been given to several humans in high dosage (10^{13} plaque-forming units [p.f.u.] subcutaneously) without incident (Cassel and Garrett, 1965). This virus was passaged in our laboratory once in pathogen-free embryonated eggs. The NDV was then concentrated from chorioallantoic fluid by ultracentrifugation and passed through a 0·45 μ cellulose acetate filter. The preparation was subjected to safety tests by standard bacteriological techniques to check for bacterial, pleuropneumonia-like organisms, or fungus contaminants, and it was inoculated into several tissue culture lines and experimental animals so that other adventitious agents could be looked for.

Our first goal was to examine the dose response curve for interferon production by NDV in humans. Patients with tumours were carefully studied after low dosages of virus had been intravenously injected in the hope that we might find a dose which would induce circulating interferon without symptomatology. If a safe dose in humans can be established we are considering study of the influence of various host factors, including splenectomy, the presence of high or low amounts of circulating white cells, various drugs or disease states, etc., on the human interferon production mechanism *in vivo*. As this virus had not been clearly associated with systemic disease in man despite the frequency with which it is handled in the laboratory and in the veterinary industry, it seemed a good candidate for this purpose. Also, we do not expect to encounter individuals with circulating antibodies directed against this virus which might interfere with its interferon-inducing capabilities. As Dr. Gresser and his co-workers (1968) will tell us, interferon is active against tumour viruses in mice, and Wheelock and Dingle (1964) and Ho and Postic (1967), amongst others, have therefore speculated on a potential oncolytic effect of interferon-inducing agents. This suggested that some advantage might come to the patients involved in this study, hence their immediate and later clinical course was followed. Patient participation in the study, however, was obtained on the basis that the results obtained might help in understanding why certain virus infections have severe courses in patients with diseases similar to theirs, rather than as a potentially curative procedure.

We are in the process of conducting this study (Waddell, Walker and Merigan, 1967), and so far have only defined the dosage necessary for interferon production, which is rather low: 10^{-5} p.f.u. When the dose is increased to 2×10^{-6} p.f.u., interferon levels are higher but associated with fever and mild influenza-like symptoms. Eleven patients have been given varying doses with, as yet, no major effects on tumour growth or significant side effects other than a transient mild leucopenia. A serological response to the virus was defined in each patient by a neutralization assay, but viraemia and viruria have not been noted, whereas the latter has been demonstrated in patients given higher doses (Cassel and Garrett, 1965).

Other investigators have followed serum interferon production after the 17D strain of yellow fever (Wheelock and Sibley, 1965) and influenza virus (Jao, Wheelock and Jackson, 1965) vaccinations, as well as during infection of infants with respiratory syncytial virus (Ray, Gravelle and Chin, 1967). In these cases circulating interferon appeared also during the period of symptomatology. Human interferon has been identified in the cerebrospinal fluid during mumps virus infection and other cases of aseptic meningitis associated with enterovirus infections (Larke, 1967). It has also been found in the pharyngeal washings of patients undergoing upper respiratory tract infections (Gresser and Dull, 1964) and has been reported in the vesicle fluid of naturally occurring chicken-pox (Wheelock, 1967) and of primary immunizations with vaccinia (Wheelock, 1964).

We have had the opportunity to study a child with mild progressive vaccinia, and an adult patient who ultimately died of disseminated herpes zoster occurring during treatment for a lymphoma. It is of interest that we were able to demonstrate interferon both in the infant's primary vaccination scab and in the cerebrospinal fluid and skin vesicle fluid of the patient with zoster, indicating that a *complete* defect in interferon synthesis did not underlie its dissemination in either of these cases (D. Waddell and T. C. Merigan, 1967, unpublished observations). Of course, a quantitative defect is still possible, as would be failure of cells to respond to interferon in a normal fashion.

Recently, we have observed interferon in the parotid gland secretions of individuals undergoing natural mumps infection (Waddell, Merigan and Wilbur, 1967), which demonstrates the ability of the infected salivary gland tissues to produce interferon as well as virus. In the patients with mumps infection and during NDV vaccination we have looked for interferon in the urine. Only with methods involving concentration of urine were we able to demonstrate a few units of human interferon despite elevated circulating interferon. It was hoped that the urine might be a source of crude human interferon for further purification, but this appears unlikely at the present time.

NON-VIRAL INDUCERS OF INTERFERON

Non-viral inducers appear preferable to live agents for the induction of endogenous interferon in man. This is because of the difficulty in both ruling out the presence of adventitious contaminants in any preparation of live agents and being assured that live agents will behave benignly in all individuals. Therefore, about a year ago, in collaboration with Drs. Sheldon Wolff and Harry Kimball of the National Institutes of Health,

Dr. Dorothy Waddell and I examined the possibility that endotoxin would act as a trigger for interferon production in man. Unfortunately, with the doses of endotoxin employed in experimental studies in man at present, no interferon production could be observed despite a good febrile response. Independently, Dr. Richard Michaels at the University of Pittsburgh has made similar observations (Ho and Postic, 1967). Clearly, agents like cycloheximide which induce interferon in animals are unlikely to be useful in inducing human interferon *in vivo*, since their parallel effect on protein synthesis appears to be irreversible and is probably directly related to their interferon-producing action. Phytohaemagglutinin might be a useful

TABLE I

INTERFERON-INDUCING CAPACITY OF VARIOUS SYNTHETIC POLYANIONS (PART I)

Polymer designation	Components*	Modification	Mol. wt.	Dose (mg./kg.)	Interferon titre in units/4 ml.†
NSC46015-C	MA/DVE	None	17,000	125	246
NSC46015	MA/DVE	None	36,000	125	185
X1308357-H6	MA/DVE	None	40,000	125 / 400	75 / 87
NSC68987	MA/DVE	None	110,000	125 / 400	97 / 480
NSC68988	MA/DVE	None	450,000	125 / 400	78 / 360
T-145	MA/VA	45% half methyl ester	> 120,000	100 / 500 / 1000	280 / 200 / +
S983	MA/VME	Ammoniated	20–30,000	100 / 500 / 1000	30 / 30 / +
AN119	MA/VME	None	250,000	500 / 1000	< 10 / 80
AN4151	MA/VME	50% amidated	250,000	500 / 1000	< 10 / 55
AN3391	MA/VME	50% methyl esterified	500,000	150 / 300	430 / 1000
AN169	MA/VME	None	1,250,000	200 / 500	< 10 / 300
AN4651	MA/VME	50% amidated	1,250,000	500 / 1000	< 10 / < 10
S810	MA/S	None	1,400	25	< 10
S-811	MA/S	None	10,000	25 / 125	< 10 / < 10
S-812	MA/S	None	70,000	25 / 75	< 10 / 30
T-148	MA/S	Ammoniated	120,000	100 / 500	< 10 / < 10

* Maleic anhydride—MA; divinyl ether—DVE; vinyl methyl ether—VME; vinyl acetate—VA; styrene—S.
† + = died.

INTER.—3

stimulus of human interferon *in vivo*, but the response appears to be only modest in the whole animal (mouse) (T. C. Merigan and L. Epstein, 1967, unpublished observations). Phytohaemagglutinin is still material obtained from natural sources and would require careful purification before large-scale use in man.

Synthetic materials of known composition prepared in the laboratory would be the simplest inducers if they were effective. Recently, synthetic copolymers of maleic acid anhydride have been observed to induce interferon production in the mouse (Regelson, 1967). We have become quite interested in this series of compounds in the past few months, studying some 35 to determine the structural requirements for their interferon-inducing action (Merigan, 1967) (Tables I and II). These studies were carried out in the mouse and utilized these compounds at several different dosage levels, despite difficulties due to their variable solubility in the aqueous buffers used for the injections. The compounds had toxic effects at high dosages and, after injection of these polymers, circulating white cells have been observed to have inclusion bodies, most probably representing phagocytized aggregates of the polymers (Regelson, 1967) (Fig. 1). The interferon production at its peak is only modest, perhaps 1/20th that observed in intravenous injection of NDV in the mouse, and 1/6th to 1/8th that observed with statolon in the mouse.

Characterization of the circulating antiviral activity induced by these polymers in the mouse has shown it to be interferon. Studies were carried out in some detail because at high concentration these materials are capable of direct polyelectrolyte interaction with most viruses. We find that after either intravenous or peritoneal injection of copolymer the antiviral activity is produced by the host and does not represent circulating copolymer for several reasons. First, several hours are required for its appearance. So far we have failed to induce interferon *in vitro* with the copolymer. The antiviral material is a protein of 70,000 molecular weight; it is somewhat acid-labile and can be inactivated with trypsin. It is cell-species-specific in its antiviral action and requires time for its action to be demonstrated in a tissue culture assay. The presence of actinomycin D will block its antiviral action in a fashion similar to virus-induced interferon. Table III summarizes the data in Tables I and II and points out what we consider at present, from studies with both the maleic anhydride/ethylene and the polyacrylic acid series, to be the structural requirements for the interferon-inducing activity of these copolymers. At present, it can be stated that the required structure appears to be a 17,000 molecular weight or greater, saturated aliphatic carbon chain with carboxylate groups on

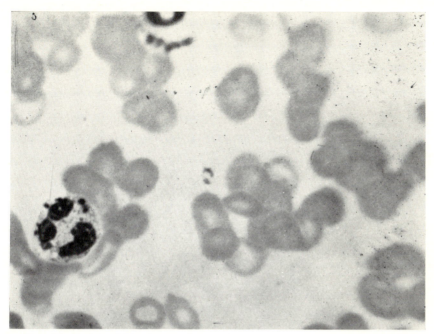

FIG. 1(*a*). Peripheral blood smear (× 320) showing polymorphonuclear leucocytes with inclusion bodies in a patient 12 days after the injection of 8 mg. of pyran/kg. body weight.

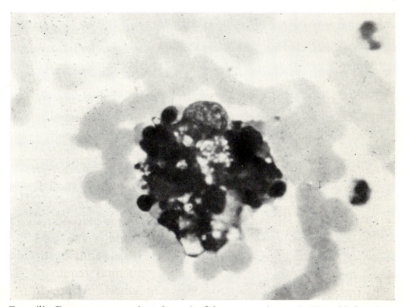

FIG. 1(*b*). Bone marrow aspirate (× 320) of the same patient as in Fig. 1(*a*) showing a histiocyte containing polymer particles.

[*To face page 54*

TABLE II

INTERFERON-INDUCING CAPACITY OF VARIOUS SYNTHETIC POLYANIONS (PART 2)

Polymer designation	Components*	Modification	Mol. wt.	Dose (mg./kg.)	Interferon titre in units/4 ml.†
S-645	E/MA		2–3,000	100 500	< 10 < 30
S-216	E/MA	Ammoniated	2–3,000	100 500	< 30 < 30
S-750	E/MA	1/2 Amide 1/2 Acid	20–30,000	100 500	48 55
T-1	E/MA	Mono methylated 1/2 amide	20–30,000	100 500	< 30 < 30
S-749	E/MA	Ammoniated	20–30,000	100 500 1000	< 30 93 +
T-16	E/MA	Para-aminobenzoic acid 1/2 amide	20–30,000	25 50 100	< 30 88 +
S-215	E/MA		60–70,000	10 50 100	151 402 +
S-730	E/MA		80–100,000	50 100 500	70 96 +
T-138	E/MA	Ammoniated	80–100,000	100 500	< 30 < 30
T-142	P/MA		20–30,000	100 500 1000	< 30 250 +
S-917	P/MA	Ammoniated	20–30,000	100 500	145 100
S-969	IB/MA	Ammoniated	60–70,000	125 500	110 +
T-13	IB/MA	Dimethylamino- propyl amine 1/2 amide	20–30,000	100 200 500 1000	< 30 < 30 < 30 < 30
T-357	MAc		116	100	< 30
T-132	PA		60–70,000	50 100 500	< 30 91 50
S-644	PA	Methyl	60–70,000	50 100 500	< 30 < 30 128
S-692	PA	Amide	60–70,000	100 500	< 30 < 30
T-564	PE	Oxide	20,000	50 100 500	< 30 < 30 < 30
T-565	PE	Oxide	Medium	100 500	< 30 +
	PE	Imine	150,000	2	< 10

* Maleic anhydride—MA; maleic acid—MAc; ethylene—E; propylene—P; polyethylene—PE; polyacrylic acid—PA; isobutylene—IB.
† + = died.

TABLE III

REQUIREMENTS FOR COPOLYMER ACTIVITY

MOLECULAR WEIGHT

(1) Random copolymers of 17,000 to 1,250,000 are active, 3,000 or less inactive
(2) Higher molecular weight materials are less active per milligram, therefore requiring more material for same response

COPOLYMER COMPONENTS

(a) Maleic acid anhydride

```
—CH————CH—
    |        |
    CO      CO
      \    /
        O
```

(1) Maleic acid seems required for best activity, but free maleic acid is inactive
(2) If 50% methyl esterified, no loss in activity
(3) 50% amidation or ammoniation may lower activity, especially if all carboxyls are modified

(b) Other

```
—CH₂—CH—
        |
        R
```

(1) Ethylene copolymer is active, without R substitution
(2) However, R can be acetate ester, methyl ether, or ethyl ether and activity is retained
(3) If R is benzene ring (e.g. styrene), then it is inactive
(4) Propylene copolymer is also active
(5) Isobutylene copolymers are also active, but poorly soluble, hence less active
(6) A polyethyleneimine polymer of 150,000 mol. wt. and a polyethylene oxide polymer of 20,000 mol. wt. are not active

OR

(a)   (b)   Polyacrylic acid

```
—CH—CH₂—CH—CH₂—
   |         |
   COOH     COOH
```

(1) Active even with methyl group substitution on the otherwise unsubstituted backbone methylene group
(2) Amidation markedly decreases activity

two out of every four or five carbons in either alternate or adjacent positions. Some substitution on the backbone carbons is possible with either methyl or ethyl groups, but not with bulky groups such as benzene. Bulky or negatively charged groups on the carboxyl groups also tend to decrease the activity of the copolymer. It is possible that the bulky groups may interfere with the interferon-inducing capacity by sterically hindering the carboxylate groups in their interaction in the cell. The importance of these groups is suggested by the fact that derivatives without them or with completely substituted carboxylate groups appear to be inactive. A few of the less active derivatives are rather thick gels which may have difficulty reaching the interferon-inducing site from the peritoneal cavity where they are injected. Hence, the solubility properties of the polymer may play an important role in limiting the number of active derivatives.

Recently we have found that animals reinjected with these anionic copolymers three to eight days after the initial injection do not respond with circulating interferon. This phenomenon of tolerance has been noted with most other inducers of interferon and would seem to limit clinical usefulness. We are now studying possibilities for overcoming this effect.

In vivo ANTIVIRAL ACTION OF SYNTHETIC INTERFERON INDUCERS

Regelson (1967) has demonstrated these anionic copolymers to be active against Friend leukaemia virus in the mouse for as long as six days at a dosage of 125 mg./kg. We have been interested in their action in the mouse against a small neurotropic RNA virus, Mengo. We have noted that dosages of 125 mg./kg. down to 1 mg./kg. will keep alive mice challenged with a lethal dose of Mengo virus. Anionic polymers from natural sources have been noted to be active against viruses in this class *in vivo* but only for a period of a few hours after their injection (Elliott and Higginbotham, 1960). Although we found that the pyran copolymer was not active against Mengo if given a day or more after the Mengo virus, when it was given between one and 32 days before the Mengo virus it significantly increased survival in contrast to that of untreated controls.

This prolonged protection, together with the knowledge that polymer persists in white blood cells for several weeks (long after circulating interferon has ceased to be detected), concerned us. It raised the possibility of either a separate direct polymer-virus interaction or continued low-level interferon production. Knowing others had observed direct interaction between Mengo and anionic copolymers, we had deliberately chosen the L strain of virus which was resistant to direct inhibition by other acidic copolymers (Campbell and Colter, 1965). However, when we incubated the pyran copolymer with our strain of Mengo virus at a concentration of 0·1 mg./ml. it decreased the infectivity and the plaque-forming units significantly. Regelson (1967) has already observed that this direct inhibition occurs with Friend virus leukaemia, and Feltz and Regelson (1962) have seen polyelectrolyte interaction with both Semliki Forest virus and ECHO 9. Recently, one of the more insoluble of these compounds has been advocated as a means of removing viruses from water by direct binding (Johnson, Fields and Darlington, 1967). Initially, we thought these compounds did not bind vesicular stomatitis virus. However, when this was re-examined at a higher concentration of polymer (0·5 mg./ml.), it was clear that some neutralization of infectivity of VSV occurred.

As we were interested in the basis of the action of these compounds *in vivo*, we decided to work with vaccinia, a virus which showed only a minimal interaction with polyelectrolytes. Incubation of vaccinia with the copolymer demonstrated that only at 5 mg./ml., which is perhaps 50-fold the concentration which would react with Mengo, would some decrease in infectivity of vaccinia occur. Therefore, with this great disparity in interaction and probably similar sensitivity of these two viruses to interferon action, we can probe the extent of antiviral protection due to interferon by measuring the effect of these polymers on vaccinia lesion formation on the tail of the mouse. Preliminary results suggest that the polymers are similarly active against vaccinia. In all cases the direct action of these polymers was dependent on their concentration and, in the absence of exact knowledge of their intracellular fate and the *in vivo* sites of virus replication, it is difficult to exclude the possible direct effects on a given virus.

COPOLYMER STUDIES IN MAN

In conclusion I would like to describe briefly the results of some studies that we are carrying out in collaboration with Dr. William Regelson (Merigan and Regelson, 1967). One of these polyanions, a pyran copolymer of 17,000 molecular weight (Fig. 2), has been approved in the United

$$-CH-CH- \qquad\qquad CH_2=CH-O-CH=CH_2$$
$$\begin{array}{cc} | & | \\ CO & CO \\ \diagdown & \diagup \\ & O \end{array}$$

Maleic anhydride   Divinyl ether

FIG. 2. Components of pyran (NSC 46015–C), an interferon-inducing synthetic anionic random copolymer of 17,000 molecular weight.

States for use in humans as an antitumour agent in studies conducted by the Eastern Solid Tumor Group. This pyran copolymer is one of the more active interferon-inducing compounds in the series, and we have undertaken study of the dosage level required in man to induce circulating interferon. It appears that a dosage very similar to that employed in the mouse is required for interferon production in humans, i.e. 12 to 15 mg./kg. The time of appearance of this antiviral material in the serum of humans is quite similar to that in the mouse at this dose, since it peaks at two days after injection and is detectable for a period of perhaps three days. The antiviral activity has been characterized in our human interferon assay (foreskin fibroblast-VSV). It behaves similarly to virus-induced interferon as it appears in the human sera, in that it is trypsin-sensitive and not sedimented by 100,000 **g** for two hours, and is species specific in its antiviral action. In the future we plan to examine the *in vivo* antiviral potential of these compounds against safe standard live virus challenges to determine what dosage of copolymer is required for protection. It is possible that the dosage required for *in vivo* protection will be, as in the mouse, much lower than that required to produce circulating interferon. As we have already observed a systemic action of interferon induced *in vivo* in the human against vaccinia with similar circulating levels of interferon (Petralli, Merigan and Wilbur, 1965*b*), I suspect these compounds will provide *in vivo* protection in man. However, it certainly remains to be seen whether this approach is as promising as that proposed by Dr. Chany and his colleagues (Falcoff *et al.*, 1966) in which interferon prepared *in vitro* is given to protect against virus infection in humans.

There is one clear disadvantage with this series of compounds—they are not readily biodegradable and they deposit in the reticuloendothelial system. Unless more biodegradable but active forms can be prepared by polymer chemists, it is still possible that such a property is essential for their interferon-inducing action. Their polyanionic character makes them intriguingly similar to polynucleotides, which, as Dr. Burke and colleagues (1968) have discussed, are the likely virus components responsible for interferon production. It is conceivable that the activity of these compounds relates to the recent observation that anionic molecules are the best stimulators of pinocytosis within macrophages (Cohn and Parks, 1967).

SUMMARY

This paper reviews results with a variety of viral and non-viral interferon inducers in man, including naturally occurring virus infection, live virus vaccines, bacterial endotoxin and synthetic anionic copolymers. The most potent and consistent stimulators of human interferon *in vivo* were found to be myxoviruses, including measles, Newcastle disease virus and mumps.

Synthetic anionic polymers have striking antiviral effects *in vivo* which may be due to their direct polyelectrolyte interaction with virus and/or their ability to induce interferon production. Certain structural requirements have been defined for the interferon-inducing abilities of these materials. One member of this series has been studied in man as an inducer of circulating interferon, and results are quite similar to those found in the mouse.

ACKNOWLEDGEMENTS

I am grateful to Dr. William Regelson for the gift of the polymers employed in these studies and for the photographs, Fig. 1a and 1b, and to the United States Public Health Service for grants to support this work (AI-05629, AI-185-06).

REFERENCES

BURKE, D., SKEHEL, J. J., HAY, A. J., and WALTERS, S. (1968). This volume, pp. 4–15.

CAMPBELL, J. B., and COLTER, J. S. (1965). *Virology*, **25**, 608–619.

CASSEL, W. A., and GARRETT, R. E. (1965). *Cancer*, **18**, 863–868.

COHN, Z. A., and PARKS, E. (1967). *J. exp. Med.*, **125**, 213–232.

ELLIOTT, A. Y., and HIGGINBOTHAM, R. D. (1960). *Tex. Rep. Biol. Med.*, **18**, 362.

FALCOFF, E., FALCOFF, R., FOURNIER, F., and CHANY, C. (1966). Personal communication. IEG No. 6, Memo 211.

FELTZ, E. T., and REGELSON, W. (1962). *Nature, Lond.*, **196**, 642–665.

GRESSER, I., COPPEY, J., FONTAINE-BROUTY-BOYE, D., FALCOFF, E., FALCOFF, R., ZAJDELA, F., BOURALI, C., and THOMAS, M. T. (1968). This volume, pp. 240–248.

GRESSER, I., and DULL, H. (1964). *Proc. Soc. exp. Biol. Med.*, **115**, 192–196.

HO, M., and POSTIC, B. (1967). In *First International Conference on Vaccines against Viral and Rickettsial Diseases of Man*, pp. 632–649. Washington, D.C.: PAHO/WHO Scientific Publication 147.

JAO, R. L., WHEELOCK, E. F., and JACKSON, G. G. (1965). *J. clin. Invest.*, **44**, 1062 (abstract).

JOHNSON, J. H., FIELDS, J. E., and DARLINGTON, W. A. (1967). *Nature, Lond.*, **213**, 665–667.

LARKE, R. P. (1967). *Can. med. Ass. J.*, **96**, 21–33.

MERIGAN, T. C. (1967). *Nature, Lond.*, **214**, 416,

MERIGAN, T. C., and REGELSON, W. (1967). *Clin. Res.*, **15**, 309 (abstract).

PETRALLI, J. K., MERIGAN, T. C., and WILBUR, J. R. (1965a). *New Engl. J. Med.*, **273**, 198–201.

PETRALLI, J. K., MERIGAN, T. C., and WILBUR, J. R. (1965b). *Lancet*, **2**, 401–405.

RAY, C. G., GRAVELLE, C. R., and CHIN, T. D. Y. (1967). *J. Pediat.*, **71**, 27–32.

REGELSON, W. (1967). *Proc. Int. Symp. on Atherosclerosis and Reticuloendothelial Systems*. In press.

WADDELL, D., MERIGAN, T. C., and WILBUR, J. (1967). In preparation.

WADDELL, D., WALKER, S., and MERIGAN, T. C. (1967). In preparation.

WHEELOCK, E. F. (1964). *Proc. Soc. exp. Med. Biol.*, **117**, 650–653.

WHEELOCK, E. F. (1967). In *First International Conference on Vaccines against Viral and Rickettsial Diseases of Man*. Washington, D.C.: PAHO/WHO Scientific Publication 147.

WHEELOCK, E. F., and DINGLE, J. (1964). *New Engl. J. Med.*, **271**, 645–651.

WHEELOCK, E. F., and SIBLEY, W. A. (1965). *New Engl. J. Med.*, **273**, 194–198.

DISCUSSION

Ho: We have been trying to prepare a stock of Newcastle disease virus which is free from extraneous agents. Did you test for the avian leucosis complex in the NDV you used in humans?

Merigan: The eggs we used to prepare our passage of the virus were leucosis-free but we cannot rule out the presence of adventitious leucosis agents from previous passages.

De Maeyer: Why did you assay the therapeutic effect on tumours? As far as I know interferon has no effect on tumour cells in tissue culture.

Merigan: That is true. However, since the provocative studies of E. F. Wheelock and J. H. Dingle (1964. *New Engl. J. Med.*, **271**, 645) on the effect of viruses inducing interferon on the course of a patient with leukaemia, there has been a certain amount of enthusiasm for this approach to human malignancy.

De Maeyer: Maybe one should first try to eliminate as many tumour cells as possible with a chemotherapeutic agent, and then use interferon in an attempt to inhibit the action of the hypothetical leukaemia virus.

Merigan: Studies in many laboratories have demonstrated that interferon is only active against tumour viruses soon after their infection of cells, and from such studies I would not expect antitumour effects. On the other hand Dr. Ho has commented recently that if such viruses cause tumours in man, successive rounds of infection might be involved, and if so, one might be able to prevent further cell transformation with interferon. However, this is speculative.

Stoker: Do the copolymers induce interferon production in cultured cells?

Merigan: We have not been able to induce interferon production in tissue culture, or even get interference with virus growth with them. This may be due to the lack of phagocytosis of these materials by tissue culture cells. We are very anxious to look at something like macrophage cultures or cultures representing cells that are more highly active in their ability to take up material than mouse fibroblast cells.

Stoker: Supposing one postulated that these agents act by lighting up a latent virus infection?

Merigan: I could not refute such a hypothesis.

Gresser: We gave four injections of statolon (100 mg.) to Swiss mice before and after inoculation of Friend virus, thinking that four injections would be preferable to one. Interferon was produced after the first injection. The spleen weight is the best criterion we have at the moment for estimating the evolution of Friend leukaemia (Rowe, W. P., and Brodsky, I. [1959]. *J. natn. Cancer Inst.*, **23**, 1239). In two experiments of this kind statolon did not inhibit splenomegaly. In fact we observed considerable toxicity after intraperitoneal inoculation of statolon. In a third experiment we gave only one injection (26 mg.) of statolon one hour after giving the Friend virus. As in the two previous experiments, interferon was present in the serum. In this experiment splenomegaly was markedly inhibited, in accord with the observations of E. F. Wheelock (1967. *Proc. Soc. exp. Biol. Med.*, **124**, 855). I don't know how to interpret these experiments but the results may be of interest to those working on statolon.

Finter: Do the granule-containing white cells from the patients injected with pyran copolymers form interferon, Dr. Merigan?

Merigan: We have only studied the serum of these patients.

Finter: We have not been able to find interferon in the urine of a number of children with measles, mumps and chicken-pox. What amounts of interferon did you find?

Merigan: We think that when, say, 100 units/ml. are found in the serum, the amount in the urine might be about $0 \cdot 1$ to 1 unit/ml.; it is really quite low and we can only get clear-cut levels by concentrating the urine by ultrafiltration.

Kleinschmidt: We have tested about 50 natural and synthetic polyanions, with negative results until recently, when we found such a polyanion, a copolymer of acrylic acid plus some hydroxyl-containing monomer, synthesized for us by Rohm and Haas. Its molecular weight is 1 million. The figure you gave was 17,000 or greater for activity as an inducer.

Merigan: I can't be precise on the minimal molecular weight for interferon-inducing activity because we studied only a few low molecular weight polymers —the largest inactive one was 3,000 mol. wt. However, those with molecular weights of 17,000 to $1\frac{1}{4}$ million were active; with the materials of higher molecular weights, that is, from 100,000 upwards, a greater weight of polymer seemed to be needed to get the interferon effect.

Kleinschmidt: The interferon produced by our synthetic polymer has the same characteristics as yours, including slight inactivation—about 25 per cent—at pH 2.

Burke: Is that unusual? I thought one of the basic dogmas was that interferon was stable at pH 2. Does this vary from species to species?

Merigan: I think it does. It might even vary from inducer to inducer. It may be related to a particular molecular species of interferon predominating in the sample.

Finter: I am sure there are no dogmas in relation to interferon!

Joklik: In the experiment where the copolymer was able to protect mice for 32 days do you think that the copolymer is only taken up by certain cells and not by other cells? You administered the challenging virus intraperitoneally. Would you expect the virus to be taken up first by those cells which would also concentrate the copolymer?

Merigan: This is the problem. Not knowing the fate within the animal of either the polymer or the virus in absolute detail, we cannot decide whether we are seeing inhibition of the virus because of direct interaction or because of interferon protection.

Joklik: You didn't try intracerebral injection of the virus in these experiments?

Merigan: No, but with our protection experiments against vaccinia, we use intravenous injection of the virus and intraperitoneal injection of the copolymer.

Wagner: In the pre-interferon days many substances, often bacterial or microbial products, most of them impure and of unknown chemical nature, were used to try to inhibit viral infections in animals. In large doses quite a few of them gave partial protection. Moreover, some were effective for as long as 32 days. The experiments are rather tricky and their interpretation may be a bit difficult, but it is worth remembering that many other factors besides interferon production could be producing the effects you see, Dr. Merigan, including the age of the animals, because after 32 days the mouse is a species of experimental animal very different from the one you started with.

Merigan: We used sham-injected or uninjected matched controls for every experiment. Elliott and Higginbotham (1960, *loc. cit.*) refer to an anionic polymer derived from a bacterial filtrate of a polysulphonated nature with which they demonstrated *in vivo* antagonism of encephalomyocarditis virus. This polymer was only active for about two or three hours; that is, the virus had to be injected either simultaneously or within a very few hours, or else no protection was obtained. My interpretation was that this could be direct inactivation, but I do not know which is the critical mechanism for the antiviral activity of our copolymer *in vivo* because I believe it is still present in the animal even at late times.

Finter: We have found that a single injection of 5,000 units of interferon can protect mice for up to five days (Finter, N. B. [1967]. *J. gen. Virol.*, **1**, 395–397), and this appears to be quite a small amount of interferon in relation to amounts formed during natural virus infections of mice. So if something like statolon, which leads to formation of quite a lot of interferon, is injected, the resulting protection observed over a long period could result simply from the interferon. It is very difficult to analyse what different factors may be involved in protection *in vivo*. Of course I agree with Dr. Wagner that factors other than interferon may be involved, but I don't think one can exclude the latter simply because of the persistence of the protection.

Tyrrell: Could chemical measures be used to determine whether these polymers really persist?

Merigan: We are going to try radioactive labelling and Regelson has histochemical studies under way.

Tyrrell: Labelled polymers could perhaps be tested in tissue cultures to see whether they really do enter cells. If they have a direct antiviral effect they may normally get inside the cells of an animal and then be able to act on the virus when that is subsequently injected, whereas in tissue cultures they may never enter the cells at all.

A SIMPLE SYSTEM FOR THE MASS PRODUCTION OF HUMAN INTERFERON: THE HUMAN AMNIOTIC MEMBRANE

Charles Chany, Françoise Fournier and Ernesto Falcoff

Institut Nationale de la Santé et de la Recherche Médicale, Groupe de Recherches sur les Virus, Hôpital Saint Vincent de Paul, Paris

The species specificity of interferon makes it necessary to search for human cells as a source for production. The regular supply of such human cells in large quantities is difficult, and restricts the possible sources essentially to two: human leucocytes and placental tissues.

In several previous studies human leucocytes were suggested as a possible source for interferon and the optimum conditions for its production were described. The alternative possibility is to use the human amniotic membrane (HAM). HAM appears to be, among the placental tissues, the most suitable for the production of interferon. In a previous study we showed that HAM simply maintained *in vitro* can be infected with viruses and that it produces interferon under certain conditions (Gresser, Chany and Enders, 1965). The fundamental substance forms a matrix around the cells which probably contains mucoproteins, and which can consequently be destroyed by myxoviruses possessing neuraminidase (Chany *et al.*, 1966).

As a result, with myxoviruses interferons can be produced in human tissue maintained *in vitro*, where large numbers of cells are available. The interferon preparations obtained have a small protein content and a high biological activity. This report will describe, in summary, the preparation, the optimum conditions for production, the biophysical properties, and the control of these HAM interferons.

PREPARATION

Placentas obtained from normal delivery or after Caesarian section from carefully controlled healthy donors are thoroughly washed in six successive baths of Hanks solution containing antibiotics. The viruses used for the preparation of interferon are myxoviruses: myxovirus para–influenza type I (Sendai), Newcastle disease virus (NDV). In most of the experiments, however, Sendai virus was employed.

In order to establish the optimum conditions for the production of interferon, the role of u.v. irradiation of Sendai virus was compared to that of live virus. The optimum multiplicity of the infection and the optimum serum concentration, pH and temperature were also determined (see Tables I and II).

TABLE I

OPTIMUM CONDITIONS FOR THE PRODUCTION OF HAM INTERFERON

Multiplicity of infection	Sendai virus, 5×256–512 HA/g. membrane
Serum concentration of the medium	2%
Temperature of incubation	37° C
pH of the medium	7·2–7·4

TABLE II

BIOLOGICAL PROPERTIES OF HAM INTERFERON

Molecular weight	160,000
Cell specificity	Yes
Conservation	−20° C
Action	Intracellular; integrity of cellular RNA and protein synthesis necessary

Effect of u.v. irradiation on the inducing virus. Radiation studies on Sendai virus show that the quantity of interferon eliminated in the medium from the infected membranes increases with the amount of radiation of the virus and appears to be maximal at 5,100 ergs/mm.². Through subsequent irradiation the interferon yield decreases. These studies are in contrast to previous studies with the same virus, when leucocytes were employed instead of the amniotic membranes. In this case irradiated virus did not induce the production of interferon.

The role of multiplicity of infection. Since non-infectious as well as infectious viruses are capable of producing interferon, the multiplicity of infection was roughly estimated by the number of haemagglutinating units (HA) present in the viral suspension per gram of tissue. The optimum ratio was about five times 256–512 HA per gram of tissue.

The minimum serum concentration in the medium which did not cause a loss in the yield of interferon was 2 per cent. Interferon could also be produced in a serum-free medium; however, the amniotic membrane always contains a small amount of deeply absorbed residual serum.

Role of pH and of the gas/liquid phase on the production of interferon. The optimum ratio between the medium and the weight of the tissue was between 3 and 6, with an optimum pH in the physiological range (pH 7·4).

The effect of temperature on the production of interferon was studied in carefully controlled conditions in an agitated water bath, adjusted to 31°, 33°, 34°, 36°, 37°, and 39° C. The results show that the optimum temperature for interferon production was 37°, which is the body temperature of the donor. At this temperature DNA and protein synthesis of the cells are at an optimum level (Vendrely and Chany, 1965, unpublished experiments).

Characterization of HAM interferon. The molecular weight of HAM interferon was estimated by the gel filtration technique on Sephadex G100 and G200. The protein concentration of the fraction was measured by u.v. absorption, using a Uvicord Spectrophotometer (2537 Å). Since there is a linear relationship between the log of the molecular weight and the volume of effluence, the molecular weight of HAM interferon can be estimated to be close to $160,000 \pm 10$ per cent.

Mode of action of HAM interferon. When HAM interferon is incubated on amnion cells with $0 \cdot 1$ μg. of actinomycin D its protective titre decreases significantly. It therefore seems very likely that, like other interferons, HAM interferon acts indirectly through the derepression of an antiviral protein in the cell.

DISCUSSION

The technique of interferon production here presented seems to be of interest from a practical as well as from a theoretical standpoint.

Cellular material derived from amniotic membranes is routinely used in many laboratories. In spite of intensive experience with the system, reports of the presence of latent viruses in amniotic cells, except in cases with rubella, are rare. Placental material is also routinely used for the mass production of gamma globulins extensively employed in human therapeutics. Screening techniques used on blood transfusion donors can also be adapted for use with HAM interferon. Placental tissues are easy to obtain in large quantities.

Live or u.v.-inactivated myxovirus produces large quantities of interferon which are eliminated in the tissue culture fluid for up to five days. A preparation of relatively high biological activity can be obtained in a medium with a low protein concentration.

In addition to its practical interest the system here presented has other remarkable properties.

First, when Sendai virus is used the u.v.-inactivated virus induces higher yields of interferon than live virus. It therefore seems very likely that u.v. irradiation destroys a part of the genome responsible for the production of substances like stimulons, antagonistic to the interferon.

Secondly, when the tissue culture medium is changed every 24 hours and the elimination of interferon is measured in the supernatant, the peak is observed not 24 but 48 hours after infection. Subsequently, the titre decreases in a linear manner and disappears completely in about five days. A new challenge after five days does not produce interferon again, although the amniotic membrane can be maintained alive for two months *in vitro*, as shown in previous experiments (Gresser, Chany and Enders, 1965).

Thirdly, the molecular weight and some basic properties of HAM interferon are strikingly different from those of interferon produced by white blood cells, in spite of the fact that the same inducer was used. The question arises of whether the inhibitor presented here can be considered as an interferon since there is at present no agreed definition for interferon. We wish to put forward the following provisory definition, which, if it is accepted, may reasonably permit us to classify the material here presented as an interferon:

(1) It is a protein.

(2) It protects cells of the same animal species; however, crosses between phylogenetically close animal species can be observed.

(3) It is not present in uninfected cells. Its synthesis is coded by the cellular genome. Consequently, in the uninfected cell interferon synthesis is repressed.

(4) It acts during the eclipse phase of intercellular viral multiplication, and needs the integrity of cellular RNA and protein synthesis. It acts through the derepression of an antiviral protein (actinomycin or puromycin blocks its action.)

(5) The antiviral protein acts on viral protein synthesis at the poly-ribosomal level.

REFERENCES

CHANY, C., GRESSER, I., VENDRELY, C., and ROBBE-FOSSAT, F. (1966). *Proc. Soc. exp. Biol. Med.*, **123**, 960.

GRESSER, I., CHANY, C., and ENDERS, J. F. (1965). *J. Bact.*, **89**, 470.

DISCUSSION

Cantell: How many interferon units do you get from one human amniotic membrane?

Chany: A whole amniotic membrane will yield about 500 ml. of interferon with an activity of 500 to 2,000 protective units per millilitre. Interferon titres of course vary very much from one laboratory to another, even when the same interferon is used in different cell systems. We have recently observed that in some instances when the cell system used for the titration of interferon contained latent virus the interferon titre went down to nil. So the use of reference interferons is absolutely necessary. The titre of the HAM interferon is about the same as that of the standard white cell reference interferon.

Rotem: Did you try to purify this material and find whether it has the same activity? Did you try to break down the high molecular weight interferon into smaller units? If so, were you able to show that these still retain the same biological effect?

Chany: We did not purify this interferon much because it is much less stable than white cell interferon. Its mode of action looks very much like that of any other interferon with intracellular species specificity. In two experiments we found that when we depolymerized the heavy interferon we also destroyed its activity. So the question is still open.

Fantes: Do you also get the high molecular weight interferon when you use amnion cells instead of amnion membranes?

Chany: Yes. Of course in general the interferon yield from cultured cells is much lower. The tissue culture cell population is a highly selected one, especially in the amniotic cells. This might explain why much less interferon is produced. On the other hand there are also far fewer cells available for the same volume of tissue culture medium than in the membrane itself.

Merigan: The amnion is certainly not the only human material capable of producing high molecular weight interferon. In our patients injected with Newcastle disease virus we see a small amount of an interferon with a molecular weight of over 100,000, as well as the major interferon species of 30,000 molecular weight, so *in vivo* in man both these species appear during a virus infection.

Chany: The virus may multiply in the blood vessels, so a high molecular weight interferon is certainly possible.

De Maeyer: What is the molecular weight of the human copolymer interferon, Dr. Merigan?

Merigan: We have not characterized its molecular weight yet in man.

Chany: We could easily separate the WBC interferon and the amnion interferon but we were not able to separate them on a density gradient—I don't know why.

Ho: In what way is this type of interferon more labile?

Chany: If it is dialysed much of the biological activity is lost. Dr. S. G. Anderson has studied accelerated inactivation of human interferon with or without stabilizers such as dextran. The inactivation rate of HAM interferon was much higher than that of white cell interferon.

Ho: This must be quite different from the interferon obtained from human amnion cells in culture, which is one of the first types of interferon we got when I was working in Dr. Enders' laboratory (Ho, M., and Enders, J. F. [1959]. *Proc. natn. Acad. Sci. U.S.A.*, **45**, 385; *Virology*, **9**, 446). It was quite stable at acid pH, at 56° and after dialysis.

Chany: Yes, but if it is kept for long periods it is less stable than the white cell interferon.

De Maeyer: We kept human amnion tissue culture interferon stable for six months at 4°.

Ho: This is of some interest because there seems to be some association between high molecular weight and lability. I suspect that Dr. Merigan's copolymer interferon, which is labile, may also be the high molecular weight type. But I am surprised that the amnion cell culture interferon with a high molecular weight is stable.

Chany: Of course the tissue culture system differs from the tissue itself. For instance, it is possible that all interferons have the same active site with different protein supports. Perhaps a difference in the protein support of the active molecule makes them stable or unstable.

Burke: The variations in molecular weight are very unsettling. We had all decided on 35,000 but now these multiple species are being produced. We agree that these molecules all have common biological activity and a few physical properties in common, but are we looking at a family of molecules, like a family of antibodies? What is really going on here? We talk about derepression, but we are talking about derepression of a wide range of physicochemical molecules and I find this hard to systematize.

Chany: The definition of interferon can only be based on its mode of action. I can visualize a heavy molecule and a light molecule having the same mode of action, but if molecules of identical molecular weight don't have the same mode of action, then they are not comparable. The molecular size is less important for the definition.

Wagner: We found different molecular species of interferon made by rabbit cells, depending on the tissue type and the inducer.

Tyrrell: The only satisfactory definition of an antibody, to my knowledge, is that it is something which combines with the antigen which has induced it. This doesn't disturb immunologists now; they have reoriented themselves and they realize that this particular property may be carried on many molecules with different charges and of varying sizes.

Crick: The point is the classification into families. In a lot of different molecules which do the same thing is there some similarity, as there is in antibodies? Have they got very similar specificities in the way that myoglobin is like haemoglobin, or are they something quite radically different? There seems to be no answer at the moment. Even things belonging to the same family are not necessarily quite the same; for example although haemoglobin and myoglobin fold up in the same way, and both take up oxygen and are clearly related, nevertheless they are distinctly different. Until more is known about these molecules, I don't think they can be classified into families.

Wagner: This is true. A few years ago we weren't much concerned by the fact that all interferons were species specific, as far as we could tell. They may not behave in the same way, and they do not necessarily have the same mode of action. I suspect that there is something radically different among the various interferons which must have some molecular basis.

Crick: The essence of a family is that the members are different but have similarities, and one has to say what these are. When the molecular structure is known you may be able to see whether in fact you have two quite radically different things which happen to overlap, or whether you have things which are really very similar and yet, like isozymes of various other sorts, give similar but not identical actions.

Fantes: There is very strong evidence that we have more than one interferon, or possibly even a series of different interferons, in fluids from chick embryo and fibroblast tissue cultures after infection with the same virus.

Stoker: Can more than one type of interferon be obtained from cloned lines of cells?

Crick: Different haemoglobins may come from one cell—from one reticulocyte, for example.

Tyrrell: After all, antibodies from different species are all different; they can be precipitated with species-specific antibodies.

Burke: Yes, but they fall into groups. The 7 S antibodies have a common pattern, for example.

Crick: That is a family with enormous variety. Haemoglobin is by far the best example if we must search for a molecular analogy.

Levy: We can develop a definition of interferon on two different bases. One is on the nature of the molecular structure. In view of Dr. Fantes' observations, to attempt such a definition at present would be difficult because we are not going to have enough interferon within the next five years to define the molecules. The second would be on the basis of its biochemical mode of action. If two "interferons" had the same mode of action would people agree that they represent families of related molecules?

Wagner: No!

Crick: What do you mean by the same? Presumably if they are different they will act slightly differently, have different absorption rates and so on, but two radically different ones could of course act at the same spot. I agree with you that an operational definition may be the best thing to go for when a structural characterization is impossible.

Cantell: Have you used the chorionic membrane, Dr. Chany?

Chany: Yes. We also tried placental fragments. Both produce small amounts of interferon. Among the placental tissues the amniotic membrane is apparently the best producer of interferon.

Merigan: A third method we have been considering as a means of preparing *in vitro* human interferon for possible clinical usage is virus stimulation of cells passaged in tissue culture, namely Newcastle disease virus infection of human foreskin fibroblasts, which we carry in large quantities. Unfortunately, as with all primary cells, these do not grow in suspension, so there is all the tedium of handling them in monolayers and so on. We can get levels approaching but not as high as those formed by the white cell. We have also looked into large-scale apparatuses for growing these cells in tissue culture on monolayers. Some of these look reasonably promising. They offer the possibility that one can at least define a particular cell line reasonably critically as far as adventitious contaminants, etc., go. It is obvious that purification of crude interferons is required to eliminate the possibility of adventitious contaminants and that is why we have been working on methods of improving yields of human interferon derived from cell culture sources in purification sequences. It is a difficult job because human interferon is much less stable than chick interferon when purified, so the yields are not as good. A large amount of starting material and improvements of present yields from purification are needed.

Burke: The increased ability to produce interferon with u.v.-irradiated Sendai virus has been found in other systems too. One doesn't have to postulate that a substance antagonistic to interferon is produced—there are other explanations. It is not an uncommon situation that as one decreases the ability to produce virus, one increases the ability to produce interferon. Dr. Isaacs once talked about opening and closing doors (1962. *Br. med. J.*, **2**, 353–355); this can't be pursued in a biochemical sense but there is a germ of truth in it. Semliki Forest virus grows rapidly at 37° and late production of interferon occurs. If one stops the SFV from growing by moving the system to 42° very much earlier production of interferon is seen. There are all sorts of explanations for this, one being that some part of the virus multiplication may somehow turn off a mechanism which is essential for the production of interferon. It is just possible that this might be a way in for the derepression mechanism that so intrigues me. Is there any clue to this in this situation in which we tend to get either interferon or virus—virus being switched off as interferon is switched on?

Chany: In our system absolutely no virus is produced, neither infectious virus nor haemagglutinin. In fact the membranes only produce interferon.

Burke: That is even more complicated.

Stoker: Are there any data on the production of interferon and virus in the same cell? Is the immunology of interferon good enough yet for immunofluorescence?

Chany: It is very difficult and it takes a very long time. Only a heterologous animal can be used for antibody production.

GENERAL DISCUSSION

INTERFERON STANDARDS

Stoker: Several people here have been involved in attempts to make standard interferon preparations. Dr. Baron, could you tell us about this?

Baron: In 1964 at a meeting in Washington people working on interferon suggested that laboratories should be able to compare their assays of interferon. A reference chick interferon preparation and a mouse interferon preparation have now been made available internationally by the NIH. Dr. Merigan, who has worked on these standards, can tell us about them.

The other important question is how reference preparations should be used to standardize assays.

Merigan: The mouse interferon standard was produced with Newcastle disease virus in L cells in tissue culture; the preparation was virus-inactivated by pH 2 treatment, neutralized, and after 0·05 per cent bovine serum was added it was put up in 1 ml. samples in glass vials, lyophilized and rubber-stoppered. The chick interferon preparation was chromatographically purified; it was initially prepared by influenza infection of embryonated eggs. Chorioallantoic fluid was collected at 72 hours, treated with perchloric acid to inactivate and remove the virus, and then chromatographed on XE-64 resin followed by carboxymethyl Sephadex, as I have described elsewhere (Merigan, T. C., Winget, C., and Dixon, C. [1965]. *J. molec. Biol.*, **13**, 679). After dialysis against tissue culture medium and addition of 0·05 per cent bovine serum albumin, it was put up in vials and lyophilized in the same way as the mouse interferon. These preparations are available through the Reference Reagents branch of the National Institutes of Health, so that laboratories may standardize their internal standards with those of other laboratories; then each laboratory could use its own internal standards for the weekly assays. Only a few thousand of these vials have been prepared in these series and each laboratory will have to relate its own standard to them rather than expect to run the primary standards frequently.

Joklik: Have you any evidence concerning their stability?

Merigan: Yes; we have assayed this in two laboratories. In our laboratory we looked at these materials for about nine months. Keeping them at −20° we found them to have similar activity, when tested periodically, to a standard which was frozen and kept continuously at −20° over the same period of time. We think that as long as they are re-run frequently in the reference laboratory we can claim relative stability for these materials.

Baron: We have not tested the stability for as long as nine months, but from past experience at least the chick interferon will probably be stable, perhaps indefinitely.

Finter: One unit of human interferon as measured in our laboratory is equivalent to about two of the units used in Dr. Chany's laboratory, and 1/14th of Dr. Cantell's units; it is about the same as Dr. Wheelock's unit. So if different people talk about apparently the same amount of interferon measured in terms of their individual units, they may be dealing in fact with very different concentrations. This means, to take only a single example, that one cannot correlate the published data from different laboratories for the amounts of interferon found in the blood of man under different circumstances. It really is important that a common potency unit should be adopted for each species of interferon as soon as possible.

Chany: Dr. S. G. Anderson at the National Institute for Medical Research at Mill Hill has five litres of human white blood cell interferon which has been tested for its stability for two years and is now available for distribution. It can withstand successive freezing and thawing even a number of times. The addition of stabilizer did not improve its stability; however, its biological titre is unchanged for years when it is kept in a lyophilized state at $-20°$; at $+4°$ the activity decreases within a few months.

Finter: It is important to be sure that after they have been freeze-dried these materials are stable at relatively high temperatures. If they are going to be shipped around the world they may, for short periods during transit, be exposed to quite high temperatures, certainly up to, say, $37°$. We prepared some mouse brain interferon, and, in collaboration with Dr. S. G. Anderson, we freeze-dried this as a possible standard. After a month at $37°$, the ampoules had lost a lot of their activity. To have stability under such conditions is a very stringent requirement. Nevertheless, are the standards proposed by the NIH group stable for a reasonable period of time under accelerated degradation conditions?

Merigan: We have not tested stability at high temperatures. Inactivation of labile interferon species might occur with such temperatures, and even under $45°$ one might get losses. We have held our materials at $4°$, and now plan provisionally to ship them refrigerated.

Pereira: For a standard to be accepted internationally the material must be put in ampoules and stored under the very precise conditions laid down by the WHO Biological Standards Committee. I have had experience of a material which was proposed as a standard; it was a good material but it had been freeze-dried in vials with rubber caps. This was not acceptable so it had to be reconstituted, re-freeze-dried in appropriate ampoules, and re-tested—which is the most laborious part of the whole exercise! With a little forethought all this could have been avoided, and this should be borne in mind here.

Tyrrell: At a meeting of the directors of the WHO Reference Laboratories and in consultation with the Biological Standards Section of WHO it was suggested that international reference preparations should be prepared according to the standards which Dr. Pereira has just mentioned. Dr. Anderson of the National Institute for Medical Research is at present organizing such preparations. Chick embryo material from Dr. Fantes has been ampouled according to WHO directions and has successfully withstood accelerated degradation at high temperatures. This material is now acceptable as an international standard. It is going to be tested further by comparative assays in different laboratories. I think it is most desirable that this standard and the U.S. standards should be tested together so that anybody who has access to either of them will be able to compare his results with anybody else's. We hope that mouse and human interferon standards will be prepared too.

My hope, which is probably shared by many others, is that from now on where the titre of interferon itself is mentioned in a paper or is of any importance whatever, the relationship between the laboratory units used and the appropriate international or NIH reference preparation titre should also be indicated.

Fantes: Dr. Anderson and I prepared a rather limited quantity of chick interferon standard last year. The material was partly purified (say 50 to 100 times) and freeze-dried in the presence of 5 ml. gelatin/ml. We could detect no deterioration whatsoever after eight months at 37° and even at 50° we only lost something like 50 per cent of the activity. Encouraged by this, we have now prepared four litres of similar material. Unfortunately, the titre of the freeze-dried material is somewhat lower than we expected—it is between 40 and 60 units/ml., when reconstituted. Dr. Merigan and I have in the past exchanged samples of chick interferon and our assays are in very close agreement. Dr. Merigan had previously exchanged samples with Dr. G. P. Lampson of the Merck Research Institute and their units were also comparable.

Stoker: I hope that the labels will also show the molecular weight!

VIRAL INDUCERS

Stoker: We have so far been discussing the production of interferon and the agents responsible for it, which seem to fall into two main groups: the complex and the even more complex phenomena. The first includes viruses and statolon, which I understand are effective in tissue culture systems, and the second the other inducers, which so far have only been found to work in animals. With reference to the viral inducers, why don't virus mutants turn up which don't induce interferon? One would have thought that they would have a great selective advantage. Their non-appearance suggests that induction of interferon is essential for virus multiplication. Does this give us any clue as to what in fact the inducer is?

Crick: There is also the fact that so many different viruses produce interferon, which may be another facet of the same thing.

Stoker: But are there any which produce no interferon?

Burke: Yes, those which turn off RNA synthesis—the viruses of vesicular stomatitis and polio, for example.

Ho: The attenuated polio strain will produce interferon, whereas the virulent ones usually will not.

Chany: This observation should be related to the cell system used. Our strain of vaccinia, for example, produces interferon in mouse cells but none in rat cells, and ten times more plaques in rat cells than in mouse cells.

Levy: Viruses may also produce mutants which are not sensitive to the action of interferon. Certainly there are strains of viruses, among the Mengo group for example, which are quite sensitive and others which are not. This is another way out for the virus.

Stoker: At the moment we have to consider the induction system rather than the sensitivity, although both these are possibilities.

Baron: Natural selection has many facets. As Sir Christopher Andrewes has pointed out, the virus cannot eat up all its food or it will have nothing left to live on; the virus must be able, therefore, to infect animals without killing them, so that virus variants which do not induce the interferon system might be selected against. Among the viruses which are poor inducers of interferon are the NDV group. Many of the virulent strains induce small amounts of interferon in chick cells, while the attenuated vaccine strains, which multiply as well as the virulent strains, induce no detectable interferon (Baron, S. [1964]. In *Newcastle Disease Virus: An Evolving Pathogen*, ed. Hanson, R. P., Madison: University of Wisconsin Press). Dr. S. Hermodsson (1964. *Acta path. microbiol. scand.*, **62**, 224) has provided an example of a virus which causes persistent infection of cells in culture but which induces no detectable interferon production. More recently J. E. Osborn and D. N. Medearis (1966. *Proc. Soc. exp. Biol. Med.*, **121**, 819) have reported that cytomegalovirus infection *in vivo*, which is also a persistent infection in the mouse, probably inhibits the ability of the infected cells to produce interferon. Many possible virus–cell combinations leading to different degrees of induction of interferon seem to exist.

Wagner: We have been warned that the relationship of inhibition of cellular RNA synthesis to the lack of ability of a virus to induce interferon is not necessarily absolute, and the point that the cell system is important should be quite obvious. Vesicular stomatitis virus does not induce interferon synthesis in ascites tumour cells, and also it very rapidly switches off cellular RNA synthesis (Wagner, R. R., and Huang, A. S. [1966]. *Virology*, **28**, 1). There seems to be, at least temporally, a good correlation between those two events, which would make one think that the inhibition of RNA synthesis is related to the inability of these cells to make interferon even when superinfected with a good inducing virus like NDV. In L cells, on the other hand, the rate of virus-induced inhibition of cellular RNA synthesis is slower, and yet they do not produce interferon either when infected with VSV. Patently, there is no absolute correlation between these observations. One obvious point, probably of limited importance and applicable to only a few virus–cell systems, is that inhibition of cellular RNA synthesis by certain viruses results in their failure to induce interferon synthesis. The cytomegalovirus is probably another case, in which there is no evidence that it switches off cellular RNA synthesis, and yet it does apparently inhibit interferon synthesis (Osborn, J. E., and Medearis, D. N. [1966]. *Proc. Soc. exp. Biol. Med.*, **124**, 347).

Joklik: There are several phases here: a virus infects a cell which is not producing interferon, then there comes a phase during which interferon production may be possible, and then inhibition of host cell RNA synthesis may occur. The length of the middle phase determines whether interferon is produced or not.

Burke: It seems that one can predict when a virus won't produce interferon but not when it will.

Crick: Has this anything to do with whether a virus is a DNA virus or an RNA virus?

Wagner: The cytomegalovirus is a DNA virus and it inhibits interferon synthesis in the mouse. VSV is an RNA virus and, at least in certain cell systems, it also inhibits interferon synthesis.

Crick: I can understand those cases where one turns off RNA synthesis and doesn't get interferon. When one doesn't turn off RNA synthesis, and where one may or may not get interferon, is this in any way correlated with whether the virus is DNA or RNA?

Wagner: We have not looked at enough combinations of viruses and cells.

Burke: But there are plenty of examples of DNA viruses producing interferon.

Stoker: On the whole the animal DNA viruses don't turn off host RNA and protein synthesis very rapidly.

Chany: But DNA viruses are usually less good producers of interferon than RNA viruses.

Joklik: The DNA viruses can be divided into two groups: the papovaviruses and the adenoviruses which do not turn off host cell biosynthetic events very rapidly, and herpes and poxviruses which do—except for certain poxviruses like fibroma virus.

Levy: By and large the papovaviruses and the adenoviruses are poor interferon producers.

STATOLON

Crick: Professor Chain and Dr. Kleinschmidt didn't make it clear whether their statolons had equal potency. Perhaps a statolon unit should be defined now.

Kleinschmidt: We feel we should get purer material before we can define one.

Burke: Has anyone established whether statolon-induced interferon production is susceptible to puromycin and actinomycin? We hope to look at this but haven't got our system set up. This may be the one case of a non-viral inducer working in tissue culture. Does it cause release of pre-formed interferon or is there *de novo* synthesis?

Levy: Irving Gordon has tested the effect of several inhibitors on the production of interferon by cells treated with statolon. He finds the same effects as with virus-induced interferon. This was in tissue cultures.

Kleinschmidt: We have preliminary results indicating that statolon-induced interferon is inhibited by actinomycin.

Burke: This means we have to accommodate statolon into our virus-induced story and consider polyanions again as perhaps the common denominator between nucleic acids and statolon. I find this unsatisfactory but there may be something in it.

Fantes: The fact that statolon induces interferon in mice much later than endotoxin does suggest that *de novo* synthesis occurs.

Crick: How many milligrams does a million units of interferon represent? It would also be very useful to know the same for statolon: do you get micrograms or grams of it?

Fantes: The most highly purified chick interferon we have prepared has a specific activity of $1 \cdot 6 \times 10^6$ units/mg. of protein, but this is definitely still impure. This specific activity is based on protein content. Should interferon be found to consist, for example, of 90 per cent carbohydrate and 10 per cent protein, then the specific activity, on a total weight basis, will of course be quite different. I have assumed that it is mainly protein.

Merigan: I have very similar figures for virus-induced interferon, but there are no data at all for statolon-induced interferon.

Crick: Could a million units correspond to as little as a microgram? Is it as impure as that?

Fantes: If the main constituent of interferon is not protein but something else, the specific activity could be much less. If, however, it is protein then pure interferon will be found to have an activity very much higher than 1·5 million units/mg.

Merigan: We have had material with approximately the same range of activity as yours, Dr. Fantes, and I have made some speculative calculations of the number of molecules required to protect a cell. By taking the molecular weight, and the weight of the purest material required for protection, one can calculate that about 1,000 molecules are required to protect a cell. Dr. Baron has observed that very little interferon from the supernatant over cells is taken up by them. It appears that in his model there is no more than 1 per cent absorption. That would push the number of molecules entering the cell for protection down to a maximum of 10 per cell. Then, from the purification data it is quite possible that 90 per cent of the most purified preparations consist of contaminants. It is therefore conceivable that only a single molecule of interferon penetrates a cell to protect it. This hypothesis is of interest in the light of the current thought that interferon acts on cells by inducing the host genome to produce another material which mediates its antiviral action. One molecule of exogenous material could affect 1,000 ribosomes by a cascade-like effect in which the host genome, once turned on by the single molecule of interferon, goes on to produce 1,000 copies of the antiviral polypeptide.

Crick: How easy is it to get 1 mg. of statolon? How many milligrams can you get of those particles you described, Dr. Kleinschmidt? This is relevant because how one characterizes a molecule depends on how much one has of it. With 10 mg. or 100 mg. one can do a lot more than with only 0·1 mg. to 1 mg. I have the impression that although people have very little interferon, Dr. Kleinschmidt has a lot of statolon.

Tyrrell: Dr. Kleinschmidt said that 10^{10} of his particles would protect a mouse, so on that basis about 1 µg. of crude statolon per mouse would be the protective dose.

Kleinschmidt: Our data indicate that there are approximately 4×10^{12} particles in 1 gram of our statolon preparation (containing glucose and $(NH_4)_2CO_3$). The weight of a statolon particle with a diameter of 30 mµ and a density of 1·2 would be $1·7 \times 10^{-11}$ µg. This would mean that 1 gram of our statolon would contain about 70 µg. of particles. So we have had milligram quantities of statolon particles in our laboratory—at the most about 70 mg.

PURIFICATION OF INTERFERONS

K. H. FANTES

Glaxo Laboratories Ltd., Stoke Poges, Bucks.

THE first publications by Isaacs and his colleagues (Isaacs and Lindenmann, 1957; Isaacs, Lindenmann and Valentine, 1957; Lindenmann, Burke and Isaacs, 1957) already indicated that interferon produced in chick chorio-allantoic membranes by treatment with heat-inactivated influenza virus was, or at least contained, protein. Many workers (e.g. Zemla and Vilcek, 1961*b*; Lampson *et al.*, 1963; Fantes and O'Neill, 1964) confirmed this for virus-induced chick interferon; others showed that virus-induced mammalian interferons obtained from mouse (e.g. Henle *et al.*, 1959; Merigan, Winget and Dixon, 1965), man (e.g. Gresser, 1961; Wheelock and Sibley, 1965), guinea pig (Friedman *et al.*, 1962), dog (Sellers and Fitzpatrick, 1963), calf (Hermodsson, 1964), rabbit (Kono and Ho, 1965), rat (Schonne, 1966), pig (Torlone, Titoli and Gialletti, 1965) and hamster (Stewart and Sulkin, 1966), as well as those obtained from a reptile (Falcoff and Fauconnier, 1965) and from fish (Gravell and Malsberger, 1965), were destroyed by proteolytic enzymes and thus consist, at least in part, of protein. This is generally accepted, but mention should be made here of somewhat different views held by a group of Japanese workers.

In a series of papers, Nagano and Kojima (1958, 1960), Nagano, Kojima and Suzuki (1960), Haneishi and co-workers (1964), Nagano (1965), Nagano and co-workers (1965, 1966) and Nagano, Kojima and Kanashiro (1966) described the isolation of an interferon-like substance from rabbit skin infected with vaccinia virus. This could be obtained, depending on purification conditions, either as a high molecular weight (sedimentation coefficient $S = 4 \cdot 7$) glycoprotein, or as a low molecular weight ($< 10,000$) protein-free polysaccharide, the latter being active only in animals, but not in tissue culture. It is postulated that the natural, active saccharide acquires stability, species specificity and *in vitro* and *in vivo* activity by its loose attachment to inert protein or proteins. Such a unifying hypothesis is thought by the Japanese workers to explain the existence of interferons of different molecular sizes and species specificities, but some of their experimental results and interpretations do not agree at all with findings by other workers in other systems. Clearly, further studies are needed to show whether these properties are uniquely those of an antiviral agent induced by vaccinia virus in the rabbit skin or whether they are of more general relevance.

Another group of proteinaceous antiviral substances has been produced in various cells by non-viral stimuli. Some of these materials have higher molecular weights, higher isoelectric points and lesser stabilities than corresponding viral interferons. Yet in biological properties they are indistinguishable from their virus-induced counterparts. This division is, however, not clear-cut since viruses can, under certain conditions, induce high molecular weight interferons, and not all non-viral interferons are macromolecular. Whether and how these substances are interrelated is not known and so far no attempts to purify other than low molecular weight, virus-induced interferons, seem to have been made. The properties of non-virus-induced interferons have recently been discussed (Ho et al., 1966) but they do not form part of this review.

PURIFICATION OF VIRUS-INDUCED INTERFERONS

Some of the terms used in this review should first be defined:

Interferon units: have been defined in different ways by individual authors, but are usually expressed as the reciprocal of the highest dilution of a sample that protects either all or half the cells against viral attack. See also page 85.

Specific activity = number of interferon units per milligram of protein.

Purification = increase of specific activity.

Purification factor = specific activity of sample : specific activity of starting material.

Protein: in our work, has been estimated by the method of Lowry and co-workers (1951), using crystalline bovine plasma albumin as the standard.

The knowledge that interferons were, or at least contained, protein has been of great value in purification studies. Most of the methods known to protein chemists have been applied in various ways and combinations to the purification of interferons. Such operations include: precipitation of interferon or of inert impurities by salts, certain acids, metal hydroxides or organic solvents; adsorptions and elutions; chromatography on ion-exchange resins, celluloses and gels; gradient centrifugation, gel filtration and electrophoresis.

PRECIPITATION METHODS

The old friend of protein chemists, ammonium sulphate, was already used in very early work by Lindenmann, Burke and Isaacs (1957), who found that chick interferon was precipitated by a saturated solution of the salt. Later workers (e.g. Wagner and Levy, 1960; Paucker, 1965) showed that lower concentrations (60 to 75 per cent saturation) of the salt sufficed. Burke (1961) attempted fractional precipitation using ammonium sulphate, without much success, but Baron, Barban and Buckler (1964) collected material precipitated at 60 per cent saturation after discarding the precipitate formed at a saturation of 40 per cent.

Other interferons (e.g. mouse, human, calf, rat) have also been precipitated by ammonium sulphate (Vilcek *et al.*, 1964; Davies, 1965*b*; Falcoff *et al.*, 1965; Hermodsson, 1964; Denys, 1963). Mouse interferon was found by Vilcek and co-workers (1964) to be precipitated only at higher (80 per cent) saturation, but this was not confirmed by Davies (1965*b*), who also showed that precipitation was facilitated in acid solution. In general, only slight purification is achieved by ammonium sulphate precipitation, but the method is useful for concentrating interferons.

Protein-precipitating acids such as trichloroacetic, sulphosalicylic, tetrametaphosphoric, perchloric, phosphotungstic, phosphomolybdic, picric, tannic, *p*-toluenesulphonic, osmic and naphthalene disulphonic have been used with varying success for concentrating or purifying chick, mouse, human, rabbit, monkey, calf and rat interferons. At low concentration some of the acids precipitate only inert protein, but at higher concentration interferon is also precipitated though it is not always recoverable. Some of the workers who have used these acids for various interferons are Zemla and Vilcek (1961*b*), Lampson and co-workers (1963), Merigan (1964*a*), Davies (1964), Schonne (1966), Fantes (1966) and Lampson (1966). The highest purification achieved was about 15-fold.

Fantes, O'Neill and Mason (1964) and Fantes (1965, 1967*a*) achieved some purification of chick interferon by precipitating inert protein in acid solution with iodide or thiocyanate. Davies (1965*b*) applied the same method with some success to mouse brain interferon, but when Schonne (1966) attempted to purify rat interferon with acid thiocyanate, all activity was lost.

Hydroxides or oxides of some metals, e.g. Zn, Co, Ca, Hg, Sr, Ba, Cd, Pb^{++}, Fe^{++}, Fe^{+++} and Cu^{++}, have been found to precipitate or adsorb chick and other interferons. Concentrated active material could usually be recovered from the precipitate by acidification and by removal of the metal ion by dialysis, or chelation. Only moderate purification has been achieved in this way, but the method is again useful for concentrating interferons (e.g. Lampson *et al.*, 1963; Lampson, 1966; Fantes and O'Neill [see Fantes, 1966]). Zinc especially has been used by many workers (e.g.

Lampson *et al.*, 1963; Merigan, 1964*a*), but Schonne (1966) was unable to recover rat interferon after precipitation with zinc or cadmium.

Organic solvents have frequently been used in protein fractionations, and several workers have used them in the concentration and purification of interferons. Burke (1961) attempted to fractionate chick interferon with cold ethanol, but activity was distributed between all fractions. Zemla and Vilcek (1961*a*) precipitated chick interferon with acetone or ethanol at $-10°$ to $-15°$ C and claimed 80-fold purification, but this seems to have been based on removal of total nitrogen, not of protein-nitrogen, and probably represented mainly elimination of amino acids from the "199" tissue culture medium. Fantes, O'Neill and Mason (1964) precipitated chick interferon with methanol, ethanol or acetone, but achieved only slight purification. Vilcek and co-workers (1964), Merigan, Winget and Dixon (1965) and Davies (1965*b*) used solvents to precipitate mouse interferon. Fantes (1965, 1967*a*) found that chick interferon was soluble in these solvents under acid conditions and could be recovered, with some purification, after neutralization. Acid ethanol was used by Davies (1964) with some success in the purification of calf interferon, but his attempts to apply the method to mouse interferon failed (Davies, 1965*b*), and Schonne (1966) was only partly successful in purifying rat interferon. The effect on chick interferon of some other solvents was investigated by Fantes and O'Neill (see Fantes, 1966): efforts to extract chick interferon from aqueous solution into *n*-butanol failed, benzyl alcohol caused loss of activity, and partitioning into and out of 80 per cent phenol gave erratic results. Homogenizing with Arcton 113 afforded only little purification.

ADSORPTION METHODS

Concentration or purification by adsorption onto and elution from a solid matrix is another method for purifying interferons. The first to adopt this procedure was probably Wagner (1960) who found that chick interferon was readily adsorbed by bentonite, but only a small proportion of the activity could be eluted. Burke (1961) achieved no significant purification of chick interferon by chromatography on hydroxyapatite. Fantes, O'Neill and Mason (1964) and Fantes (1966, 1967*a*) investigated a number of materials for their ability to adsorb chick interferon reversibly. Of these, two synthetic sodium-aluminium silicates, Doucil-25 and Alusil-165 (J. Crosfield and Sons, Warrington) were found to be most suitable. Adsorption of crude interferon at pH 5 onto 3 to 5 mg. of either of the substances per millilitre, followed by elution with 0.5 to 0.7 M-phosphate buffer at pH 7.5, reduced the volume fivefold to tenfold and increased the specific activity threefold to fivefold. Potassium thiocyanate was later used as eluant instead of phosphate (Fantes, 1965), as it offered two advantages in subsequent purification: (a) it precipitated inert protein on acidification, and (b) it was soluble in aqueous methanol. Davies (1965b) found that Alusil adsorbed mouse interferon irreversibly. He concentrated calf interferon by adsorption onto glass (ballotini) beads and eluted activity with a mixture of butanol, pyridine, acetic acid and water (Davies, 1965a).

NON-SPECIFIC CONCENTRATION METHODS

Most of the methods so far mentioned did not produce very highly purified interferons, but they were useful in reducing the large bulk of crude fluid to small volumes, which were then better suited for handling by other more selective processes. Before these are discussed several non-specific concentration methods may also be briefly mentioned; some of them also lead to slight incidental purification by denaturing inert protein. Such operations include pressure dialysis (e.g. Lindenmann, Burke, and Isaacs, 1957; Merigan, Winget and Dixon, 1965), freeze-drying (e.g. Sutton and Tyrrell, 1961; Davis, 1964), pervaporation (e.g. Paucker, 1965; Kreuz and Levy, 1965), dialysis against solutions of high molecular weight substances (e.g. Chany, 1961; Boudreault and Pavilanis, 1964; Falcoff et al., 1965) and distillation under reduced pressure (Davies, 1965a).

ION-EXCHANGE CHROMATOGRAPHY

Much greater purification factors were achieved, after initial disappointing results, when synthetic ion-exchange materials were used to fractionate interferon-containing solutions. The use of ion-exchange resins was first described by Burke (1961) who, however, was unable to purify chick interferon significantly by chromatography on the carboxylic Amberlite IRC-50 resin. Lampson and co-workers (1963) mentioned, without giving details, two other cation exchangers, Amberlite XE54 and Permutit H70; Merigan, Winget and Dixon (1965) were able to increase appreciably the specific activities of chick, mouse and human interferons by chromatography on Amberlite XE64.

Ion-exchange celluloses were first used by Wagner and Levy (1960), and by Burke (1960, 1961). The former reported irreversible adsorption of chick interferon by DEAE- and CM-celluloses. Burke too found CM-cellulose unsuitable, but achieved twofold to threefold purification after chromatography on DEAE-cellulose at pH 4·5 (interferon not retained) or at pH 6·6 or pH 5·8 (retention of interferon at 0·01 M-phosphate, but elution at increased molarity). DEAE-cellulose was also used by Fantes,

O'Neill and Mason (1964) who achieved substantial further purification of partly purified chick interferon (in o·01M-phosphate, pH 7·5; interferon retarded but not retained). Davies (1964) found that calf interferon resembled chick interferon (Burke, 1961) in its behaviour on DEAE-cellulose at pH 4·5 and at pH 5·8, and Schonne (1966) and Cocito, Schonne and De Somer (1965) confirmed the same for rat interferon on chromatography at pH 4·5. Davies (1965b) achieved marginal purification of mouse brain interferon by the batchwise use of the exchanger. Lampson and co-workers (1963)—unlike Wagner and Levy (1960) and Burke (1960, 1961)— used CM-cellulose very successfully; they were able to increase the specific activity of partly purified chick interferon over 100-fold by twice chromatographing on this exchanger (adsorption from o·01 M-phosphate at pH 6·0, elution, after washing, with o·01 M-phosphate/o·1 M-sodium chloride at pH 8). Schonne (1966) and Cocito, Schonne and De Somer (1965) applied the same technique successfully to the purification of rat interferon, but Davies (1965b) recovered only little mouse-brain interferon after CM-cellulose chromatography. SM-cellulose was used only by Burke (1961) who was able, by chromatography at pH 2, to double the specific activity of chick interferon.

Ion-exchange gels instead of celluloses have been used for interferon purification by several workers. The first to do so was Merigan (1964a) who adsorbed partly purified chick and mouse interferon on CM-Sephadex C25 columns from o·01M-phosphate solution at pH 6; he then removed much inert protein by washing with the same buffer and he finally eluted active material by means of a o·1 M-phosphate gradient of rising pH. Fantes (1965, 1967a) also used this exchanger (but the C50 grade) for chick interferon, eluting either stepwise or by means of a gradient, and Cantell and co-workers (1965) followed the elution pattern of Lampson and co-workers (1963), but they too substituted CM-Sephadex C50 for CM-cellulose. Recently Falcoff and co-workers (1966) have raised the specific activity of human leucocyte interferon 40-fold by the batchwise use of CM-Sephadex C50.

GEL FILTRATION

Gel filtration has been used with moderate success by several workers in attempts to raise the purity of interferons, but the main application of this method has been for molecular weight determinations. Kreuz and Levy (1963) purified chick interferon about tenfold by passage through a Sephadex G100 column, and similar purifications were achieved by Phillips and Wood (1964) and by Merigan, Winget and Dixon (1965). The latter group and Davies (1965*b*) used the method with some success for mouse interferon, but Polson and Vargosko (1965) could not purify calf interferon significantly on Sephadex G75.

GRADIENT CENTRIFUGATION

Another method that has been used much more frequently for molecular weight determinations than for purification purposes is gradient centrifuging. The only instance where increased specific activity seems to have been recorded was a threefold purification of partly purified mouse interferon on high-speed spinning in a sucrose gradient (Vilcek *et al.*, 1964).

ELECTROPHORESIS

Some data are available on the purification achieved by electrophoresis of interferons, a method more commonly used for isoelectric point determinations or as an analytical tool. Burke (1961) and Phillips and Wood (1964) separated chick interferon from other proteins by starch gel electrophoresis at pH 8·9 and pH 7·6 respectively, and Lampson and co-workers (1963) were able to raise the specific activity of highly purified chick interferon from 95,000 units to 236,000 units per milligram of protein by electrophoresis in Pevikon (Stockholm Superfosfat Fabriks A.B., Stockholm) at pH 8·9. Zone electrophoresis in a sucrose gradient at pH 9 removed some inert protein from chick interferon (Bodo and Jungwirth, 1964) and Merigan, Winget and Dixon (1965) further purified partly-purified chick interferon threefold to fivefold by electrophoresis at pH 4·3 on cellulose acetate and on acrylamide gel.

MULTIPLE-STEP PURIFICATIONS

Several groups of workers, by combining various processes described above, have obtained highly purified interferons. The first to attempt multi-step purification of chick interferon was Burke (1960, 1961). His starting material, induced in chorioallantoic membranes by interaction with the u.v.-inactivated Melbourne strain of influenza A virus, had a higher specific activity than is usually found in allantoic interferon. It was purified 22-fold, in 60 per cent yield, by these steps:

(1) Precipitation by ammonium sulphate (73 per cent saturation) and pressure dialysis;
(2) Chromatography on SM-cellulose at pH 2;
(3) Re-concentration by pressure dialysis and chromatography on DEAE-cellulose at pH 6·6;
(4) Passage through DEAE-cellulose at pH 4·5.

Burke's best material had a specific activity of about 4,400 units/mg. protein.*

Substantial progress was made by Lampson and co-workers (1963) who purified allantoic chick interferon 1,830 times (4,500 times after electrophoresis) by these operations:

(1) Precipitation of virus and inert protein with 0·15 N-perchloric acid;
(2) Concentration in two stages by precipitation with zinc hydroxide;
(3) Chromatography on CM-cellulose (adsorption from 0·01 M-phosphate solution at pH 6·0 followed by washing, and elution at pH 8 with 0·01 M-phosphate/0·1 M-sodium chloride);
(4) Re-concentration with zinc hydroxide;
(5) Re-chromatography on CM-cellulose;
(6) Re-concentration with zinc hydroxide;
(7) Electrophoresis in Pevikon at pH 8·9.

The recovery of interferon up to the electrophoresis step was 7·2 per cent and it had a specific activity of 95,000 units/mg. protein. Electrophoresis raised it further to 236,000 units/mg. protein. In a later paper, the same authors (Lampson et al., 1965) showed that at least the first stages of their process could also be applied to the purification of interferon derived from chick embryo tissue culture cells.

Merigan (1964a, b) and Merigan, Winget and Dixon (1965) obtained material of even higher purity by modifying Lampson's methods. They used CM-Sephadex C25 instead of CM-cellulose and they eluted the active material by a rising pH gradient, not stepwise. Their best material obtained without electrophoresis was purified 6,500 times and had a specific activity of 293,000 units/mg. protein.

Fantes, O'Neill and Mason (1964) and Fantes (1965, 1966, 1967a) developed methods whereby the specific activity of allantoic fluid and of tissue culture interferon was raised to $1·6 \times 10^6$ units/mg. protein, which for allantoic interferon represented nearly 20,000-fold purification. These steps gave an overall recovery of 7 per cent of tissue culture interferon:

(1) Adsorption onto the sodium aluminium silicate Doucil at pH 5 and elution with 0·5 M-KSCN at pH 7·5;
(2) Precipitation of inert protein by acidification to pH 3·5 and then to pH 2·0;

---

* An "interferon unit" has been defined differently by different authors. Merigan and Lampson, and Merigan and Fantes have assayed identical samples and have concluded that their "units" were similar. With certain assumptions the titre of Burke's interferon could be expressed in similar units (see Fantes, 1966).

(3) Precipitation of inert protein by addition of methanol (five volumes) at pH 2;

(4) Precipitation of interferon by neutralization of the acid methanol solution;

(5) Extraction of interferon from the precipitate with $0 \cdot 01\text{M}$-phosphate buffer pH $7 \cdot 5$ and passage of the solution through DEAE-cellulose.

(6) Adsorption onto CM-Sephadex-C50 at pH $5 \cdot 9$ from $0 \cdot 1$ M-phosphate solution and elution by a rising pH gradient, sometimes followed by readsorption onto CM-Sephadex and direct elution in one step.

Two other groups of workers (Cantell *et al.*, 1965; Pokidova *et al.*, 1965) used modifications of Lampson's method (Lampson *et al.*, 1963) to purify chick interferon. Merigan, Winget and Dixon (1965) found that the methods used by them to purify chick interferon were also suitable for human and mouse interferons.

Schonne (1966) and Cocito, Schonne and De Somer (1965) purified rat tissue culture interferon by this series of steps:

(1) Concentration by ultrafiltration;

(2) Passage through DEAE-cellulose ($0 \cdot 01$ M-acetate, pH $4 \cdot 5$);

(3) Adsorption by CM-cellulose from $0 \cdot 01$ M-phosphate solution, pH $5 \cdot 8$, and elution, after washing, with $0 \cdot 01$ M-phosphate/$0 \cdot 1$ M-sodium chloride at pH 8 (or with $0 \cdot 01$ M-acetate/$0 \cdot 42$ M-sodium chloride at pH $4 \cdot 2$).

The purified interferon had a specific activity of 50,000 units/mg. protein.

PURITY OF INTERFERONS TO DATE

Work on the purification of interferons has been in progress for six to seven years. High purification factors and specific activities have been achieved, and several workers thought at times that they had obtained a homogeneous product. Burke (1961), for example, thought that his chick interferon was pure, but Burke and Ross (1964, 1965) later realized that their material, compared with that of Lampson and co-workers, was still relatively impure. Lampson and his colleagues (1963) found that their own most highly purified chick interferon gave only one band on Pevikon electrophoresis at pH $8 \cdot 9$ and, since they published physical and chemical data, they presumably assumed purity, although this was not claimed. Merigan, Winget and Dixon (1965), on the other hand, found by acrylamide gel electrophoresis at pH $4 \cdot 3$ that their presumably best material was far from homogeneous. Schonne's (1966) purified rat interferon produced only one protein band on acrylamide gel (electrophoresis conditions were not stated), and Fantes (1965, 1966) interpreted results obtained with chick interferon on pH 8·9 electrophoresis in acrylamide gel and on pH 7·05 electrophoresis in a sucrose gradient as implying at least substantial purity.

RECENT ELECTROPHORESIS RESULTS

Fantes and I. G. S. Furminger (see Fantes, 1966, 1967b) investigated acrylamide gel electrophoresis of purified chick interferon further. Originally, separate columns were used for staining proteins and for demonstrating activity, but, in order to avoid possible errors due to different migration rates, the same columns were later used for both purposes. After electrophoresis, the column was cut lengthwise. One half was stained with amido black and the other half was cut into small equal pieces, each of which was individually eluted with 0·5 M-phosphate buffer, pH 7·5, containing bovine plasma albumin (500 μg./ml.) and Tween 80 (20 μg./ml.), and assayed for interferon content.

At first the alkaline method of Davis (1964) was used. One rather diffuse stained protein zone was observed and it seemed to coincide with activity. Overall recovery of activity was however poor, but some activity was always found in the spacer and sample gels. When these were omitted, and the samples applied directly to the small-pore gel in sucrose, recoveries improved and the stained zone appeared to be sharper. When the most highly purified interferon so far obtained by us (specific activity $1·6 \times 10^6$ units/mg. protein) was subjected to electrophoresis in this way, a very sharp double zone of protein was formed, coinciding exactly with the activity peak. However, since the region of activity extended over a wider zone than the stained protein, it was suspected that the correspondence of activity and stain could have been fortuitous. Electrophoresis at pH 4·3 (Reisfeld, Lewis and Williams, 1962) was therefore tried, but it invariably resulted in total or nearly total loss of activity. The cause was found to be the presence of persulphate, used by both Davis and Reisfeld to catalyse the polymerization of the small-pore gels. Incubation (18 hours, 4°) of crude or purified interferon, with and without ammonium persulphate (0·0064 M, the concentration used by Reisfeld) at pH 8·9 and pH 4·3, showed that acid persulphate, but none of the other treatments, destroyed the activity. When gels were later polymerized in the presence of riboflavin instead of persulphate, electrophoresis of the highly purified interferon at pH 4·3 gave good recoveries, but the activity now lay between two protein zones and did not seem to be related to either.

Staining of gels, after electrophoresis, with dyes normally used to reveal neutral or acidic polysaccharides has so far led to inconclusive results, and paper chromatography of an acid hydrolysate (of material before electrophoresis) followed by spraying with aniline phthalate did not produce any spot due to a sugar. This does not prove the absence of carbohydrate, since the tests may not have been sufficiently sensitive.

Electrophoresis has shown that the most highly purified interferon so far prepared by us (specific activity $1 \cdot 6 \times 10^6$ units/mg. protein) is probably still far from pure. The biological activity—assuming the major component of interferon to be protein—of even such impure material, however, is equalled only by few other substances. The very low level of protein associated with high activity could perhaps explain why interferon was considered a poor antigen (Paucker and Cantell, 1962) and why Burke and Walters (1966) failed to find a messenger RNA that codes for interferon.

HETEROGENEITY OF PURIFIED CHICK INTERFERON

Antiviral activity after gel electrophoresis was never confined to a very narrow band but usually occupied a fairly wide zone of the column. It is considered unlikely that this was solely due to diffusion of interferon, since electrophoresis of ribonuclease, a smaller protein, gave rise to a much narrower and better defined band of activity. Adsorption, however, could have played some part.

There is strong evidence that the active component in the purified interferon does not behave as a homogeneous substance: whenever the interferon was eluted from a CM-Sephadex column by means of a rising pH gradient and when early and late eluate fractions were readsorbed on two separate gel columns, the "early" material could always be re-eluted at a lower pH than could the "late" material, suggesting heterogeneity of either molecular weight or electric charge. It is not clear from these results whether the active material itself is heterogeneous or whether heterogeneity is caused by association of a homogeneous molecule with two or more different substances.

At one time we thought that dissolving interferon in acid methanol, one of our purification steps, could have caused partial methylation of the molecule and thus artificially created moieties with different isoelectric points. In order to test this hypothesis, two samples of purified interferon were prepared from the same starting fluid, but only one of them was exposed to acid methanol during purification. Both samples, however, eluted from CM-Sephadex in an identical manner and we therefore think it unlikely that the heterogeneity is an artifact.

PHYSICOCHEMICAL PROPERTIES OF VIRUS–INDUCED INTERFERONS

Although several groups of workers, including ourselves (e.g. Wagner, 1960; Burke, 1961; Lampson *et al.*, 1963; Davies, 1965*a*; Fantes, 1966), have published analytical figures on interferons, we no longer believe, in view of our recent electrophoretic results, that these data have much relevance, since they were probably obtained from impure materials.

In the absence of pure materials, all that is known about other properties of interferons has been learnt from work with crude or partly purified preparations. The nature and concentration of the impurities may well have influenced some results (e.g. Burke, 1962), and they may also have been the reason for some as yet unresolved contradictions. Nevertheless many of the observations have led to similar conclusions and an overall picture is emerging.

Purification studies and other researches into the physicochemical nature of interferons have so far not revealed any remarkable properties. Most of the interferons induced by viruses in a great variety of animal cells have several features in common. They are neutral or near-neutral proteins or protein-containing substances of molecular weight about 25,000–35,000. They are remarkably stable to acid and alkali and they are more heat-resistant than many other proteins. They are destroyed by reagents known to oxidize or reduce disulphide bonds, and chick interferon at least seems to need one or more free amino groups for antiviral activity (Fantes and O'Neill, 1964; Merigan, 1964*b*; Merigan, Winget and Dixon, 1965; Schonne, 1966). Their biological properties, on the other hand, make interferons fascinating and potentially very useful substances.

FUTURE OUTLOOK

As far as further purification studies are concerned, the first aim is still the isolation of at least one interferon as a pure substance. To prepare enough for determination of its structure will not be an easy task and the possibility of synthesizing an interferon or an active fragment of it seems still far away.

SUMMARY

Methods used for purifying the low molecular weight (about 30,000) interferons, induced by viruses in a variety of animals, are discussed. Some interferons, especially from chick cells, have been purified several thousand-fold and specific activities of over one million units/mg. protein have been obtained, interferons thus being placed among the most active biological substances. Yet even the most highly purified samples are probably still far from pure, and it seems unlikely that the structure of even one interferon will become known in the near future.

REFERENCES

BARON, S., BARBAN, S., and BUCKLER, C. E. (1964). *Science*, **145**, 814.

BODO, G., and JUNGWIRTH, C. (1964). *Biochem Z.*, **340**, 56–59.

BOUDREAULT, A., and PAVILANIS, V. (1964). *Revue can. Biol.*, **23**, 277–283.

BURKE, D. C. (1960). *Biochem. J.*, **76**, 50P.

BURKE, D. C. (1961). *Biochem. J.*, **78**, 556–564.

BURKE, D. C. (1962). In *Drugs, Parasites and Hosts*, pp. 294–319, ed. Goodwin, L. G., and Nimmo-Smith, R. H. London: Churchill.

BURKE, D. C., and ROSS, J. (1964). Fed. Europ. Biochem. Socs., Abstracts of Communications, 1st Meeting, London, 47.

BURKE, D. C., and ROSS, J. (1965). *Nature, Lond.*, **208**, 1297–1299.

BURKE, D. C., and WALTERS, S. (1966). *Biochem. J.*, **101**, 25–26P.

CANTELL, K., VALLE, M., SCHAKIR, R., SAUKKONEN, J. J., and UROMA, E. (1965). *Annls Med. exp. Biol. Fenn.*, **43**, 125–131.

CHANY, C. (1961). *Virology*, **13**, 485–492.

COCITO, C., SCHONNE, E., and DE SOMER, P. (1965). *Life Sci.*, **4**, 1253–1262.

DAVIES, A. (1964). *Biochem. J.*, **90**, 29P.

DAVIES, A. (1965a). *Biochem. J.*, **95**, 20P.

DAVIES, A. (1965b). Personal communication.

DAVIS, B. J. (1964). *Ann. N.Y. Acad. Sci.*, **121**, 404–427.

DENYS, P. (1963). *Lancet*, **2**, 174.

FALCOFF, E., FALCOFF, R., FOURNIER, F., and CHANY, C. (1966). *Annls Inst. Pasteur, Paris*, **111**, 562–584.

FALCOFF, E., and FAUCONNIER, B. (1965). *Proc. Soc. exp. Biol. Med.*, **118**, 609–612.

FALCOFF, E., LEVY, H., COLIN, J., and CHANY, C. (1965). *C. r. hebd. Séanc. Acad. Sci., Paris*, **260**, 5405–5407.

FANTES, K. H. (1965). *Nature, Lond.*, **207**, 1298.

FANTES, K. H. (1966). In *Interferons*, pp. 119–180, ed. Finter, N. B. Amsterdam: North-Holland Publishing Co.

FANTES, K. H. (1967a). *J. gen. Virol.*, **1**, 257–267.

FANTES, K. H. (1967b). *2nd Int. Symp. Med. Appl. Virol.*, Ft. Lauderdale.

FANTES, K. H., and O'NEILL, C. F. (1964). *Nature, Lond.*, **203**, 1048–1050.

FANTES, K. H., O'NEILL, C. F., and MASON, P. J. (1964). *Biochem. J.*, **91**, 20P.

FRIEDMAN, R. M., BARON, S., BUCKLER, C. E., and STEINMULLER, R. I. (1962). *J. exp. Med.*, **116**, 347–356.

GRAVELL, M., and MALSBERGER, R. G. (1965). *Ann. N.Y. Acad. Sci.*, **126**, 555–565.

GRESSER, I. (1961). *Proc. Soc. exp. Biol. Med.*, **108**, 303–307.

HANEISHI, T., SHIRASAKA, M., OKAZAKI, H., NAGANO, Y., and KOJIMA, Y. (1964). *C. r. Séanc. Soc. Biol.*, **158**, 1433–1436.

HENLE, W., HENLE, G., DEINHARDT, F., and BERGS, V. V. (1959). *J. exp. Med.*, **110**, 525–541.

HERMODSSON, S. (1964). *Acta path. microbiol. scand.*, **62**, 133–144.

HO, M., FANTES, K. H., BURKE, D. C., and FINTER, N. B. (1966). In *Interferons*, pp. 181–201, ed. Finter, N. B. Amsterdam: North-Holland Publishing Co.

ISAACS, A., and LINDENMANN, J. (1957). *Proc. R. Soc. B*, **147**, 258–267.

ISAACS, A., LINDENMANN, J., and VALENTINE, R. C. (1957). *Proc. R. Soc. B*, **147**, 268–273.

KONO, Y., and HO, M. (1965). *Virology*, **25**, 162–166.

KREUZ, L. E., and LEVY, A. H. (1963). *Nature, Lond.*, **200**, 883–884.

Kreuz, L. E., and Levy, A. H. (1965). *J. Bact.*, **89**, 462–469.

Lampson, G. P. (1966). United States patent 3,256,152.

Lampson, G. P., Tytell, A. A., Nemes, M. M., and Hilleman, M. R. (1963). *Proc. Soc. exp. Biol. Med.*, **112**, 468–478.

Lampson, G. P., Tytell, A. A., Nemes, M. M., and Hilleman, M. R. (1965). *Proc. Soc. exp. Biol. Med.*, **118**, 441–448.

Lindenmann, J., Burke, D. C., and Isaacs, A. (1957). *Br. J. exp. Path.*, **38**, 551–562.

Lowry, O. H., Rosebrough, N. J., Farr, A. L., and Randall, R. J. (1951). *J. biol. Chem.*, **193**, 265–275.

Merigan, T. C. (1964a). *Science*, **145**, 811–813.

Merigan, T. C. (1964b). In *Int. Symp. on Non-specific Resistance to Virus Infection, Interferon and Viral Chemotherapy*, Bratislava.

Merigan, T. C., Winget, C. A., and Dixon, C. B. (1965). *J. molec. Biol.*, **13**, 679–691.

Nagano, Y. (1965). *Jap. J. exp. Med.*, **35**, 21P.

Nagano, Y., and Kojima, T. (1958). *C. r. Séanc. Soc. Biol.*, **152**, 1627–1629.

Nagano, Y., and Kojima, Y. (1960). *C. r. Séanc. Soc. Biol.*, **154**, 2172–2175.

Nagano, Y., Kojima, Y., Haneishi, T., and Shirasaka, M. (1966). *Jap. J. exp. Med.*, **36**, 535–541.

Nagano, Y., Kojima, Y., and Kanashiro, R. S. (1966). *Jap. J. exp. Med.*, **36**, 477–480.

Nagano, Y., Kojima, Y., Shirasaka, M., and Haneishi, T. (1965). *Jap. J. exp. Med.*, **35**, 133–140.

Nagano, Y., Kojima, Y., and Suzuki, T. (1960). *C. r. Séanc. Soc. Biol.*, **154**, 2166–2168.

Paucker, K. (1965). *J. Immun.*, **94**, 371–378.

Paucker, K., and Cantell, K. (1962). *Virology*, **18**, 145–147.

Phillips, A. W., and Wood, R. D. (1964). *Nature, Lond.*, **201**, 819–820.

Pokidova, N. V., Furer, N. M., Zapozhnikova, G. A., and Ermolieva, Z. V. (1965). *Antibiotiki*, **10**, 713–717.

Polson, A., and Vargosko, A. J. (1965). Unpublished results.

Reisfeld, R. A., Lewis, U. J., and Williams, D. E. (1962). *Nature, Lond.*, **195**, 281–283.

Schonne, E. (1966). *Biochim. biophys. Acta*, **115**, 429–439.

Sellers, R. F., and Fitzpatrick, M. (1963). *Res. vet. Sci.*, **4**, 151–159.

Stewart, W. E., and Sulkin, S. E. (1966). *Proc. Soc. exp. Biol. Med.*, **123**, 650–654.

Sutton, R. N. P., and Tyrrell, D. A. J. (1961). *Br. J. exp. Path.*, **42**, 99–105.

Torlone, V., Titoli, F., and Gialletti, L. (1965). *Life Sci.*, **4**, 1707–1713.

Vilcek, J., Tomisova, J., Sokol, F., and Hana, L. (1964). *Acta virol., Prague*, **8**, 76–79.

Wagner, R. R. (1960). *Bact. Rev.*, **24**, 151–166.

Wagner, R. R., and Levy, A. H. (1960). *Ann. N.Y. Acad. Sci.*, **88**, 1308–1318.

Wheelock, E. F., and Sibley, W. A. (1965). *New Engl. J. Med.*, **273**, 194–198.

Zemla, J., and Vilcek, J. (1961a). *Acta virol., Prague*, **5**, 129.

Zemla, J., and Vilcek, J. (1961b). *Acta virol., Prague*, **5**, 367–372.

DISCUSSION

Crick: Why do you lose so much activity in the last step of your purification, when it goes down from 21 per cent to 7 per cent?

Fantes: The purer interferon becomes, the more readily it adsorbs onto all sorts of things. Lampson (Lampson and co-workers, 1963, *loc. cit.*) says it is not adsorbed onto polypropylene so we store all our highly purified material in polypropylene, not in glass. But we invariably find that our very highly purified interferon loses activity on being kept either in frozen or liquid form. Dr.

Merigan thought that freezing was not a good thing for very highly purified interferon, but we seem to lose the activity whatever we do.

Burke: Is re-running the material off the polyacrylamide gel feasible? If so, does it still show the heterogeneity you observed?

Fantes: We have not re-run it yet. In the experiments which gave the best recoveries we had a very potent and highly purified interferon. Now we are working with interferon of similar purity but lesser potency, so we don't get these nice pictures and we don't get such good recovery from the gel. If we had more of the purified interferon we could do much more. At the moment our stocks of this highly purified material are 2 to 3 ml. of material containing 8 μg. protein/ml.

Pereira: Interferon activity might depend on the presence of two different proteins, and in the acrylamide gel fractionation the activity might be in the area where the two are mixed.

Fantes: We don't think that is very likely. With the present interferon material, which has only 8 μg. protein/ml., the band is much weaker and we only see one faint zone of protein, not two.

Burke: But you could mix some of the different fractions from the polyacrylamide gel and get more activity.

Martin: It seems unlikely that the interferon activity is due to two proteins, and occurs only where they overlap, since you are getting about 60 per cent recovery of the activity you put onto the gel in the active band.

Fantes: Another thing which makes life difficult is that we elute the interferon from the acrylamide gel (and I think it is necessary to do this) with bovine plasma albumin and Tween. So if this should be re-run, additional difficulties will be created. I don't think much active material would be eluted if the gel pieces were just suspended in phosphate buffer.

Tyrrell: If you accept Nagano's theory, what you are getting in between the peaks may be an interferon which doesn't require protein to stabilize it, at least while it is being run on electrophoresis. Is it still susceptible to proteolytic enzymes when it comes out?

Fantes: I don't know. Several items in Nagano's work are difficult to understand. For instance, nobody else has ever found an interferon with a molecular weight of less than 10,000, though many people have determined molecular weights of many interferons. Again, Nagano's polysaccharide is inactive in tissue culture (Nagano *et al.*, 1965, *loc. cit.*), but all our assays are done in tissue culture, so this differentiates our material quite clearly from his. Nagano (Nagano, Y., Kojima, Y., Sawa, I., Hagihara, B., Kobayashi, S., Shirasaka, M., and Haneishi, T. [1967]. *Jap. J. exp. Med.*, in press) claims that unlike chick interferon, for example, both the polysaccharide and the glycoprotein inhibit oxidative phosphorylation, not only in rabbit cells but also in rat liver cells. He finds that dialysis of the glycoprotein against 0·01 M phosphate buffer at pH 7·2 slightly denatures the material, which then loses much of its species specificity and is active even in chick cells (Nagano, Kojima and Kanashiro, 1966, *loc. cit.*). We found on the other hand (in collaboration with Dr. N. B. Finter and Dr. R. D. Andrews) that the further we purified chick interferon the more species specific it became. During the purification we dissolve the material—and store it sometimes for long periods—in 0·01 M buffer (pH 7·5) under conditions claimed by Nagano to make the material non-specific, but we find it is much more specific than the crude material. The theory has many attractions, but is it correct?

Merigan: As I understand it, the Japanese workers used the low molarity buffer as a means of dissociating the carbohydrate from the protein. Their study of its non-species-specific nature was based on what diffused through the dialysis bag. Their interpretation of its *in vivo* antiviral action was that if they put the active carbohydrate back into another animal it could find a carrier protein of that species and thereby become active as an interferon.

Fantes: This is part of the story, but the material that goes through the cellophan is a polysaccharide which is altogether inactive *in vitro*, though active *in vivo*. It is the partly denatured non-dialysable glycoprotein material which is active *in vitro* in chick cells and which has lost its species specificity.

Joklik: It seems you will have to start off with an amount of interferon that gives you a reasonable chance of finishing up with about 1 mg. of pure material.

Fantes: From about 20 litres of starting fluid we end up with 10 ml. of material containing, say, 10 μg. protein/ml. At one time we were able to get supernatant fluids from influenza vaccine manufacturers, but this source has now dried up. We have to make every drop ourselves and it takes a long time to collect 20 litres.

Joklik: Does anybody have a tissue culture system using suspension cells or is it all made from monolayers? Twenty litres of suspension culture is nothing and a drug company could scale this up without any trouble.

Fantes: We use, for other purposes, BHK cells in suspension and those are available in large amounts, but most of our interferon work is done with chick material.

Wagner: Instead of trying to get tremendous amounts of interferon, perhaps one should try to label it radioactively and look for this as the marker, together with the biological activity. Tissue culture cells could then be used fairly well as confluent monolayers and these may not be making nearly as much extraneous protein as your chick system, Dr. Fantes. By timing the period in which, say, uniformly labelled [14C]amino acids were pulsed into the system, one could probably get a relatively specific labelling. There would be a lot of extraneous proteins and other substances, but the material could then be purified so that a radioactive band was obtained at the site where the biological activity of interferon peaks on, for example, polyacrylamide. Certain studies could be done under these conditions that cannot be done with the material you have now—and it may not be possible to purify your material any further.

It may be time to get away from the chick system. Other systems can give much higher levels of interferon to start with, so that losses during purification would be less significant. This might provide the opportunity to go much further towards characterization and analysis of interferons.

Fantes: What interferon would you suggest as having a much higher activity?

Wagner: I shall be telling you about that shortly, but the initial titres of rabbit interferons can be up to a hundredfold greater than you started with, with far less protein in the material. That is a tremendous purification step right at the beginning.

Finter: The mouse L cell in suspension is a good source of interferon. With our laboratory strain of NDV we get a titre of about 200 to 300 units/ml.

Tyrrell: A. Polson and A. J. Vargosko did some work (unpublished) in which they seemed to be separating, by zone electrophoresis of relatively crude chick material, more than one substance with interferon-like properties. You mentioned earlier, Dr. Fantes, that there were other things in allantoic fluid which weren't interferon, or at least the sort of interferon you purify. Could you say a little more about this?

Fantes: My colleague Dr. R. D. Andrews (1961. *Br. med. J.*, **1**, 1728) showed that several materials other than rabbit interferon prevent the formation of vaccinia lesions in rabbit skin. Certainly crude chick interferon is a very potent material in this respect. We have since done some further experiments with Dr. Finter, who found that our crude chick interferon had some activity in his mouse assay, but this activity decreased very rapidly with purification. We had partly purified material which was 20 times more active in chick cells than the crude preparation, yet the former was much less active in mouse cells than the crude material, implying that there is some non-specific activity which is removed during purification. The same happened in human embryonic lung cells challenged with HGP virus: the crude chick material appeared to have some activity in this system but the more purified material had not. After electrophoresis of crude chick interferon Dr. Polson found three peaks, but not all of these were active against the two viruses he used. Do you mean, Dr. Tyrrell, that these other two materials, which are eliminated during purification, explain the low recoveries we get?

Tyrrell: We may be able to simplify this by saying that what you are purifying is interferon. But is there in fact something else present as a result of virus infection which gets thrown away in the course of the purification procedures you use?

Fantes: I am sure that is so. The mere fact that crude interferon has some activity in mouse and human cells while more concentrated and partly purified interferon, with a higher chick titre, has not, would suggest that there is something else.

Burke: There is also the stimulator of oxidative phosphorylation which is obviously produced in virus-infected cells but is removed during purification of interferon. Then there are Dr. Chany's stimulon and Dr. Isaacs' blocker too.

ON THE APPARENT HETEROGENEITY OF RABBIT INTERFERONS

Robert R. Wagner and Thomas J. Smith*

Departments of Microbiology, University of Virginia, Charlottesville, and The Johns Hopkins University, Baltimore

The original aim of these experiments was to determine the capabilities of mammalian leucocytes in the production of interferon. The long-range objective was and is to evaluate the potential role of macrophages in host defences against viral infection. Leucocytes, and particularly mononuclear leucocytes, seemed to be good candidates for such a study for several reasons, among them: (1) they have long been considered as prominent participants in viral inflammatory responses (Mims, 1964; Gresser and Lang, 1966); (2) macrophages appear to have an important function in cellular immunity to certain bacterial infections (Mackaness, 1964); and (3) several investigators have demonstrated quite conclusively that leucocytes from various sources are capable of producing interferons in response to viral and non-viral stimulation (Glasgow and Habel, 1963; Wheelock, 1965; Gresser and Lang, 1966). In fact, very recent studies have shown that human blood leucocytes may provide one of the richest sources of interferons for potential therapeutic purposes (Falcoff *et al.*, 1966).

We chose the rabbit as our experimental animal for several reasons: (1) considerable work has been done with rabbit peritoneal leucocytes in our department (Bornstein, Bredenberg and Wood, 1963); (2) the rabbit produces very large amounts of circulating interferon in response to intravenous injection of virus or bacterial endotoxin (Ho and Kono, 1965) and a single animal can be bled repeatedly with great ease; and (3) rabbit renal epithelium provides an excellent tissue for comparative studies of interferon production as well as for assay of interferons. In many respects the rabbit exceeded our highest hopes as an experimental model because of the ease with which tissue could be obtained for these studies and the extraordinarily rapid production of interferons in very large amounts both *in vitro* and *in vivo*. The basic observations are reported in two papers that have just been published (Smith and Wagner, 1967*a*, *b*).

* Present address: Walter Reed Army Institute of Research, Washington, D.C.

The protocols for these experiments were quite simple and the results, at least initially, were straightforward and consistent with those from previous studies with cells of other animal species (Wagner and Huang, 1965). However, it soon became apparent, as we should have anticipated, that the results could not be wrapped up neatly in a single interpretative package. The experiments provided some answers but raised many more questions. We believe that the way in which these questions are framed can influence the course of at least two related aspects of research on interferons: their nature and their cellular sites of synthesis. Therefore, we are taking the liberty of proposing a number of hypotheses, some of which can be tested experimentally by available techniques whereas others require considerable refinement of these techniques or an entirely new methodology. It is our contention that future progress in research on interferon synthesis hinges on the solution of these technical problems.

SYNTHESIS OF RABBIT MACROPHAGE INTERFERONS

Virus-induced interferon synthesis

The most obvious first step in these experiments was to determine whether rabbit leucocytes can synthesize interferon in response to viral infection. As anyone who has worked with leucocytes knows, and as we learned, the first problem is to separate and identify the respective cell types from whatever source. This is no mean task. Methods are available for obtaining relatively homogeneous populations of morphologically similar cells (Wheelock, 1966), but we have not done this as yet. Instead, we resorted to a technique that provides leucocyte suspensions which are predominantly, but not exclusively, polymorphonuclear or mononuclear in their morphology (Bornstein, Bredenberg and Wood, 1963). The method is relative simple and consists of inducing a mild and sterile peritonitis by means of intra-abdominal instillation of 0·1 per cent glycogen in non-pyrogenic physiological saline solution. This irritant causes marked transudation of fluid rich in polymorphonuclear (PMN) leucocytes by 24 hours, following which much of the fluid is absorbed, leaving by 48–72 hours a relatively dry inflammatory exudate which contains about 90 per cent macrophages. About 5×10^7 macrophages can be obtained uniformly from the peritoneal cavity. These cells suspended in a medium of lactalbumin hydrolysate with 5 per cent calf serum attach readily to glass or plastic surfaces and form a fairly homogeneous layer. Cell cultures of early and late peritoneal exudates produce very large amounts of interferon when infected with 3×10^8 plaque-forming units (p.f.u.) of Newcastle disease virus (NDV) at input multiplicities ranging from 5 to 0·1 p.f.u./cell. The interferon yields per millilitre of medium were consistently 5,000–20,000 plaque-depressing doses (PDD_{50}/ml.) as assayed on rabbit kidney (RK) cell cultures with vesicular stomatitis virus (VSV) as the test virus.

One striking finding was that about 8×10^7 cells in macrophage-rich 72-hour exudates consistently made three to four times more interferon than about 8×10^8 cells in PMN-rich 24-hour exudates. In fact, the amount of interferon produced by cells in early exudates was always related to the degree of contamination with macrophages. We cannot exclude the possibility that PMN leucocytes make interferon but we are fairly confident that the macrophage is the primary competent cell in peritoneal exudates. This also holds true for alveolar macrophages and for explanted spleen cells which have the morphological appearance of macrophages and which produce large amounts of interferon after infection with NDV. Very recent studies by Kono (1967) also indicate that macrophages are the competent interferon-synthesizing cells in cultures of bovine blood leucocytes and that this function increases with maturation. We leave to the histologists and immunologists the problem of defining a macrophage, but we shall take the liberty of using this designation to mean the predominant cell type in 72-hour peritoneal exudates. The reservation of obvious cellular inhomogeneity is implicit.

It was of interest, nevertheless, to compare the interferon-synthesizing capacity of peritoneal macrophages with that of a completely different cell type, renal tubular epithelium, in the same animal. Once again, RK cells are by no means pure populations but there seems little doubt that the method of preparing the cultures favours the growth of epithelial cells. Clear-cut results were obtained by careful comparative studies of the kinetics of interferon synthesis by RK cells and macrophages. Both cell types produced interferon in comparable amounts at virtually identical rates. In each case the lag period after viral induction was one hour or slightly longer, after which the interferon activity of the culture media increased linearly to a peak of 5,000–20,000 PDD_{50}/ml. by six hours.

Perhaps a more precise comparison of the kinetics of NDV-induced interferon synthesis by RK cells and macrophages can be made by using actinomycin and puromycin to delineate and time the events. As had been shown previously in studies of chick embryo and mouse cells (Wagner, 1964; Wagner and Huang, 1965), actinomycin inhibits interferon production during the first four hours after viral induction, presumably by switching off cellular messenger RNA (mRNA) synthesis. Once the hypothetical interferon-specific mRNA is transcribed by the cells, interferon synthesis and release continue even in the presence of actinomycin. Similar results were obtained with rabbit cell cultures except for the fact that mRNA appears to be transcribed much more rapidly than it is in chick and mouse systems. Interferon synthesis by rabbit macrophages was found to be inhibited by actinomycin only during the first hour after viral induction, whereas in RK cells the transcriptive event requires two hours to reach completion. Although this finding indicates a significantly greater rate of transcription of interferon-specific mRNA in macrophages, the difference is not profound nor does it signify necessarily any major variation in the mechanism of interferon synthesis by the two rabbit cell types. As expected (Wagner and Huang, 1965), puromycin was found to shut off interferon synthesis by both cell types at any stage of the cycle.

None of these experiments provides any secure basis for distinguishing between the interferon-synthesizing machinery of macrophages and RK cells. Moreover, similar kinetics of interferon production were noted in rabbits injected intravenously with NDV except for the possibly significant fact that serum interferon ordinarily appears earlier (by one hour) and titres peak sooner (by four hours) than in any *in vitro* system. It is not possible from these experiments to rule out macrophages, or for that matter renal epithelium and other parenchymal cells, as the source of circulating interferon in intact rabbits infected with NDV.

Interferon synthesis by uninfected macrophages

To serve as controls for the foregoing studies of virus-induced interferon synthesis, media were removed from uninfected cultures of peritoneal macrophages and tested for interferon content by plaque inhibition of VSV plated on RK cells. Much to our surprise appreciable amounts of a viral inhibitor appeared in these presumably uninfected cultures merely on incubation at 37° C directly after the cells were plated. Cells disrupted by ultrasound or by freezing and thawing yielded no interferon even after incubation at 37°, a finding which suggested that the inhibitor is made *de novo* rather than being preformed and released. Nor did macrophages incubated at 4° produce interferon. A useful trick, however, was to hold the cultures at 4° for 24–48 hours, during which time no interferon was formed, and then to warm them to 37°, which resulted in a slightly but significantly augmented yield. This increase in temperature served in lieu of an inducing agent and permitted us to time the rate of synthesis of this "spontaneously produced" interferon. These kinetic experiments revealed that interferon could first be detected in media of macrophage cultures between one and two hours after being warmed from 4° to 37°; the titres then increased linearly to a peak at six hours in a manner entirely analogous to that of NDV-induced macrophage interferon. However, the total yields of "spontaneously produced" interferon were only about 1 per cent of that resulting from viral induction. In addition, both interferons could be made sequentially in the same macrophage cultures, but of course there was no way of determining whether the same cells made both the "spontaneous" and virus-induced interferons.

We also sought to determine whether the glycogen used to stimulate sterile peritonitis served as an inducer of interferon synthesis by macrophages present in 72-hour peritoneal exudates. This turned out not to be the case since sterile, pyrogen-free suspensions of fine glass beads caused an identical peritonitis and the mobilized macrophages were equally competent as interferon producers. Nagano and co-workers (1966) have also shown that peritoneal exudates induced in rabbits by injection of liquid paraffin contain macrophages which make interferon "spontaneously".

We also tested macrophages normally present in the abdominal cavity of rabbits without peritonitis and found them to be far less efficient producers of "spontaneous" or endotoxin-induced interferon than macrophages present in inflammatory exudates. This latter finding suggests that mobilization and maturation of macrophages result in development of interferon-synthesizing capability in a manner resembling the enhanced metabolic activity and lysozomal enzyme formation which occurs on maturation of these cells (Cohn and Benson, 1965).

The fly in the ointment of these experiments was our inability to exclude pyrogens from the media used to cultivate the macrophages. Despite all our efforts, each batch of serum and commercial media from several suppliers caused fever when intravenously injected into rabbits, suggesting strongly contamination with bacterial endotoxin.

Other investigators have shown that interferons rapidly appear in the serum of rabbits or other animals injected with bacterial lipopolysaccharides (Ho and Kono, 1965). We found that *Escherichia coli* lipopolysaccharide added to the media of macrophage cultures caused an increase in interferon yields five- to sixfold greater than that of "spontaneously produced" interferon, although this augmentation effect required the extremely large dose of 10 μg./ml. and was not evident with 1 μg./ml. Therefore, the question of whether endotoxin is necessary for induction of interferon synthesis by uninfected macrophages must be held in abeyance. We are inclined to believe, without concrete evidence, that endotoxin is not required but that these cells can produce interferon "constitutively", i.e. without inducer. Whatever the mechanism, it seems likely that this property of non-viral-induced or "spontaneous" interferon synthesis is restricted to macrophages, because RK cells, spleen cells and PMN leucocytes produced no interferon spontaneously or on exposure to large amounts of endotoxin.

Quite obviously, additional evidence was required to determine whether the interferons produced by uninfected macrophages are synthesized *de novo* or are preformed and merely released on incubation at 37° or on exposure to endotoxin. This latter possibility has been suggested by Ho and Kono (1965) and by Youngner, Stinebring and Taube (1965) as the mechanism of endotoxin-induced interferon production in intact rabbits and mice on the basis that the response could not be inhibited by prior administration of actinomycin, puromycin or cycloheximide. Negative results such as these are, of course, rather difficult to interpret, particularly in a system as complex as the intact animal. Therefore, we re-examined these alternative hypotheses (*de novo* synthesis versus release of preformed interferon) by using uninfected macrophage cultures, a system which offers a better basis for discrimination. The results, in brief, showed that actinomycin (10 μg./ml.) completely blocked "spontaneous" or endotoxin-induced formation of interferon, but only during the first 30 minutes after induction. By one hour, the interferon-synthesizing potential of the macrophages was unaffected by actinomycin, which is quite analogous to what happens in virus-induced synthesis of interferon by the same cells. One can legitimately criticize these experiments on the basis of the very large doses of actinomycin used, which can cause dissolution of polysomes and which probably affect cell functions other than RNA transcription, but we point out again that the same dose of actinomycin was completely ineffective by one hour after non-viral induction.

Further evidence for *de novo* synthesis of interferon by uninfected macrophages was provided by studying the effect of puromycin. As predicted, "spontaneous" and endotoxin-induced synthesis of interferon was interrupted at any stage when cell cultures were exposed to puromycin (50 μg./ml.). The experiments would have been even more conclusive if the puromycin effect could have been completely reversed by washing out the drug, but this turned out to be possible only to a limited extent. Nevertheless, 25 per cent of expected interferon yields could be achieved after changing to puromycin-free medium in puromycin-blocked cultures.

These experiments indicate that mature macrophages in late peritoneal exudates, in contrast to other cultured rabbit cells, can synthesize interferon *de novo* either "spontaneously" or on induction by bacterial endotoxin. These results do not, of course, rule out the possibility of release of preformed interferon or activation of interferon precursors by endotoxin injection in intact animals. In common with other cell systems, however, interferon synthesis by uninfected macrophages appears to require sequential transcriptive and translational events.

COMPARATIVE PROPERTIES OF RABBIT INTERFERONS

Virus-induced interferons from macrophages, RK cells and serum, as well as "spontaneous" and endotoxin-induced interferons of macrophages, all met the usual criteria for classification as interferons. The biological activity of each preparation was (1) trypsin-sensitive, (2) non-sedimentable at 100,000 g, (3) non-dialysable, (4) inactive in cell cultures of species other than rabbits, (5) not virus-specific, and (6) not virucidal. In general, each of these interferons was relatively acid-resistant but several exhibited suggestive quantitative differences in this property, as well as apparent variations in sensitivity to inactivation by heat, depending, apparently, on tissue source and nature of inducer.

Other investigators have reported that serum or leucocyte interferons induced by endotoxin (Ho, 1964) or phytohaemagglutinin (Wheelock, 1965) are considerably more labile to heat and acid treatment than are virus-induced interferons produced by cells of the same animal species. Our studies indicate that these distinguishing characteristics hold true only to a limited extent for rabbit interferons. It might be worth recounting the pitfalls we encountered in trying to make such comparisons. Initially, we found that non-virus-induced macrophage interferons lost 75–80 per cent antiviral activity when heated to 56° for one hour or when dialysed for 24 hours at 4° against HCl at pH 2. Under identical conditions NDV-induced macrophage or RK interferon was completely stable. It finally occurred to us, however, that the conditions of these tests were hardly comparable for the two kinds of interferons since the acid–dialysis step used routinely to process virus-induced interferons could easily have destroyed heat-labile as well as acid-labile components. This turned out to be the case. When only prolonged ultracentrifugation was used to rid macrophage interferons of inducing NDV, 50 per cent of the antiviral activity was lost at 56° or at pH 2. In fact, NDV-induced serum interferon was found to be even more labile: comparable exposure to heat or acid caused loss in activity of 75 per cent or greater. It is clear that virus-induced rabbit interferons from various sources contain at least one labile component, which is not residual virus, as is shown by lack of antiviral activity on chick cells and by failure of potent anti-NDV antibody to neutralize antiviral activity for rabbit cells. Moreover, the acid-stable component was found to be, for the most part, heat-stable.

These studies raise the question of the validity of the crude tests, such as those described above, which are in common use for characterizing and comparing interferons from different sources. Stability of interferons is also undoubtedly influenced by the presence of contaminating, biologically inactive proteins, as shown clearly by the purification studies of Lampson and co-workers (1963). Despite these reservations, our experiments seem to reveal certain differences in lability of interferons from different sources and in those induced by different agents, which suggested the presence of more than one molecular component in several of the preparations.

ESTIMATIONS OF MOLECULAR WEIGHTS

Although Ke, Ho and Merigan (1966) had clearly identified the presence of two distinct molecular components by Sephadex gel filtration of interferons in sera of rabbits previously injected either with NDV or bacterial endotoxin, we were still quite unprepared for the surprising degree of heterogeneity found among our preparations of rabbit interferons examined by the same technique. We took considerable pains in our experiments to design and carefully calibrate a Sephadex G100 column with high resolving power—one which would also afford dependable reproducibility even when loaded with relatively large volumes of each sample. Effluent fractions were each assayed by plaque inhibition on at least three replicate plates and peak antiviral activity was compared with peak elution of five marker proteins of known molecular weight. The techniques have been described in detail elsewhere (Smith and Wagner, 1967b; Wagner, Levy and Smith, 1967). Repeated examinations were made of rabbit interferons from the following four sources: RK and macrophage cultures infected with NDV, serum collected after intravenous injection of NDV, and macrophages exposed to *E. coli* lipopolysaccharide. The significant data from these studies are summarized in Table I.

TABLE I

SEPHADEX FRACTIONATION OF RABBIT INTERFERONS AND ESTIMATED MOLECULAR
WEIGHTS OF IDENTIFIABLE COMPONENTS

Source	Inducer	$\sim$ Mol. wt. classes,* $\times 10^3$
Kidney	NDV	45 ($\pm$ trace > 134)
Macrophages	NDV	45; 37 ($\pm$ trace > 134)
Serum	NDV (i.v.)	>134; 51; $\pm$ 45
Macrophages	Endotoxin	>134; 77; $\pm$ 45; 37; $\pm$ 30

* Molecular weight rules are based on discrete peaks of VSV plaque-inhibiting activity in effluent fractions from a Sephadex G100 column compared with peak elution of proteins of known molecular weight.

Despite obvious difficulties in interpreting these results of gel diffusion studies, several basic points stand out and are worth noting. (1) *NDV-induced kidney interferon* is predominantly a single, homogeneous molecular species with a molecular weight of 45,000. (2) *NDV-induced macrophage interferon* also contains a prominent component with a molecular weight of about 45,000 but, in addition, another distinct component with a molecular weight of about 37,000 is present in comparable amount. This latter component appeared to be more labile than the former. (3) *NDV-induced serum interferon* may also contain a component with a molecular weight of about 45,000, although the resolving power of the column was insufficient to establish this point unequivocally. By far the predominant interferon activity in serum peaks at molecular weight equivalent to 51,000 daltons and about 10 per cent of the antiviral activity is excluded from the gel (mol. wt. $\geqslant$ 134,000). This high molecular weight component was found to be extremely heat- and acid-labile, whereas the more slowly diffusing factors were relatively stable. This pattern of Sephadex filtration appears to rule out circulating macrophages as the primary source of serum interferon made in response to intravenous injection of NDV. (4) *Endotoxin-induced macrophage interferon* is polydisperse with respect to diffusion through Sephadex G100, but one component, which is consistently present, resembles the interferon of molecular weight of about 37,000 found in media of macrophage cultures infected with NDV.

INTERPRETATIONS AND HYPOTHESES

The data presented in this report can be analysed in at least two different ways, depending somewhat on whether one tends to be a scientific "splitter" or a "lumper". To the "splitter" the results of the Sephadex filtration studies might appear to indicate that rabbit interferons are hopelessly heterogeneous—which could, of course, be a function of heterogeneity of cells in primary cultures, to say nothing of those in intact animals. Tissue culture techniques being what they are, it will undoubtedly be a long time before an experiment can be designed to determine whether the interferons of molecular weight of about 45,000 and 37,000 present in virus-infected macrophage cultures are produced by the same or different cells. What does seem likely, however, is that the bulk of virus-induced serum interferon with a molecular weight of about 51,000 and of 134,000 or more is made by cells other than macrophages. A valid hypothesis based on these data might be that four or more rabbit genes can direct the synthesis of NDV-induced interferons with similar antiviral activity. Alternatively, it is of course conceivable that NDV induces synthesis in all cells of a single molecular species of interferon which is bound in varying degrees to biologically inert proteins or other substances; such complexes would be expected to exhibit different diffusional and other physical properties. In fact, there is no assurance that diffusion rates are purely a function of molecular size as measured by the sieving properties of the gel. Nevertheless, it seems more likely that we are dealing with interferons truly differing in molecular weight and which are produced by different cells or even by different genes in a single cell, such as the macrophage. It is tempting to think in terms of designing future experiments on the assumption that macrophages subserve a special function in defence against viral infections by virtue of being equipped with more than one interferon gene. It even seems possible that maturation of macrophages in inflammatory exudates (Cohn and Benson, 1965) results in the switching on of cistrons which are ordinarily repressed.

This latter hypothesis is even more appealing when one considers interferon synthesis by mature macrophages in the apparent absence of viral infection. It does not seem too far-fetched to predict the existence of a constitutive state in mature, but not in immature, macrophages which permits interferon synthesis in the absence of specific inducer. This theory would not seem to be severely compromised by our inability to rule out contaminating endotoxin as inducer or by the fact that large amounts of endotoxin augment interferon yields in macrophage cultures. However, the polydispersity on gel diffusion of endotoxin-induced interferon is more difficult to reconcile with our postulate of a simple constitutive state. One could assume that macrophages carry many different genes for interferon synthesis, but this borders on genetic chaos. More likely, there are a few interferons, or interferon subunits, which polymerize or form complexes with biologically inert proteins, resulting in altered diffusional properties of endotoxin-induced interferons. The somewhat greater lability to acid and heat compared with virus-induced interferons might be consistent with such a hypothesis.

From the viewpoint of the "lumper" the most significant aspect of these studies would seem to be the evidence for similarities in mechanisms of interferon synthesis regardless of tissue source or nature of inducer. The actinomycin and puromycin experiments clearly suggest sequential transcriptive and translational events. The data, as they now stand, cannot be logically interpreted in any way other than as being consistent with *de novo* synthesis of interferons by macrophages at comparable rates both with and without viral induction. This finding appears to simplify, or at least to unify, this aspect of interferon research. It is no longer necessary to postulate that bacterial endotoxin or other non-viral stimuli merely promote release of preformed interferon or activation of interferon precursors.

Conceivably, endotoxin could act *in vivo* merely by augmenting spontaneous production or mobilizing interferons that are continuously made in small quantities by competent cells of the uninfected animal. However, the macrophage studies place the burden of proof on those who postulate that the mechanism of interferon production in response to non-viral stimuli is fundamentally different from that of virus-induced interferons.

These hypotheses and unabashed speculations are all well and good but the real question is whether they are testable. The answer is that they are probably not, at least by present methodology, which is being stretched to the limit of its usefulness. Newer approaches and techniques are required. One procedure that seems worthy of intensive effort is an attempt to produce radioactively labelled interferon. In this regard it is worth noting that rabbit kidney and macrophage cultures appear to exhibit marked contact inhibition. Such cells might be ideal for specific labelling of interferon if $[^{14}C]$amino acids were pulsed in at a time of maximal interferon synthesis but minimal synthesis of extraneous proteins. This technique might also afford a greater degree of purification of interferon than any physical or chemical methods currently in use. If labelled interferons were to become available, physical and chemical characterization could obviously be accomplished with greater ease and assurance than is the case with relatively crude bioassay techniques. One other lead that would be worth following up is the preliminary report by Merigan, Winget and Dixon (1965) of the use of polyacrylamide gel electrophoresis for identifying and comparing interferons. This procedure is now being refined to the point where it gives much greater resolution than chromatographic or electrophoretic techniques alone, particularly when coupled with radioactive labelling of proteins for radioautography to enhance sensitivity. By these and similar means it may be possible to test some of the hypotheses posed in this discussion, and to open up new areas of investigation concerning interferon synthesis and characterization.

SUMMARY

Although no experimental model is wholly satisfactory, the rabbit seems to be the most suitable and convenient host for analysing systematically the tissue sources of interferons made in response to different inducers. Comparatively large amounts of interferon are produced consistently at an extremely rapid rate in response to NDV infection of intact rabbits or of primary cultures of rabbit kidney (RK) cells or peritoneal macrophages. Adequate amounts are also produced "spontaneously" by cultured macrophages or on stimulation of these cells by bacterial endotoxin.

No profound differences could be detected in biological activity or physicochemical reactivity of these various rabbit interferons, at least not by the crude tests in common use, and each satisfies the general criteria for classification as an interferon. Moreover, the kinetics of synthesis and sensitivity to actinomycin or puromycin appear to be virtually identical in each *in vitro* system. We find no evidence for a "preformed" interferon or an interferon precursor in rabbit macrophages. However, a surprising degree of heterogeneity was noted among rabbit interferons from different sources as determined by filtration rates through a column of Sephadex G100 with high resolving power. All tissue sources showed two or more sharply delineated peaks of interferon activity in effluent fractions, but the major components of each were as follows: NDV-induced RK cells, molecular weight $\simeq$ 45,000; NDV-induced macrophages, molecular weights $\simeq$ 45,000 and 37,000; NDV-induced serum interferon, molecular weights $\simeq$ 51,000, $\geqslant$ 134,000 and (?) 45,000. Endotoxin-induced macrophage interferon was polydisperse by Sephadex diffusion but exhibited two relatively consistent peaks equivalent to molecular weights of 37,000 and $\geqslant$ 134,000.

REFERENCES

BORNSTEIN, D. L., BREDENBERG, C., and WOOD, W. B., JR. (1963). *J. exp. Med.*, **117**, 349.

COHN, Z. A., and BENSON, B. (1965). *J. exp. Med.*, **121**, 153.

FALCOFF, E., FALCOFF, R., FOURNIER, F., and CHANY, C. (1966). Personal communication.

GLASGOW, L. A., and HABEL, K. (1963). *J. exp. Med.*, **117**, 149.

GRESSER, I., and LANG, D. J. (1966). *Prog. med. Virol.*, **8**, 62.

HO, M. (1964). *Science*, **146**, 1472.

HO, M., and KONO, Y. (1965). *Proc. natn. Acad. Sci. U.S.A.*, **52**, 220.

KE, Y. H., HO, M., and MERIGAN, T. C. (1966). *Nature, Lond.*, **211**, 541.

KONO, Y. (1967). *Proc. Soc. exp. Biol. Med.*, **124**, 155.

LAMPSON, G. P., TYTELL, A. A., NEMES, M. M., and HILLEMAN, M. R. (1963). *Proc. Soc. exp. Biol. Med.*, **112**, 468.

MACKANESS, G. B. (1964). *J. exp. Med.*, **120**, 105.

MERIGAN, T. C., WINGET, C. A., and DIXON, C. B. (1965). *J. molec. Biol.*, **13**, 679.

MIMS, C. A. (1964). *Bact. Rev.*, **28**, 30.

NAGANO, Y., KOJIMA, Y., ARAKAWA, J., and KANASHIRO, R. (1966). *Jap. J. exp. Med.*, **36**, 481.

SMITH, T. J., and WAGNER, R. R. (1967a). *J. exp. Med.*, **125**, 559.

SMITH, T. J., and WAGNER, R. R. (1967b). *J. exp. Med.*, **125**, 579.

WAGNER, R. R. (1964). *Nature, Lond.*, **204**, 49.

WAGNER, R. R., and HUANG, A. S. (1965). *Proc. natn. Acad. Sci. U.S.A.*, **54**, 1112.

WAGNER, R. R., LEVY, A. H., and SMITH, T. J. (1967). In *Methods in Virology*, vol. 3, ed. Maramorosch, K., and Koprowski, H. New York: Academic Press.

WHEELOCK, E. F. (1965). *Science*, **149**, 310.

WHEELOCK, E. F. (1966). *J. Bact.*, **92**, 1415.

YOUNGNER, J. S., STINEBRING, W. R., and TAUBE, S. E. (1965). *Virology*, **27**, 541.

DISCUSSION

Gresser: In 1962 Dr. Chany and I (see Gresser, I., and Lang, D. J. [1966]. *Prog. med. Virol.*, **8**, 89) wondered whether leucocytes obtained from individuals with diseases such as infectious hepatitis or infectious mononucleosis might liberate interferon when maintained *in vitro*, thus indicating the presence of a virus within these cells. Leucocytes from patients with illnesses such as infectious hepatitis, infectious mononucleosis, acute leukaemia and unknown febrile disorders, were suspended in a culture medium *in vitro*. In over 50 per cent of the cases we obtained a factor which possessed a number of the properties of interferon. However, we also recovered this substance from about 50 per cent of "normal" individuals. The titres were about 1:2 to 1:8, or in other words about 0·1 to 1 per cent of the amount one might expect had one infected these cells with a virus such as Sendai or NDV. We also observed that extraction by freeze-thawing of the white cells did not release this factor. It was necessary to place the white cells under conditions of cell culture. Although we didn't do precise kinetic studies, we found that the factor was not present a few minutes after placing the white cells in culture, but was present 24 hours later.

Thus we concluded that the release of this substance seemed to be related to the environmental conditions. We did not feel that "normal" leucocytes were latently infected. We really didn't know what to make of the findings at the time but they were certainly repeatable. I wonder whether it may not be related to the destruction of neutrophils or perhaps to the changes which lead to the transformation of cells into macrophages.

One more finding may be apposite. In 1964 Dr. Naficy and I (Gresser, I., and Naficy, K. [1964]. *Proc. Soc. exp. Biol. Med.*, **117**, 285) found that the presence of an interferon-like inhibitor in the cerebrospinal fluid of patients with aseptic meningitis seemed to be related to the number of leucocytes in the CSF. We suggested the possibility that *uninfected* leucocytes released this substance *in vivo* in the patient or *in vitro* in the tube containing the CSF. This hypothesis was prompted by the above observations in 1962 and by the finding that the titres of the interferon-like substance were low and surprisingly uniform, suggesting that viruses which vary in their interferon-inducing ability may not have been the direct cause of the liberation of this interferon-like substance.

Chany: With Dr. Gresser we found the spontaneously appearing interferon-like substance in the leucocyte system but we also found it in the amniotic system which I have described here. It appeared in the diffusate when the amniotic membrane had been kept in suspension for several days at room temperature. However, we never found this type of inhibitor in a tissue culture system, only in organ suspensions—if by extension the leucocyte can be considered as an organ. The question arises of whether the inhibitor comes from the cell or from the fundamental substance of the tissues; does it act in the cell or on the cell surface? In the leucocyte system we found that actinomycin did not block the action of the spontaneously-appearing interferon-like inhibitor.

Ho: Your excellent titering system may be the secret of your findings with this material, Dr. Wagner. The only difference between your system and ours appears to be that you use kidneys from rabbits two or three weeks old and we use rabbit embryos. We have certainly been unable to get anything near your indicated titres with peritoneal or peripheral leucocyte material.

Have you tried to characterize endotoxin-induced interferon *in vivo*, that is to say serum material from rabbits inoculated with endotoxin (Ke, Y. H., Ho, M., and Merigan, T. C. [1966]. *Nature, Lond.*, **211**, 541)?

Wagner: No.

Ho: Does medium depleted of the nutrients or simple basic salt solutions seem to stimulate the spontaneous release of interferon from macrophages, as indicated by Nagano and his co-workers (Nagano, Y., Kojima, Y., Arakawa, J., and Kanashiro, S. [1966]. *Jap. J. exp. Med.*, **36**, 481)?

Wagner: Just the opposite—we seem to get less, which fits in with our hypothesis that the "spontaneous" interferon is actively synthesized by the macrophages.

Ho: You postulate that macrophages spontaneously release this type of interferon and that the increased titre is accounted for by macrophages as opposed, for example, to polymorphonuclear leucocytes. Taking this into account, wouldn't you expect cells from tissues rich in macrophages, e.g. liver, spleen or even peripheral blood, to produce some spontaneous interferon? The point at issue here is obviously the possibility that peritoneal leucocytes stimulated by your method are already "induced".

Wagner: Alveolar macrophages produce just trace amounts of interferon and with spleen cells we found none. We attribute this, possibly wrongly, to the fact that a maturation process following the inflammatory response and macrophage mobilization is required for them to have the optimum capacity to make interferon spontaneously.

De Maeyer: The mouse macrophages I referred to earlier (p. 36) were obtained from normal peritoneal cavities just by rinsing with culture fluid, not from inflammatory cavities.

Tyrrell: How many millilitres of fluid, of what titre, do you get from the washings from one rabbit, Dr. Wagner?

Wagner: A culture prepared from one rabbit has about 80 million cells suspended in 10 ml. of fluid, and titres of 20,000 to 50,000 PDD_{50}/ml. can be readily obtained after viral induction, i.e. a total of half a million units/culture, which is getting close to the biological activity of the highly purified material that Dr. Fantes talked about.

Tyrrell: Could the fluid phase of your washings contain something which would stimulate the cells still further? Something is stimulating the outpouring of these cells and maybe the same thing makes them produce interferon.

Wagner: We didn't find that anything we added stimulated the cells further; also, they were thoroughly washed before they were put into culture. Sterile glass beads were as good as glycogen for mobilizing these interferon-producing macrophages.

Tyrrell: When you take out the washings you take out the proteins, the peptides and all sorts of things from the peritoneal cavity; if you allowed the supernatant to react with the cells a bit more, would you get more stimulation?

Wagner: No.

Merigan: In the past both our laboratory and several others have found that a species of interferon with a molecular weight of 30,000 predominates after NDV stimulation of the mouse. Both our group and Hallam and Youngner have recently also noticed heavier species occurring—one of perhaps 55,000 and one of 90,000 molecular weight—after NDV stimulation in the mouse. I think we shall only understand the cellular origin of interferons *in vivo* if we can do what you are doing and attempt to distinguish species with grossly different molecular weights; it is only by following their separate kinetics and so on that we can really get any idea about what is happening during *in vivo* stimulation of the animal. Different sites may release different species at different rates, and we should follow their kinetics separately.

Wagner: That is a very important idea, but it is a lot of work.

Andrewes: What was the molecular weight of the spontaneous interferon?

Wagner: The problem there is that the titres were fivefold or sixfold lower than the endotoxin-induced interferon, which was not good enough to get adequate recovery from the column. We could try to concentrate it and do it over again. It looked as if the "spontaneous" interferon was about the same as the endotoxin-induced interferon by other criteria, but it was not as reliable as studying the induced material. We cannot be certain that we are getting the same molecular species from the endotoxin-induced materials as from the spontaneous material because we haven't, for technical reasons, been able to do the experiment properly.

Fantes: What was the recovery rate from your Sephadex columns?

Wagner: It was not very good—probably 25 to 50 per cent or less. This is due partly to the lability of some of these preparations.

STUDIES ON THE MECHANISM OF ACTION
OF INTERFERON

WOLFGANG K. JOKLIK

Department of Cell Biology, Albert Einstein College of Medicine,
Yeshiva University, New York

THE history of the first decade of interferon bears a remarkable resemblance to that of bacteriophage. Just like the discovery of Twort and d'Herelle, the discovery of Isaacs has been followed by intensive efforts to implement a practical application. However, it has become abundantly apparent that the action of interferon in preventing virus multiplication poses questions of fundamental interest from the point of view of molecular biology. There are two reasons why we are beginning to obtain answers to these questions only now, some ten years after the first description of the interferon phenomenon. The first is the extraordinarily high biological activity of interferon, which for some time misled workers regarding the purity of their preparations. As a consequence, some of the effects attributed to interferon, both on non-infected and infected cells, were due not to interferon itself, but to impurities which made up the overwhelming portion of the preparations used. Secondly, it is only now that it is becoming apparent which are the best virus-cell systems for studying the mode of action of interferon.

Let us examine briefly the requirements for such a system. First, it is clear that interferon inhibits the multiplication of both RNA and DNA viruses. Unless one envisages the unlikely situation that these two classes of viruses are inhibited at entirely different stages of the viral growth cycle, one is led to predict that the reaction affected would be the one *common* to the growth cycles of the two classes of viruses, that is, the translation into polypeptide chain sequences of the genetic information in the viral genome, and, in particular, in the *parental* viral genome (Joklik, 1965). The system we are looking for should thus be one in which this early information translation can be observed with clarity. This requirement immediately rules out a number of systems. For instance, although the patterns of macromolecular biosynthesis during the growth cycles of small enteroviruses such as poliovirus and Mengo virus have been worked out in considerable detail, the fate of the incoming viral genome, which here acts as its own messenger RNA, is very difficult to observe. It is not at all clear how much of the information of the parental genome is translated. Is only that cistron which codes for a new RNA polymerase translated? Or are inhibition of the transcription of host cell messenger RNA and of host cell DNA replication, disaggregation of host cell polyribosomes, and accelerated synthesis of phospholipid, due to proteins translated from the parental genome (Willems and Penman, 1966; McCormick and Penman, 1967)? Or is the entire parental genome perhaps immediately translated as one polycistronic message? None of these early functions can be assayed easily or unambiguously, and one would not therefore expect a system such as this to yield answers concerning their possible inhibition by interferon. Similarly, one would not choose cell-virus systems involving either herpes or adenoviruses. Although such systems are quite well characterized in molecular terms, the fact that these viruses multiply in the nucleus makes it difficult to observe the transcription of messenger RNA from parental genomes. The ideal system should indeed involve a DNA virus, since, instead of observing the fate and functioning of a relatively small number of parental RNA genomes which act as their own messengers, we can then follow the transcription and translation of a number of messenger RNA molecules derived from each parental genome. Further, it should involve a DNA virus multiplying in the cytoplasm, since one can then observe the formation and subsequent functioning of messenger RNA very precisely.

The ideal system in which to study the mechanism of action of interferon is the vaccinia-virus-infected cell. Not only does this system have all the desirable attributes just discussed, but the vaccinia virus growth cycle in general has also been investigated most intensively: a large body of knowledge is available concerning the uncoating of the parental genomes, the induction of the synthesis of a number of early enzymes, the transcription and translation of both early and late messenger RNA, the replication of the viral genome, and the synthesis of structural viral proteins. We have taken advantage of this favourable system and will discuss here the effect of interferon on macromolecular biosynthesis in mouse L fibroblasts infected with vaccinia virus strain WR.

DESCRIPTION OF THE SYSTEM INVESTIGATED

The interferon used was prepared by Dr. T. C. Merigan of Stanford University from L cells infected with NDV. All experiments were carried out with L cells grown in suspension culture. Interferon was applied for a period of 16 hours before infection. The interferon preparations were of such potency that at a dilution of 1 in 100 they reduced the 24-hour yield of vaccinia virus after infection at an adsorbed multiplicity of about 200 particles per cell by about 95 per cent (Joklik and Merigan, 1966).

The interferon preparations used here had no detectable effect on the course of the vaccinia virus multiplication cycle in HeLa cells. This is in line with the demonstrated absolute species specificity of interferon and, further, provides conclusive evidence that the effects to be described below are due to interferon and not to some non-specific inhibitor.

It is becoming evident now that the synthesis of interferon can be provoked by a number of stimuli besides infection with virus and, further, that multiple forms of interferon exist. The significance of the existence of these multiple forms of interferon is not yet clear. From the point of view of the virus, the existence of more than one form of interferon may not matter very much, since interferon itself is probably not the protein which inhibits virus multiplication; rather it appears that interferon induces the synthesis of a protein, which in turn is responsible for the inhibition (Taylor, 1964; Friedman and Sonnabend, 1964). Interferon is thus to be regarded as a derepressor which can be transferred from cell to cell. Nothing is yet known concerning the *nature* of this postulated inhibitory protein; what we are concerned with here is its *function*.

THE EFFECT OF INTERFERON ON THE TRANSCRIPTION OF VACCINIA MESSENGER RNA

In L cells, as in all mammalian cells, all RNA is transcribed in the nucleus. (A possible exception is a very small amount of RNA transcribed from mitochondrial DNA.) Three types of this RNA are transported to the cytoplasm where they function: 4 S transfer RNA; ribosomal RNA, which in L cells consists of 28 S (mol. wt. $1 \cdot 3 \times 10^6$), 16 S (mol. wt. 6×10^5) and 5 S RNA; and messenger RNA, which ranges in size from 8 to rather more than 20 S. Vaccinia messenger RNA on the other hand is transcribed in the cytoplasm, and, as we shall see below, has a sedimentation coefficient of about 10 to 12 S during the early stages of the infection cycle. The problem is how to identify it in the presence of the host cell RNAs which function in the cytoplasm. We here take advantage of the fact that these various species of host cell RNA do not appear in the cytoplasm immediately after they are synthesized, but only after an interval of time characteristic of each class. Transfer RNA reaches the cytoplasm within about five minutes after it is formed; however, because of its small and distinctive size, it is always readily identified and does not interfere with the identification of vaccinia messenger RNA. 28 S and 16 S ribosomal RNA, which account for about 98 per cent of the total RNA in ribosomes, reach the cytoplasm independently, the former as a component of 60 S ribosomal subunits, the latter as a component of the smaller 40 S ribosomal subunit. 16 S ribosomal RNA is first detected in the cytoplasm about 25 minutes after its formation (unless radioactive label of extremely high specific activity is used): 28 S RNA only appears after about 60 minutes (Joklik and Becker, 1965a). Cell messenger RNA does not appear in the cytoplasm in significant amounts before about 15–20 minutes after its transcription (Girard et al., 1965). It is clear therefore that it is possible to identify vaccinia messenger in the cytoplasm as the only radioactively labelled RNA (apart from the distinctive 4 S transfer RNA) provided that pulses of radioactive precursor of not longer than ten minutes are administered. The fact that this RNA really is vaccinia messenger RNA is readily shown by base ratio analysis, which shows 36 per cent guanine plus cytosine (GC), the same as in vaccinia virus DNA, and by specific hybridization with vaccinia virus DNA (Joklik and Becker, 1964; Oda and Joklik, 1967).

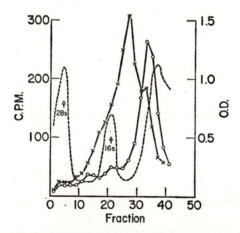

Fig. 1. Newly-labelled RNA species in the cytoplasm of uninfected L cells (o—o) and L cells infected with vaccinia virus (×—×). Cells were pulse-labelled with [¹⁴C]uridine for 10 minutes at 1·5 hours after infection at a multiplicity of 300 virus particles adsorbed per cell. ------: optical density at 260 mμ. Cytoplasmic fractions derived from 2×10⁷ cells were rendered 1 per cent with respect to sodium dodecyl sulphate (SDS) and centrifuged on 15–30 per cent sucrose–SDS density gradients for 18 hours at 25,000 rev./min. at 27°C.
(Joklik and Merigan, 1966.)
C.P.M.: counts per minute.
O.D.: optical density.

In L cells a very rapid burst of early vaccinia messenger RNA transcription occurs (Oda and Joklik, 1967). Fig. 1 shows a typical sucrose-sodium dodecyl sulphate density gradient profile of the newly-labelled RNA species in the cytoplasm of L cells infected at a multiplicity of 300 virus particles per cell, as well as in the cytoplasm of non-infected cells. The viral RNA forms a sharply defined band with a sedimentation coefficient of 10–12 S. As the multiplicity is reduced, the rate of early vaccinia messenger RNA transcription decreases rapidly; at a multiplicity of 100, very little

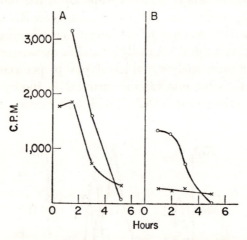

FIG. 2. Rate of formation of vaccinia messenger RNA in normal and interferon-treated cells. Each point was derived from summation of the appropriate areas of sucrose–SDS density gradient profiles obtained as described in the legend for Fig. 1. A: Multiplicity of infection, 750; B: multiplicity, 150. ×—×, no interferon; ○—○, interferon-treated. (Joklik and Merigan, 1966.)

messenger is formed. Pretreatment of cells with interferon increases the rate of transcription of vaccinia messenger RNA, the effect being more marked at low than at high multiplicities. This is illustrated in Fig. 2 (Joklik and Merigan, 1966). At a multiplicity of 750, interferon increases the rate of transcription of vaccinia messenger RNA by about 50 per cent; at a multiplicity of 150 by about 400 per cent. At both multiplicities, as infection proceeds the rate of transcription decreases more rapidly in the presence than in the absence of interferon. This is due in part to the fact that interferon-treated cells disintegrate far more rapidly after infection than cells normally infected (see below). The size of the vaccinia messenger RNA transcribed in interferon-treated cells is the same as that transcribed in control cells, and the messenger RNA transcribed in interferon-treated cells hybridizes with vaccinia DNA with the same efficiency as vaccinia messenger RNA from normally infected cells.

The conclusion is that pretreatment with interferon does not inhibit the transcription of early vaccinia messenger RNA; on the contrary, it enhances it. The reason for this effect is not clear at this time. It has recently been found in a number of laboratories that under certain conditions some early vaccinia messenger RNA may be transcribed from parental vaccinia DNA before it is uncoated as judged by sensitivity to digestion by deoxyribonuclease (Kates and McAuslan, 1967; Woodson, 1967; Joklik, 1967); however, this situation has not yet been worked out completely and further speculation is pointless at this time.

RATE OF SYNTHESIS OF DNA POLYMERASE

The activity of DNA polymerase increases at about one hour after infection of L cells with vaccinia virus. In all probability this represents the functioning of one of the early vaccinia messenger RNAs (Jungwirth and Joklik, 1965). Fig. 3 illustrates the kinetics of the synthesis of this enzyme in L cells infected normally and after pretreatment with interferon (Joklik and Merigan, 1966). Under the conditions used here, pretreatment reduces the

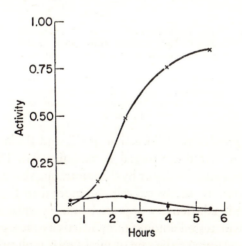

Fig. 3. Synthesis of DNA polymerase in normal and interferon-treated L cells infected with vaccinia virus. Multiplicity, 500. Activity is expressed as mµmoles [³H]-thymidine triphosphate rendered acid-insoluble/mg. protein per 30 minutes at 37°. x—x, no interferon; ●—●, interferon-treated. (Joklik and Merigan, 1966.)

amount of DNA polymerase formed to no more than one-twentieth of that formed in control cells. Early vaccinia messenger RNA is thus evidently not able to express itself.

VACCINIA VIRUS DNA REPLICATION

Replication of vaccinia virus DNA can be followed by pulse-labelling infected cells with [^{14}C]thymidine for ten minutes, breaking open the cells and measuring the amount of radioactivity incorporated into acid-insoluble

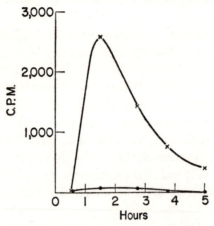

FIG. 4. Replication of vaccinia DNA in L cells infected with vaccinia virus. ×—×, no interferon; ●—●, pretreated with interferon. Cells were pulse-labelled for 10 minutes with [^{14}C]thymidine at each time point. Multiplicity, 500. The radioactivity incorporated into cytoplasmic fractions was measured.

material in the cytoplasmic cell fraction (Joklik and Becker, 1964). It can readily be shown that this material is vaccinia virus DNA, either by determining its buoyant density or by demonstrating that it is incorporated into mature virions. In uninfected cells, no more than 1–3 per cent of the total incorporated radioactivity appears in the cytoplasmic fraction. In infected cells, the increased amount of radioactivity incorporated into this fraction gives a measure of the rate of viral DNA replication. Under the conditions used here, the maximum rate occurs at between 1·5 and 2·5 hours after infection. In cells pretreated with interferon the rate of viral DNA replication is at the most 5 per cent of that in control cells (Fig. 4). Inhibition of the synthesis of the virus-coded DNA polymerase thus entails absence of viral DNA replication. It follows that no transcription of late vaccinia messenger RNA occurs in such cells; since most structural viral proteins are translated from late vaccinia messenger RNA, the formation of mature virions is impossible.

It has been reported that a given concentration of interferon inhibits virion formation to a greater extent than the synthesis of DNA polymerase. This, of course, is precisely what we would expect. It is unlikely, and in fact evidence to the contrary is presented below, that only the messenger RNA coding for DNA polymerase is unable to express itself. Since the formation of DNA polymerase requires the expression of only one, or at the most of a few cistrons, whereas the formation of virions presumably requires the expression of *all* genetic information in the viral genome (of the order of 500 cistrons), it follows that synthesis of the enzyme will be less sensitive to interferon than the formation of mature virus particles.

RATE OF PROTEIN SYNTHESIS

Infection of L cells is followed by a decrease in the rate of protein synthesis. This decrease increases with increasing multiplicity of infection: at a multiplicity of 500 virus particles adsorbed per cell, it amounts to some 60 per cent. This decrease is due to the disaggregation of polyribosomes formed by host cell messenger RNA (see below) and the recruitment of some, but not all, of the liberated ribosomes by early viral messenger RNA. This decrease is then followed by a period when the rate of protein synthesis increases again, which coincides with the time when late vaccinia messenger RNA is formed and when the synthesis of most of the structural viral proteins commences.

Although pretreatment with interferon does not decrease the rate of transcription of early vaccinia messenger RNA, there is a dramatic decrease in the rate of protein synthesis in cells pretreated with interferon (Fig. 5)

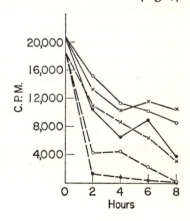

Fig. 5. Rate of protein synthesis in normal and interferon-treated L cells infected with vaccinia virus. Each point represents the amount of radioactivity incorporated into the cytoplasmic fraction of $1 \cdot 35 \times 10^7$ cells in Eagle's medium containing one-tenth of the usual concentration of amino acids, pulsed for 4 min. with 15 μc of a uniformly ^{14}C-labelled amino acid mixture ($1 \cdot 5$ mc/mg.) Continuous curves, no interferon; broken curves, interferon-treated. Crosses, multiplicity of infection 50; open circles, multiplicity 150; closed circles, multiplicity 500. (Joklik and Merigan, 1966.)

(Joklik and Merigan, 1966). This decrease is already clearly evident at one hour after infection. The higher the multiplicity, the more pronounced is this inhibition; however, it is detectable even at multiplicities as low as 50 virus particles adsorbed per cell.

We conclude that it is not only the early vaccinia messenger RNA coding for DNA polymerase which cannot express itself in cells pretreated with interferon, but that, most probably, none of the early viral messenger RNA molecules are translated.

OCCURRENCE OF POLYRIBOSOMES

Polyribosomes are readily detectable in normal L cells. Most are free or attached to the endoplasmic reticulum in a tenuous fashion only, since the number of polyribosomes found in the cytoplasm after disruption of cells in buffer and in buffer plus sodium deoxycholate is almost the same. On infection with vaccinia virus there is some decrease in the number of polyribosomes, which corresponds to the decrease in the rate of protein synthesis (see above); however, polyribosomes are readily demonstrable in L cells infected with vaccinia virus for the first six hours or so of the infection cycle. Infection of cells pretreated with interferon, however, leads to a rapid disaggregation of polyribosomes (Fig. 6). Even at one hour after infection no polyribosomes are usually detectable in cells pretreated with interferon (Joklik and Merigan, 1966). The higher the multiplicity of infection, the more rapid is this disaggregation, which is still observable at multiplicities as low as 50. It should be pointed out here that the polyribosome patterns in uninfected cells pretreated with interferon are indistinguishable from those in control cells, and that the rate of protein synthesis in such cells is likewise perfectly normal. Exposure to interferon thus has no detectable effect on protein synthesis in uninfected cells, but it drastically inhibits protein synthesis when cells are infected with virus.

We considered the possibility that pretreatment with interferon might set up a mechanism, triggered by viral infection, which accelerated disaggregation of host cell polyribosomes. This hypothesis cannot be tested in cells infected with vaccinia virus, since in such cells disaggregation of host cell polyribosomes is immediately counterbalanced by polyribosome re-formation on early viral messenger RNA. A more suitable system is the L cell infected with Mengo virus. In such cells, host cell polyribosomes break down over a period of about two hours, and the liberated ribosomes are only recruited for polyribosome re-formation after this time, when progeny viral RNA begins to be formed in appreciable amounts. Further, polyribosomes formed by Mengo virus RNA are considerably larger than host cell polyribosomes, and are readily differentiated from them by density gradient centrifugation. Accordingly, the effect of pretreatment with interferon was determined on the polyribosome patterns in L cells infected with Mengo virus. There was no difference in the polyribosome patterns for the first two hours after infection between normal L cells and cells pretreated with interferon. After two hours large

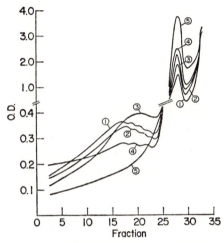

FIG. 6. Polyribosomes in normal and interferon-treated L cells infected with vaccinia virus. Each profile was derived from a 15–30 per cent sucrose density gradient charged with the cytoplasmic fraction of 5×10^7 L cells; 2 hours centrifugation at 25,000 rev./min. at 2°. Multiplicity of infection, 50. Curve 1, uninfected cells, normal or interferon-treated; curves 2, 3, and 4, normal cells infected for 1, 2, and 4 hours, respectively; curve 5, interferon-treated cells infected for 1, 2, or 4 hours. (Joklik and Merigan, 1966.)

Mengo virus polyribosomes appeared in cells infected normally, whereas there was no detectable re-formation of polyribosomes in L cells pretreated with interferon. Interferon treatment therefore does not *per se* accelerate virus-induced disaggregation of polyribosomes.

We may conclude that infection with vaccinia virus itself causes rapid disaggregation of polyribosomes and that under conditions of normal infection this breakdown is largely masked by re-formation of polyribosomes by early viral messenger RNA, whereas in the interferon-treated cell this re-formation does not occur, and disaggregation of host cell polyribosomes is therefore unmasked.

ATTACHMENT OF VACCINIA MESSENGER RNA TO POLYRIBOSOMES

We have seen that in L cells pretreated with interferon large amounts of vaccinia messenger RNA are formed, but that no polyribosomes are found as early as one hour after infection. This suggests that in interferon-treated cells messenger RNA is unable to attach to ribosomes to form polyribosomes.

The initiation of polyribosome formation is not yet clear. It has been found that in the normally infected cell newly-transcribed vaccinia messenger RNA molecules sediment at a rate suggesting combination with the smaller of the two ribosomal subunits, the 40 S subunit (Joklik and Becker, 1965b). More recently several observations have been made which support the concept that the first step in polyribosome formation is combination between messenger RNA and the smaller ribosomal subunit: thus parental RNA molecules of bacteriophage MS 2 combine with the smaller of the

TABLE I

PERCENTAGE OF VACCINIA MESSENGER RNA ASSOCIATED WITH POLYRIBOSOMES IN NORMAL AND INTERFERON-TREATED CELLS

Duration of pulse (min.)	No interferon	Interferon-treated
4	41	16
9	57	17
15	66	18

ribosomal subunits in *Escherichia coli* (Godson and Sinsheimer, 1967); native ribosomal subunits of *E. coli* are capable of re-forming ribosomal monomers in the presence of messenger RNA (Nakada and Kaji, 1967); initiation of haemoglobin synthesis by ribosomes *in vitro* is stimulated by the presence of ribosomal subunits (Bishop, 1966); and newly-formed ribosomal subunits of HeLa cells, which are transported to the cytoplasm as separate entities, combine in the cytoplasm to form ribosomal monomers attached to messenger RNA, not free ribosomal monomers (Joklik and Becker, 1965a). In the light of these findings it is of interest to inquire into the fate immediately after formation of the vaccinia virus messenger RNA which is transcribed in L cells pretreated with interferon.

Accordingly, vaccinia messenger RNA was labelled with [14C]uridine and cytoplasmic cell fractions containing this messenger were analysed on sucrose density gradients centrifuged in such a manner as to reveal any attachment of messenger either to 40 S ribosomal subunits or to polyribosomes. No attachment to 40 S subunits was found, and incorporation of messenger into polyribosomes was far less in cells pretreated with interferon than in control cells (Table I) (Joklik and Merigan, 1966). In the latter, a gradually increasing proportion of newly-transcribed messenger RNA molecules was found associated with polyribosomes as the duration of the pulse was increased; this proportion rose from 41 to 66 per cent by 15 minutes. In cells pretreated with interferon, the proportion of label found in polyribosomes remained at a constant low level (about 17 per cent); the fact that the proportion did not increase suggests that what was being observed was non-specific, rather than specific, association.

We conclude from this experiment that pretreatment with interferon prevents the attachment of vaccinia messenger RNA to ribosomes.

Destruction of cells

There is one further clearly discernible effect of pretreatment with interferon. Interferon-treated cells disintegrate rapidly from about three hours after infection with vaccinia virus. This phenomenon is illustrated in Fig. 7 (Joklik and Merigan, 1966). The number of cells that can be identified visually as "intact" decreases somewhat when normal L cells are infected with high multiplicities of vaccinia virus; this decrease depends on the density of the cell population and may amount to as much as 35 per cent

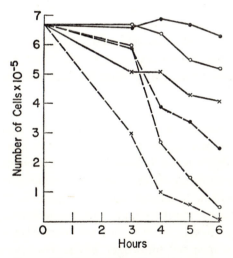

FIG. 7. Number of "intact" cells in cultures of normal and interferon-treated L cells infected with vaccinia virus. Continuous curves, normal cells; broken curves, interferon-treated cells. Crosses, multiplicity of infection, 500; open circles, multiplicity 200; closed circles, multiplicity 100. Cell destruction was somewhat less when the initial cell concentration was $2 \cdot 5 \times 10^5$ cells/ml. (Joklik and Merigan, 1966.)

at six hours after infection at a multiplicity of 500 virus particles per cell. However, at a multiplicity of 100 this effect is virtually absent. The situation is different when cells pretreated with interferon are infected. Cell destruction is then virtually complete by six hours post-infection at multiplicities greater than 200; and even at a multiplicity as low as 50, up to 50 per cent of the cells have by then been converted to "ghosts". Interferon thus certainly does not protect against infection with virus: there ensues an abortive infection cycle resulting in the early destruction of the cell.

DISCUSSION AND CONCLUSION

The work described here demonstrates that exposure of cells to interferon abolishes the ability of viral messenger RNA and ribosomes to combine. As a result virus-coded proteins are not synthesized.

It has recently been suggested, on the basis of work with a cell-free system consisting of Sindbis virus RNA and chick cell ribosomes, that the basis of interferon action is inhibition of movement of ribosomes along the messenger RNA molecule, rather than inhibition of their combination (Marcus and Salb, 1966). It is difficult to relate this result obtained *in vitro* with the results obtained within the cell which I have just described, and more work will be needed before the reason for the discrepancy is explained. However, there is no doubt that in L cells pretreated with interferon and infected with vaccinia virus no polyribosomes occur, so that combination of messenger RNA and ribosomes is certainly inhibited, and there is no evidence for inhibition of translationary movement.

We do not know as yet whether the inability of viral messenger RNA to combine with ribosomes is due to an alteration in the messenger RNA or in the ribosomes. One may weigh the alternatives as follows: on the one hand the work of both Marcus and Salb (1966) and of Carter and Levy (1967) has suggested that treatment with interferon alters ribosomes by attaching to them a protein which, either sterically or by the induction of a conformational change at the requisite site, prevents the attachment (or translation) of viral messenger RNA, while having no effect *whatever* on attachment (or translation) of host cell messenger RNA. However, it is difficult to envisage that such altered ribosomes perform their normal functions and behave normally in the cell, for there is no evidence that a cell treated with interferon is in any way unable to perform normally, and certainly an animal rapidly making interferon is a perfectly normal animal. On the other hand, there is little doubt that there must exist a fundamental difference, most probably chemical in nature, between viral messenger RNAs and cellular messenger RNAs. It is conceivable therefore that interferon induces a mechanism which in some way specifically modifies viral messenger RNAs, thereby rendering them unable to combine with ribosomes. The most likely site of such an alteration would be at the beginning of the messenger RNA molecule, where one would expect the configuration to favour initiation of meaningful translation. A great deal of careful work will be necessary before it will be possible to decide which of these alternatives is operative.

The reason for the marked disruption of cells treated with interferon and infected is not known at this time. Certainly no protein, or only very little, is synthesized in such cells. However, inhibition of protein synthesis is plainly not the reason for the disintegration, since cells treated with puromycin or cycloheximide preserve their integrity for far longer than the six hours within which infected interferon-treated L cells break up. Further, since it is unlikely that *any* virus-coded message is translated in such cells, cellular disintegration is probably not due to a virus-coded protein (and incidentally, it is also unlikely that the disruption of host cell polyribosomes is due to a virus-coded protein synthesized after infection). One explanation which ought to be explored is that infection with vaccinia virus causes damage to cellular membranes, such as lysosomal membranes, cell surface membranes, etc.

The net effect of exposure to interferon is to convert cells into virus-inactivating structures within which invading virus particles are uncoated, but in which no formation of mature viral progeny is possible. Interferon thus does not protect cells against infection: on the contrary, cells pretreated with interferon are killed and disintegrate. However, unless the number of infectious virus particles exceeds the number of cells, uninfected members of the cell population profit from the presence of interferon, since virus is effectively eliminated during the abortive infection cycle.

SUMMARY

Infection of L cells with vaccinia virus leads to the rapid disaggregation of most of the host cell polyribosomes, and to the re-formation of polyribosomes by vaccinia messenger RNA. In cells pretreated with interferon the disaggregation occurs, but the re-formation does not take place. A similar situation holds in L cells infected with Mengo virus: disaggregation of host cell polyribosomes proceeds at the same rate both in the presence and the absence of interferon, but no virus-specific polyribosomes appear in the cells treated with interferon. As a result of this disaggregation of polyribosomes, protein synthesis is inhibited. The re-formation of polyribosomes in interferon-treated cells infected with vaccinia virus is not due to an inhibition of the transcription of early vaccinia messenger RNA; on the contrary, the transcription of this messenger RNA in interferon-treated cells exceeds that in normal cells. The reason for the absence of the formation of virus-specific polyribosomes is that in interferon-treated cells the ability of viral messenger RNA and ribosomes to combine is greatly impaired. As a result of this inability of viral messenger RNA to express itself, virus-coded DNA polymerase is not synthesized and no progeny vaccinia virus DNA is formed. The abortive vaccinia virus multiplication cycle in interferon-treated cells results in complete cell destruction by five to six hours after infection.

REFERENCES

BISHOP, J. O. (1966). *Biochim biophys. Acta*, **119**, 130.

CARTER, W. A., and LEVY, H. B. (1967). *Science*, **155**, 1254.

FRIEDMAN, R. M., and SONNABEND, J. A. (1964). *Nature, Lond.*, **203**, 366.

GIRARD, M., LATHAM, H., PENMAN, S., and DARNELL, J. E. (1965). *J. molec. Biol.*, **11**, 187.

GODSON, G. N., and SINSHEIMER, R. L. (1967). *J. molec. Biol.*, **23**, 495.

JOKLIK, W. K. (1965). *Prog. med. Virol.*, **7**, 44.

JOKLIK, W. K. (1967). Unpublished results.

JOKLIK, W. K., and BECKER, Y. (1964). *J. molec. Biol.*, **10**, 452.

JOKLIK, W. K., and BECKER, Y. (1965a). *J. molec. Biol.*, **13**, 496.

JOKLIK, W. K., and BECKER, Y. (1965b). *J. molec. Biol.*, **13**, 511.

JOKLIK, W. K., and MERIGAN, T. C. (1966). *Proc. natn. Acad. Sci. U.S.A.*, **56**, 558.

JUNGWIRTH, C., and JOKLIK, W. K. (1965). *Virology*, **27**, 80.

KATES, J. R., and McAUSLAN, B. R. (1967). *Proc. natn. Acad. Sci. U.S.A.*, **57**, 314.

McCORMICK, W., and PENMAN, S. (1967). *Virology*, **31**, 135.

MARCUS, P. I., and SALB, J. M. (1966) *Virology*, **30**, 502.

NAKADA, D., and KAJI, A. (1967). *Proc. natn. Acad. Sci. U.S.A.*, **57**, 128.

ODA, K., and JOKLIK, W. K. (1967). *J. molec. Biol.*, **27**, 395.

TAYLOR, J. (1964). *Biochem. biophys. Res. Commun.* **14**, 1447.

WILLEMS, M., and PENMAN, S. (1966). *Virology*, **30**, 355.

WOODSON, B. (1967). *Fedn Proc. Fedn Am. Socs exp. Biol.*, **26**, No. 2, 450.

DISCUSSION

Mécs: If interferon treatment modifies the structure of virus messenger RNA, how do you explain the species specificity of interferon on this basis? Doesn't this mean that some common structure must be present in all inhibitory protein induced by interferon in any cell?

Joklik: The problem is whether the inhibitory protein proposed by Taylor (Taylor, J. [1964]. *Biochem. biophys. Res. Commun.*, **14**, 447) and by Friedman and Sonnabend (1964, *loc. cit.*) is induced; in that case the mouse interferon would not act as a derepressor for the synthesis of this inhibitory protein in chicken cells, for instance. There is no reason to suppose that a derepressor which is specific for one cell is able to cause derepression of a protein with a similar function in another cell. I can well imagine that there is profound species specificity.

Chany: Could you comment further on your very unusual observation that interferon treatment of the cell does not prevent the cytopathic effect of the virus? In general we find the contrary.

Joklik: In general one would miss this effect. If one puts 100 plaque-forming units of virus on a plate containing, say, 10^6 cells, and the plate is treated with interferon and no plaques appear, one cannot see the disappearance of the 100 cells which are infected.

Chany: If you use multiplicities which are high enough to infect the whole cell population, then you should be able to appreciate differences in CPE as compared to the control.

Joklik: Lockart has also commented that destruction of interferon-treated infected cells occurs provided that one has a cell population every member of which is infected. He found that with Mengo virus (Gauntt, C. J., and Lockart, R. [1966]. *J. Bact.,* **91**, 176).

We don't in fact use very high multiplicities. I measure in terms of virus particles adsorbed per cell, and 100 particles adsorbed constitutes two plaque-forming units. Not many biochemical studies in the literature use multiplicities as low as that.

Stoker: Dr. Chany's point raises the question of whether you are dealing with a situation which only applies to vaccinia or whether there is a difference in the techniques.

Joklik: It also happens with Mengo virus.

Martin: In EMC-infected Krebs ascites cells we get exactly the same sort of thing, i.e. we can inhibit virus production by 50 per cent with Dr. Baron's mouse serum interferon, and yet see no effect on cell death: all the cells still die. In this case there was a multiplicity of about three to six plaque-forming units or 30 to 60 particles per cell.

Gresser: Part of the discrepancy between your observations and Dr. Chany's, Dr. Joklik, may be due to the fact that there may be two cytopathic effects, one a toxic effect of the virus which acts perhaps on the cell membrane, and the other due to viral multiplication within the cell. We showed (see Gresser, I. [1961]. *Proc. Soc. exp. Biol. Med.,* **108**, 303) and Dr. Levy also showed (1964. *Virology,* **22**, 575) that interferon-treated cells can be protected only with considerable difficulty against the toxic effect of a virus, but they can easily be protected against the cytopathic effect. One has to distinguish therefore between the toxic effect of the virus, which is a rapid destruction of cells occurring within a matter of hours, and the cytopathic effect, which occurs much later.

Joklik: The toxic effect with vaccinia virus becomes operative at multiplicities of about 1,000 particles per cell. It is certainly not operative at about 100.

Under natural conditions the number of virus particles causing infection is not 100 per cell but one. That cannot be studied in any biochemical way. But as soon as the multiplicity is over one, what I have described here holds.

Levy: In Mengo infection in L cells, as you said, interferon gives no protection against the death of the cell. The synthesis of cell protein cuts off just as rapidly in the protected cells as in the non-protected cells. I think that this increased disintegration of the cells that you see in the vaccinia is probably specific for vaccinia —at least we don't see it in Mengo.

Baron: Many of us have observed that cells which have been pretreated with large doses of interferon and infected with very high multiplicities of viruses other than Mengo and vaccinia are protected against cell death. VSV is a good example: interferon gives virtually complete protection of an entire cell sheet. Protection against CPE is also true for equine encephalitis viruses (Lockart, R. Z., and Horn, B. [1963]. *J. Bact.*, **85**, 996). So I think that CPE in interferon-protected cells probably occurs with certain viruses and not with many other viruses.

Joklik: It could of course well be true that the introduction of some viruses into cells does *not* lead to degradative or disruptive changes. If interferon then prevents the expression of viral functions, such cells might not show cytopathic effects. Whether such cells could still divide is not known.

Baron: Evidence has been provided in other systems that infectious RNA is inhibited by interferon pretreatment of cells; a block of absorption has thereby been excluded as a mechanism of action of interferon.

De Maeyer: Your working hypothesis, Dr. Joklik, is that interferon induces a certain inhibitory protein which then somehow either changes the viral messenger RNA so that it cannot combine with the ribosomes or changes the ribosomes directly. If this protein changes the viral messenger RNA, wouldn't this imply that a certain common structure is shared by all viral messenger RNAs? It would certainly be hard to believe that the same interferon would induce different inhibitory proteins for each viral messenger RNA.

Joklik: I think there is indeed something "different" about all viral messenger RNAs. We are going to start looking at the end groups of some of them.

Cocito: You presented a graph (Fig. 4) showing that viral DNA is not formed in interferon-treated virus-infected cells. How did you separate viral from cellular DNA?

Joklik: Vaccinia DNA is in the cytoplasm.

Crick: As I understand it, you are postulating that there is a change in the messenger or in the ribosomal protein which prevents the attachment. Another hypothesis, which is very similar to yours, would be that what is missing is the initiation step of protein synthesis. Unfortunately we don't know what the initiation mechanism is in mammalian cells, but we do know there is a special mechanism in bacterial cells. An extension of your hypothesis would therefore be to say that perhaps you alter a transfer RNA which is concerned with initiation.

Burke: What is the situation with regard to the polymerase that makes the messenger RNA? Its production is clearly a stage that is not blocked by interferon production.

Joklik: That is what everybody wants to know. We have tested whole virus and, in particular, viral cores for this enzyme. A very small amount of RNA polymerase activity is associated with cores. The difficulty is in deciding whether this is something specific or not. I would say offhand that it is not sufficient to account for the rapid rate of vaccinia messenger RNA transcription, but the enzyme might be altered in some way once it is in the cell, and it might become activated.

Levy: We incubated ribosomes from interferon-treated cells and ribosomes from control cells under suitable conditions with rapidly labelled cellular RNA and with Mengo virus RNA. The ribosomes from control cells bind and become associated with both the normal cell RNA and the Mengo RNA, while the ribosomes from the interferon-treated cells bind normal cell RNA and do not bind Mengo RNA. This is in a system where there is no question of alteration of the virus.

Stoker: If the virus messenger is different, why is it that synthesis of polyoma or SV40 T antigens in transformed cells is insensitive to interferon?

Joklik: The *initial* induction, immediately after infection of T antigen, *is* sensitive to interferon. I can only say that in transformed cells this messenger RNA might acquire characteristics which make it a host cell messenger RNA.

Baron: Studies by Dr. M. N. Oxman at the National Institutes of Health relate to Dr. Stoker's question (Oxman, M. N., Rowe, W. P., and Black, P. H. [1967]. *Proc. natn. Acad. Sci. U.S.A.*, **57**, 941–948). Not only does the synthesis of SV40 T antigen become insensitive to the action of interferon in transformed cells, but in cells infected with adenovirus-SV40 hybrid viruses, where SV40 and adenovirus DNA's are physically linked, the synthesis of SV40 T antigen also becomes resistant to interferon. Dr. Oxman speculates that the acquired resistance to interferon observed in these two systems may be due to the linkage of the messenger RNA for SV40 T antigen to interferon-resistant RNA of the host cell (SV40 transformed cells) or of the adenovirus (cells infected with adenovirus-SV40 hybrid viruses).

Stoker: So if you "integrate" the DNA virus either into another virus or into a host cell the messenger becomes insensitive.

THE MODE OF ACTION OF INTERFERON

P. De Somer and C. Cocito

Rega Institute, University of Louvain, Belgium

Since the discovery of interferons (Isaacs and Lindenmann, 1957; Isaacs, Lindenmann and Valentine, 1957) numerous authors have furnished for these inhibitors definitions based on the experimental data currently available. In the review articles which have appeared (cf. e.g., Isaacs, 1959, 1961, 1962, 1963; Wagner, 1960, 1963, 1965; De Somer, 1962, 1964; Baron, 1963; Hilleman, 1963; Ho, 1964; Baron and Levy, 1966) the reader may follow the evolution of the "concept" of interferon.

The definition we propose in this paper reflects our way of thinking about these inhibitors at the present time: "Interferons are protein components of animal cells, which are either released, or synthesized and excreted, under a variety of stimuli and make other cells of the same species incapable of replicating viruses." Implicit in this definition are several basic concepts which will be discussed in this attempt to interpret the mode of action of interferon.

First, cells under physiological conditions might be able to synthesize interferon and interferon-like substances: what is their physiological role in the absence of viruses? Secondly, the release of interferon and interferon-like substances might be a physiological reaction to many changes in environmental conditions: why are such proteins excreted under these conditions? Thirdly, in cells incubated with interferons, secondary reactions occur which make some metabolic pathways no longer available for virus formation: what are the molecular bases and functions of these secondary reactions and of the block that follows? Finally, since interferon halts the replication of DNA and RNA viruses, and similar types of metabolic blocks can be expected to occur in uninfected as well as in infected cells, one may ask whether there exists a common basis for interferon action under all conditions.

This particular way of thinking about interferon leads one to consider virus-infected cells merely as tools for investigating a more general mechanism of interferon activity—precious tools, however, because viruses either shut off or slow down many of the numerous pathways of the host cells, while magnifying a few specific metabolic ways. As a result, the schema of macromolecule formation becomes more accessible to an experimental approach.

The aim of this paper is to summarize and interpret old and recent data on the mode of action of interferon. Findings concerning interferon action in virus-infected cells will be discussed first. Observations on uninfected cells will then be presented. Finally, an attempt will be made to interpret all these data on a common basis.

THE MECHANISM OF ACTION OF INTERFERON IN CELLS INFECTED WITH RNA VIRUSES

Several lines of evidence have been presented that interferon halts the replication of RNA viruses by interfering with some steps of the eclipse phase. Since incubation with interferon does not alter the kinetics of adsorption of viruses on cells, on the one hand (Isaacs and Burke, 1959; De Somer et al., 1962) and, on the other hand, virus precursor nucleic acids and proteins are not synthesized under these conditions (Cocito, De Maeyer and De Somer, 1962a; De Somer, 1962; Lockart, Sreevalsan and Horn, 1962; Cocito, 1963; Levy, Snellbaker and Baron, 1963; Levy, 1964; Taylor, 1965), the conclusion can be drawn that treatment with interferon makes the cells incapable either of transcribing the genetic message of a virus or of replicating and translating it.

The sequence of events believed to take place in cells infected with RNA viruses is as follows: (1) "early" cistrons are transcribed first, and (2) then translated into "early" enzymes, e.g. RNA-dependent RNA polymerase; (3) viral RNA next replicates through formation of a "replicative form"; (4) finally, translation of "late" cistrons occurs, which brings about formation of viral proteins (Erikson and Franklin, 1966; Baltimore, Girard and Darnell, 1966; Delgarno et al., 1966; Horton et al., 1966; Plagemann and Swim, 1966). If interferon mediated a block of the first two steps, no virus-specific polymerases would be formed. If the third step were involved, no replicative forms and no progeny viral RNA would appear. Finally, if only the fourth step were prevented, viral RNA, but no viral proteins, would accumulate in interferon-treated cells.

Since no actinomycin-resistant RNA was found in interferon-treated cells infected with RNA viruses (Taylor, 1965), it is clear that the interferon-mediated block must precede the third step of the above sequence. Action of interferon must, then, be restricted to the steps involved in the formation and action of virus-specific "early" enzymes such as the RNA-dependent RNA polymerases.

It has been reported that incubation with interferon greatly reduces the activity of RNA polymerases with respect to control cells infected with Mengo virus (Miner, Ray and Simon, 1966) and Semliki Forest virus (Sonnabend et al., 1966). Control experiments, however, have proved that homogenates of interferon-treated cells do not alter the enzyme activity in vitro. Hence the conclusion can be drawn that synthesis, and not the activity, of RNA-dependent RNA polymerase is the target.

The formation of viral polymerase can be stopped either at the transcriptional or at the translational level. An experimental model for the first type of block was proposed by us some years ago: methylated albumin combines in vitro with poliovirus RNA, yielding a nucleoprotein complex which enters a cell without infecting it (Cocito, Prinzie and De Somer, 1962). Conversely, a block in translation could be the result of either a blocked formation or an altered function of polyribosome complexes. Evidence has been provided recently that ribosomes from interferon-treated chick cells have a reduced ability to combine with Sindbis virus RNA to form polyribosome complexes. In addition, viral polyribosomes which form in the presence of interferon do not break down, as normal polyribosomes do, when polypeptide chains are synthesized (Marcus and Salb, 1966; Mécs, Sonnabend and Martin, 1966).

Finally, upon incubation with interferon some modifications occur in cell ribosomes which make the particles incapable of forming polysome complexes with viral RNA and, therefore, of synthesizing viral polymerases. This is why no virus-specific enzymes are synthesized in the presence of interferon. Consequently, no infectious RNA or replicative forms are made under these conditions.

Unfortunately, conclusions reached with RNA viruses do not help much in understanding the more general role of interferon, because cells under physiological conditions do not seem to harbour enzymes similar to the RNA-dependent RNA polymerases which can be found in cells infected with RNA viruses and which are the target of interferon. In this respect, DNA viruses can be regarded as a more useful tool, for the process of viral DNA translation mimics that of cellular DNA translation.

THE MECHANISM OF INTERFERON ACTION IN CELLS INFECTED WITH DNA VIRUSES

The adsorption of virulent DNA viruses into mammalian cells determines the following succession of events: (1) "uncoating" of viral DNA; (2) "early" transcription of DNA, with formation of "early" messenger viral RNA and its translation into "early" proteins; (3) synthesis of viral

DNA; (4) formation of "late messenger" and capsid proteins; and finally (5) assembly of complete particles (Joklik *et al.*, 1966).

In several DNA-virus systems it has been shown that interferon mediates a block which occurs during the first half of the eclipse phase, i.e. before formation of progeny viral DNA (Ghosh and Gifford, 1965; Levine *et al.*, 1966). Consequently, a decision must be made as to whether "early" transcription or "early" translation is blocked. In the first case "early" messenger RNA will not be formed, while in the second case the "early" messenger will be synthesized but not the "early" proteins.

It has been shown recently that incubation of L cells with interferon before infection with vaccinia virus does not appreciably decrease the synthesis of messenger viral RNA (Joklik and Merigan, 1966). Conversely, the rate of protein formation and the synthesis of thymidine kinase, an "early" enzyme of the vaccinia replicating cycle, are greatly reduced under these conditions (Ghosh and Gifford, 1965; Levine *et al.*, 1966). This indicates that translation, and not transcription, is blocked by interferon. The reason for the block of translation has been furnished by the observation that polyribosome complexes do not form in cells which were incubated with interferon before infection (Joklik and Merigan, 1966). Since treatment with interferon alone does not cause normal cell polysomes to disaggregate, and a breakdown of cell polysomes accompanies, instead, infection with both RNA and DNA viruses, the conclusion can be drawn that interferon prevents the re-formation of polyribosomes with viral messenger. The rapidity with which polyribosomes disappear from the cytoplasm of interferon-treated virus-infected cells may explain the inhibition of the formation of DNA polymerase and, consequently, of viral DNA.

Summarized data account also for the common basis of interferon action on the replication of DNA and RNA viruses. The metabolic pathways of replication of the two types of viruses share one step: the early translation of viral genetic message. Messenger viral RNA and viral RNA have, in fact, a similar structure, and both may perform a messenger function *in vitro* by directing the formation of polypeptide chains in cell-free systems. And it is this function of the two types of RNA that is blocked by interferon (Fig. 1).

If at this point one asks again whether these findings may help in understanding a more general mode of action of interferon on animal cells, the answer is still doubtful. Viruses have a common feature: they cause disaggregation of normal complexes of cellular messenger RNA and ribosomes, and induce the formation of a new kind of viral messenger with

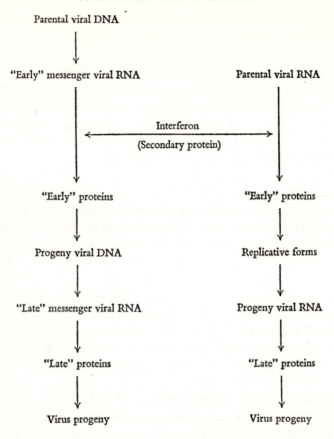

FIG. 1. The block mediated by interferon of the synthetic pathways
of DNA and RNA viruses.

which ribosomal particles form viral polysomes. Interferon mediates a
block in the formation of viral polysomes but does not cause normal
complexes to break down. Hence, these findings cannot be extrapolated to
uninfected cells. In this respect a study of oncogenic viruses might be more
advantageous: transformation of cells involves a sequence of events which
does not basically alter the metabolic pathways of the host cells.

MODE OF ACTION OF INTERFERON IN CELLS INFECTED WITH
ONCOGENIC VIRUSES

Infection of cells with tumour viruses may follow one of two alternative
pathways: virus replication and malignant transformation. Replication of
tumour viruses does not differ basically from the multiplication of non-
oncogenic particles: in both cases the viral cycle ends with the death of the

host cells. Conversely, malignant transformation leads to production of cells capable of an unlimited growth process, insensitive to physiological controls. What causes susceptible cells to decide between the two alternatives is unknown. On the other hand, there are cell species which carry this decision encoded in their genotypes and are able to undergo malignant transformation without replicating the virus.

Consequently, three possible inhibitory activities of interferon on tumour virus-host cell systems must be considered: (1) block of virus multiplication; (2) prevention of malignant transformation in cells capable of replicating viruses; (3) a similar effect in cell lines which are transformable but unable to replicate the viruses. Cases (2) and (3) must be considered separately, since a combined effect of replication and transformation must be expected in cells that are susceptible to both processes: the replication of tumour viruses increases the number of available particles, the percentage of infected cells in the population, and the chance of malignant transformation.

Let us consider first the action of interferon on the multiplication of tumour viruses in susceptible cells. Along these lines a report must be mentioned which shows that mouse lung interferon delays the onset of the cytopathic effect and reduces virus yield in mouse embryo cells infected with polyoma virus (Allison, 1961). Avian tumour viruses were also proved to be sensitive to interferon. Chick interferon obtained by use of several inducers decreases the yield of free virus in chick embryo fibroblasts infected with Rous sarcoma virus (Bader, 1962). Conversely, there are some recent reports claiming that murine leukaemia viruses are insensitive to interferon action. Data obtained in our laboratory indicate that high doses of interferon do not exert any protective effect on the splenomegalic response of mice inoculated with Rauscher leukaemia virus (Vandeputte et al., 1967). Unfortunately, the molecular basis of interferon action on sensitive cells is unknown. Yet an attempt at progressing along these lines has been made recently in our laboratory. Some characteristic alterations in nucleic acid metabolism which take place in cells infected with polyoma virus before the appearance of progeny particles (Cocito, Vandeputte and De Somer, 1965) are prevented by incubation with interferon. In fact, the latter prevents the early increase of DNA and RNA synthesis which occurs in the host cells during the first day of the polyoma replication cycle. As a consequence, virus precursor DNA (which is distinguishable from cellular DNA by chromatography on columns of methylated albumin, and can be found intracellularly six to 12 hours after infection) does not appear within three days after removal of the inhibitor. Conversely, preliminary data seem to indicate that early viral messenger RNA (RNA labelled with pulses of uridine during the first hours of the virus cycle and hybridized with polyoma DNA) still forms in cells incubated with interferon (Cocito, Vandeputte and De Somer, experiments in progress).

When cell lines capable of replicating tumour viruses and of undergoing transformation are employed, it is difficult to separate the action of interferon on the two processes. With this objection in mind, the report that interferon reduces the incidence and size of tumours caused by Rous sarcoma virus in chorioallantoic membranes (Strandström and Chany, 1960) must be considered. The incidence of tumours after injection of polyoma virus was also reduced *in vivo* by treatment of newborn hamsters with interferon (Atanasiu and Chany, 1960).

The action of interferon on malignant transformation can be dissociated from its action on virus replication when special cell lines capable of undergoing transformation without replicating viruses are employed. One such system is that of 3T3 cells and virus SV 40. Under conditions of high multiplicity of infection (about 1,000 particles per cell), this line undergoes malignant transformation with an efficiency of 50 per cent. In this system it has been found that exposure to interferon before infection reduces the frequency of transformation. The effect is proportional to the time of incubation with the inhibitor: a 50 to 75 per cent reduction occurs when interferon is given three hours before the virus, and a 90 per cent reduction when administration of interferon precedes by one day the infection with SV 40 (Todaro and Baron, 1965; Oxman and Black, 1966). These results indicate that interferon blocks one or several of the unknown steps which are essential for cell transformation.

EFFECTS OF INTERFERON PREPARATIONS IN UNINFECTED CELLS

The search for a possible action of interferon in uninfected cells has been unsuccessful so far. Nevertheless, worthy of mention are a few early publications in which morphological alterations (Gresser, 1961) and metabolic changes (Sonnabend, 1964) have been described in human amnion cells and in rat embryo fibroblasts incubated *in vitro* with given preparations of interferon. Crude preparations of interferon have also been proved to inhibit the synthesis of macromolecules in primary cultures and continuous cell lines (Cocito, De Maeyer and De Somer, 1962b; Sonnabend, 1964) and to act as uncoupling agents (Isaacs, Klemperer and Hitchcock, 1961).

Today it is generally accepted that most, if not all, the metabolic effects observed in the past with different interferon preparations were probably due to contaminants. Thus, for example, the finding that crude preparations of interferon contain basic proteins which possess an uncoupling activity (Lampson *et al.*, 1963) may explain early work tending to prove that interferon acts as an uncoupling agent. Likewise, the demonstration that purified rat interferon still contains a factor which can be distinguished from interferon and is able to repress the incorporation of labelled precursors into cellular nucleic acids (Cocito, Schonne and De Somer, 1965) may explain earlier findings with crude preparations.

Highly purified interferon obtained in two different laboratories had a powerful antiviral activity without appreciable uncoupling action (Lampson *et al.*, 1963) or inhibitory effect on nucleic acid formation in normal cells. Upon incubation of such a purified interferon with L cells, polyribosomes were isolated which were indistinguishable from those of control cells. Messenger RNA from uninfected cells apparently combines equally efficiently with ribosomes from uninfected and from interferon-treated cells (Joklik and Merigan, 1966).

In conclusion, no metabolic activity has been proved to be associated with the antiviral principle of interferon preparations.

Several lines of indirect evidence suggest that interferon does not exert its antiviral action directly but acts through a hypothetical substance, probably a protein (Friedman and Sonnabend, 1964; Lockart, 1964). Moreover, there are data indicating that a cell messenger RNA, carrying from the cell genome information for the synthesis of such a hypothetical secondary protein, might be formed in the cells upon incubation with interferon. It seems possible, in fact, to prevent with actinomycin D the transcription of cistrons of cell genome coding for the interferon-mediated response (Heller, 1963; Taylor, 1964).

It is logical, therefore, to suppose that the synthesis of the intermediary protein and of the corresponding messenger RNA might be the only metabolic responses of normal cells to interferon. If this is the case, the efforts to demonstrate a metabolic effect of interferon on cells have failed because the only action is to induce the synthesis of a protein which is still unidentified and of trace amounts of a long-lived messenger RNA. Obviously, the isolation of such a protein and the investigation of its activity in living cells and in cell-free extracts would be the clue to the problem.

DISCUSSION AND CONCLUSIONS

Although contributions from several laboratories have shed some light on the mode of action of interferon in virus-infected cells, many problems concerning this inhibitor are still unsolved. We shall put forward some hypotheses to answer some of the questions raised.

Are interferons normal cell components? We can only rely on indirect data: the wide variety of inducers and the structure of some of them (Merigan, 1966) preclude the possibility that new genetic information is required for interferon formation. Then the so-called "inducers of interferon synthesis" either act as "derepressors" or merely cause the excretion of interferon already present intracellularly. Though some *in vivo* experiments (Youngner, Stinebring and Taube, 1965) seem to demonstrate the

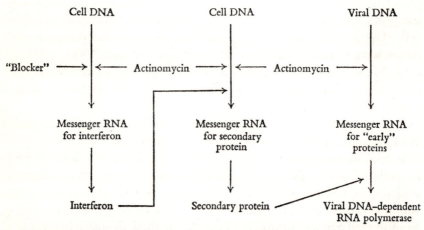

Fig. 2. Postulated action of interferon, secondary protein, blocker and actinomycin D on transcription and translation of cellular and viral DNA.

existence of interferon in animal tissues under physiological conditions, several lines of evidence have been presented that interferon is made *de novo* upon induction. Thus, for example, it has been possible to block interferon formation upon induction either by actinomycin D (Heller, 1963) or by u.v. irradiation (Cogniaux-Le Clerc, Levy and Wagner, 1966) or by inhibitors of protein synthesis (Buchan and Burke, 1966). In this connexion, the finding that crude preparations of interferon contain a factor which is resistant to proteolytic enzymes and capable of inhibiting interferon formation may be mentioned (Isaacs, Rotem and Fantes, 1966). This factor, for which the term "blocker" was proposed, could be considered as the physiological repressor of genes coding for interferon. Viruses and non-viral inducers might act by determining a release of the blocker, hence a derepression of interferon cistrons (Fig. 2).

Is interferon adsorbed by homologous cells? Most attempts to demonstrate an uptake of interferon *in vitro* by cells from nutrient fluid have failed

One must, then, admit that undetectable amounts of interferon penetrate inside the homologous cells, yet they are sufficient to induce the secondary reaction responsible for the antiviral effect. This could explain why interferon *per se* has no direct activity, but acts indirectly through a "magnifying" reaction.

Which is the target of interferon itself in the cell? Actinomycin experiments indicate that the cell genome is the target and that genetic information from cell DNA must be transcribed and translated to make interferon action effective.

How does interferon act on the cell genome? We may borrow from the bacterial world the repressor-derepressor model to formulate a derepressor hypothesis for interferon. The cistrons, which code for the hypothetical secondary protein, are controlled by an operator gene. It is with the product of this operator gene, a repressor, that interferon combines. Derepressed cistrons can thus be transcribed and translated, secondary protein being the hypothetical product of the whole reaction (Fig. 2).

How can this secondary reaction account for protection against DNA and RNA viruses? Some particular proteins, possibly basic in nature, might be able to combine with some functional site of cell ribosomes, making them incapable of aggregating and forming polysomes with both messenger viral RNA and viral RNA. Yet the most puzzling problem is how the hypothetical complexes formed by the secondary protein with ribosomes are able to distinguish between cellular messenger RNA and viral messenger.

What about the protection afforded by interferon on oncogenic transformation? The steps of such transformation are unknown. Bacterial transformation requires a series of events only partly known, such as replication of donor and recipient DNA, integration of donor cistrons into a recipient chromosome, and a delayed expression of the acquired genes. Interferon or secondary protein, or both, might interfere with similar steps occurring during the transformation of animal cells by oncogenic viruses.

Finally, one may ask why, under physiological conditions, the secondary protein cistrons are repressed. If their product has the unique ability to render ribosomes capable of distinguishing between cellular and viral messenger, during evolution these genes should have been established as dominant genes essential for the protection of cells against surrounding viruses. But perhaps we are climbing a step of evolution in which viruses have already developed their parasitic functions fully, while cells are just developing their defence mechanism. A full expression of the latter, the dominance of secondary protein genes, would begin a new step in the evolution of mammalian cells and render cells insensitive to viruses.

SUMMARY

Interferons are protein components of animal cells which are either released or synthesized and excreted under a variety of stimuli. Live and inactivated viruses, polysaccharides, and microbial toxins are the best "inducers" known of such release.

Incubation of homologous cells with interferon renders them incapable of replicating viruses. However, interferons have no direct inhibitory activity on virus synthetic pathways: they mediate a series of intermediary reactions which involve exclusively normal cell components. The cell genome carries the genetic information necessary for making the antiviral activity of interferon effective. It is presumed that, under the influence of undetectable amounts of interferon, cellular cistrons which are repressed under physiological conditions become transcribed. A specific messenger RNA is then formed and translated into hypothetical "intermediary proteins". This may account for a "magnifying" reaction (which, in turn, explains the failure to demonstrate an uptake of interferon by sensitive cells) and also for the dependence of the antiviral activity both on DNA-dependent RNA synthesis and on protein formation.

By combining with the active sites of cell ribosomes, intermediary proteins make these particles incapable of aggregating with both messenger viral RNA (which originates from early transcription of viral DNA) and viral RNA itself. Since virus-specific polyribosomes are not formed, a block at the "early" translation step occurs: thus, no virus-specific enzymes or viral precursors can be synthesized. A block at this step, which is shared by DNA- and RNA-synthesizing pathways, explains why most DNA and RNA viruses are sensitive to interferon. For the same reason, replication of most oncogenic viruses is prevented by interferon.

Conversely, formation of normal polyribosome complexes with cellular messenger RNA remains unchanged, upon incubation of uninfected cells with interferon. This could be a reason for the failure to disclose metabolic activity of purified interferon in uninfected cells.

Interferon also prevents the neoplastic transformation of homologous cells by some tumour viruses. The molecular basis for this action of interferon is unknown.

An attempt is made to interpret all these data on a common basis and to offer a general view of the mode of action of interferon.

REFERENCES

ALLISON, A. C. (1961). *Virology*, **15**, 47.

ATANASIU, P., and CHANY, C. (1960). *C. r. hebd. Séanc. Acad. Sci. Paris*, **251**, 1687.

BADER, J. P. (1962). *Virology*, **16**, 436.

BALTIMORE, D., GIRARD, M., and DARNELL, J. E. (1966). *Virology*, **29**, 179.

BARON, S. (1963). *Adv. Virus Res.*, **10**, 39.

BARON, S., and LEVY, H. B. (1966). *A. Rev. Microbiol.*, **20**, 291.

BUCHAN, A., and BURKE, D. C. (1966). *Biochem. J.*, **98**, 530.

COCITO, C. (1963). *Biochemical Properties and Metabolism of the Nucleic Acids of Viruses, Cells, and Virus-Infected Cells.* Louvain: Fonteyn.

COCITO, C., DE MAEYER, E., and DE SOMER, P. (1962a). *Life Sci.*, **1**, 753.

COCITO, C., DE MAEYER, E., and DE SOMER, P. (1962b). *Life Sci.*, **1**, 759.

COCITO, C., PRINZIE, A., and DE SOMER, P. (1962). *Experientia*, **18**, 218.

COCITO, C., SCHONNE, E., and DE SOMER, P. (1965). *Life Sci.*, **4**, 1253.

COCITO, C., VANDEPUTTE, M., and DE SOMER, P. (1965). *Arch. ges. Virusforsch.*, **15**, 402.

COGNIAUX-LE CLERC, J., LEVY, A. H., and WAGNER, R. R. (1966). *Virology*, **28**, 497.

DELGARNO, L., MARTIN, E. M., LIU, S. L., and WORK, T. S. (1966). *J. molec. Biol.* **15**, 7.

DE SOMER, P. (1962). *Proc. R. Soc. Med.*, **55**, 726.

DE SOMER, P. (1964). *Proc. Int. Symp. on Non-Specific Resistance to Virus Infection*, Smolenice.

DE SOMER, P., PRINZIE, A., DENYS, P., and SCHONNE, E. (1962). *Virology*, **16**, 63.

ERIKSON, R. L., and FRANKLIN, R. M. (1966). *Bact. Rev.*, **30**, 267.

FRIEDMAN, R. M., and SONNABEND, J. A. (1964). *Nature, Lond.*, **203**, 366.

GHOSH, S. N., and GIFFORD, G. E. (1965). *Virology*, **27**, 186.

GRESSER, I. (1961). *Proc. natn. Acad. Sci. U.S.A.*, **47**, 1817.

HELLER, E. (1963). *Virology*, **21**, 652.

HILLEMAN, M. R. (1963). *J. cell. comp. Physiol.*, **62**, 337.

HO, M. (1964). *Bact. Rev.*, **28**, 367.

HORTON, E., LIU, S. L., MARTIN, E. M., and WORK, T. S. (1966). *J. molec. Biol.*, **15**, 62.

ISAACS, A. (1959). *Symp. Soc. gen. Microbiol.*, **9**, 102.

ISAACS, A. (1961). *Perspectives in Virology*, **2**, 117.

ISAACS, A. (1962). *Cold Spring Harb. Symp. quant. Biol.*, **27**, 343.

ISAACS, A. (1963). *Adv. Virus Res.*, **10**, 1.

ISAACS, A., and BURKE, D. C. (1959). *Br. med. Bull.*, **15**, 185.

ISAACS, A., KLEMPERER, H. G., and HITCHCOCK, G. (1961). *Virology*, **13**, 191.

ISAACS, A., and LINDENMANN, J. (1957). *Proc. R. Soc. B*, **147**, 258.

ISAACS, A., LINDENMANN, J., and VALENTINE, R. C. (1957). *Proc. R. Soc. B*, **147**, 268.

ISAACS, A., ROTEM, Z., and FANTES, K. H. (1966). *Virology*, **29**, 248.

JOKLIK, W. K., JUNGWIRTH, C., ODA, K., and WOODSON, B. (1966). Personal communication. IEG. No. 7, Memo 505.

JOKLIK, W. K., and MERIGAN, T. C. (1966). *Proc. natn. Acad. Sci. U.S.A.*, **56**, 558.

LAMPSON, G. P., TYTELL, A. A., NEMES, M. M., and HILLEMAN, M. R. (1963). *Proc. Soc. exp. Biol. Med.*, **112**, 468.

LEVINE, S. (1964). *Virology*, **24**, 586.

LEVINE, S., MAGEE, W., HAMILTON, R., and MILLER, O. (1966). Personal communication. IEG No. 6, Memos 170 and 269.

LEVY, H. B. (1964). *Virology*, **22**, 575.

LEVY, H. B., SNELLBAKER, L. F., and BARON, S. (1963). *Virology*, **21**, 48.

LOCKART, R. Z. (1964). *Biochem. biophys. Res. Commun.*, **15**, 513.

LOCKART, R. Z., SREEVALSAN, T., and HORN, B. (1962). *Virology*, **18**, 493.

MARCUS, P., and SALB, J. (1966). *Virology*, **30**, 502.

MÉCS, E., SONNABEND, J., and MARTIN, E. (1966). Personal communication. IEG No. 6, Memo 208.

MERIGAN, T. C. (1966). Personal communication. IEG No. 6, Memo 202.

MINER, N., RAY, W. J., and SIMON, E. H. (1966). *Biochem. biophys. Res. Commun.*, **24**, 264.

OXMAN, M. N., and BLACK, P. H. (1966). *Proc. natn. Acad. Sci. U.S.A.*, **55**, 1133.

PLAGEMANN, P. G. W., and SWIM, H. E. (1966). *Bact. Rev.*, **30**, 267.

SONNABEND, J. A. (1964). *Nature, Lond.*, **203**, 496.

SONNABEND, J. A., MARTIN, E., MÉCS, E., and FANTES, K. (1966). Personal communication. IEG No. 6, Memo 209.

STRANDSTRÖM, H., and CHANY, C. (1960). *C. r. hebd. Séanc. Acad. Sci., Paris*, **251**, 1687.

TAYLOR, J. (1964). *Biochem. biophys. Res. Commun.*, **14**, 447.

TAYLOR, J. (1965). *Virology*, **25**, 340.

TODARO, G. J., and BARON, S. (1965). *Proc. natn. Acad. Sci. U.S.A.*, **54**, 752.

VANDEPUTTE, M., DE LAFONTEYNE, J., BILLIAU, A., and DE SOMER, P. (1967). *Arch. ges. Virusforsch.*, **20**, 235.

WAGNER, R. R. (1960). *Bact. Rev.*, **24**, 151.

WAGNER, R. R. (1963). *A. Rev. Microbiol.*, **17**, 285.

WAGNER, R. R. (1965). *Am. J. Med.*, **38**, 726.

YOUNGNER, J. S., STINEBRING, W. R., and TAUBE, S. E. (1965). *Virology*, **27**, 541.

DISCUSSION

Ho: Some years ago you reported (Cocito, De Maeyer and De Somer, 1962*a, b, loc. cit.*) that in the Sindbis virus–rat cell system interferon acted primarily by inhibiting early viral messenger RNA. Do you believe that polyoma virus is acted on by interferon in a different manner from Sindbis?

Cocito: In that paper we reported that interferon inhibits the formation of rapidly labelled RNA in rat embryo cells infected with Sindbis virus. It was argued, however, that our determinations of eclipse-RNA overlapped a period in which actinomycin-resistant viral RNA had already accumulated in control infected cells (Levy, H. B., Snellbaker, L. F., and Baron, S. [1963]. *Virology*, **21**, 48). It is therefore possible that treatment with interferon prevents the formation of precursor viral RNA in cells infected with RNA viruses. Likewise, in the case of polyoma, we believe that viral DNA, rather than virus-specific messenger RNA, is inhibited by interferon.

De Maeyer: You said that the length of the replicating cycle in your experiment with polyoma virus was about one week. Isn't that a very long cycle?

Cocito: In mouse embryo fibroblasts progeny particles appear intracellularly about 18 hours after infection with 10 $TCID_{50}$ of polyoma virus. Both free virus and total (free+cell-associated) virus increase linearly for about 30 hours and reach a plateau which lasts for at least three days (Cocito, Vandeputte and De Somer, 1965, *loc. cit.*).

De Maeyer: Is your mouse interferon made in tissue culture or *in vivo*?

Cocito: In vivo.

De Maeyer: With interferon prepared *in vivo* don't you have to be quite sure that the mouse doesn't contain polyoma antibodies, especially since you don't work with purified interferon?

Cocito: First of all the mouse colony employed was proved to be polyoma-free by the haemagglutination-inhibition test. In addition, the preparation used as a control fluid for interferon was obtained from animals coming from the same source. This is sufficient to exclude the presence of polyoma antibodies in our interferon preparations.

Stoker: If I understand your hypothesis correctly, interferon prevents synthesis of both the viral peak and the other peak of DNA?

Cocito: The appearance of viral DNA is prevented when monolayers of mouse embryo cells are incubated with interferon for 18 hours before infection. On the other hand, incorporation of tritiated thymidine into cell DNA is reduced by impure interferon preparations, but this effect apparently is not due to interferon itself. Contaminating proteins, which are physiological cell components and behave like interferon during purification, are responsible for it (Cocito, Schonne and De Somer, 1965, *loc. cit.*).

Stoker: A technical difficulty some people have found in the stimulation of cell DNA synthesis is due to the fact that in stationary cultures DNA synthesis is stimulated by minor manipulations. For example if one removes the medium and carries out a mock infection one also stimulates DNA synthesis. So it is extremely easy to induce DNA synthesis in cultures in a way which has nothing to do with the virus at all. One would not expect this DNA synthesis to be interferon-sensitive, but it would produce a background of DNA synthesis in your experiments which would mask the viral action. Do you find an increase in DNA synthesis in the dummy-infected controls?

Cocito: No.

Martin: You have shown that interferon blocks viral DNA replication without seemingly affecting the synthesis of viral specific messenger RNA. This result depends on the validity of your hybridizing technique.

Cocito: We have followed essentially the technique of hybridization on DNA membranes (Gillespie, D., and Spiegelman, S. [1965]. *J. molec. Biol.*, **12**, 829). The difficulty, however, is to make good preparations of linear single strands of polyoma DNA which can be anchored on membranes, i.e. to convert the closed circular form to the heat-denaturable form of polyoma DNA. When the DNase-heat denaturation procedure (Vinograd, J., Lebowitz, J., Radloff, R., Watson, R., and Laipis, P. [1965]. *Proc. natn. Acad. Sci. U.S.A.*, **53**, 1104; Benjamin, T. L. [1966]. *J. molec. Biol.*, **16**, 359) is applied, low molecular weight DNA and low efficiency of hybridization are frequently obtained. The background that we had with purified messenger RNA was absolutely negligible.

Martin: Is it possible to use a technique other than the methylated albumin-Kieselguhr (MAK) columns to distinguish polyoma DNA from host cell DNA?

Cocito: We have used only chromatography on MAK columns.

Stoker: There is an important implication here in relation to the problem of whether a specific viral polymerase has to be made in order to replicate the viral DNA. Many enzymes are induced after infections and all the experiments so far suggest that these are host cell enzymes—there are anyway too many of them to be all viral coded enzymes—and this includes a polymerase. But this doesn't solve the question of whether the virus requires a specific viral coded polymerase, which is present but not detectable in the large amount of cell polymerase made. If your results show that only viral DNA synthesis is inhibited by interferon it may imply that there is a virus-specific function which is needed and which is blocked because of the interferon-sensitivity of the viral messenger, whereas the cell-induced enzymes are not sufficient to replicate the viral DNA.

Joklik: The detection of early polyoma messenger RNA is very difficult. Have you done a time course experiment?

Cocito: No.

Joklik: You seem to have no difficulty in getting plenty of counts hybridized.

Cocito: In fact the efficiency of hybridization was low. We did not do saturation curves.

Joklik: How much DNA have you on the membrane?

Cocito: We did not measure it directly. We know that during the conversion of circular into linear DNA and subsequent denaturation some DNA is broken down and will not stick to the membrane.

STUDIES ON INTERFERON ACTION

J. A. SONNABEND, E. M. MARTIN AND E. MÉCS[*]

National Institute for Medical Research, Mill Hill, London

THE antiviral action of interferon can be usefully divided into two stages—the acquisition of resistance to virus growth by the uninfected cell, and the expression of this resistance after infection (Sonnabend and Friedman, 1966). Our work has been mainly concerned with the latter aspect of interferon action, and has been an attempt to define the step in the growth of an RNA virus that is sensitive to the antiviral effect of interferon. This work was done in collaboration with Dr. Karl Fantes of Glaxo Laboratories, who purified the interferon used in the experiments.

We have studied the effects of interferon on the synthesis of viral RNA and of a specific viral protein in chick embryo fibroblasts (CEF) infected with Semliki Forest virus (SFV). This system, which was originally developed by Taylor (1965), has several advantages. The virus is highly sensitive to interferon, and, although it stimulates the production of interferon in chick cells, the amount produced in a single cycle of virus growth is low and unlikely to complicate the interpretation of the observations on the effects of exogenous interferon. The growth of SFV·is not affected by actinomycin D. Since this antibiotic inhibits cellular but not viral RNA synthesis, its use has made it possible to study the effects of interferon on the synthesis of viral RNA. The use of actinomycin D has the additional advantage of inhibiting interferon production (Heller, 1963).

VIRUS GROWTH AND SYNTHESIS OF VIRAL RNA

When chick cells are infected with SFV at a multiplicity of 20–40 p.f.u./cell in the presence of 2 µg. actinomycin D/ml., virus production begins four hours later, and a single cycle of virus growth is completed by eight hours after infection. The rate of actinomycin-resistant RNA synthesis reaches a maximum at about 5·5 hours after infection, but as early as three hours, at a time before progeny virus can be detected, it has reached values of 30 to 40 per cent of the maximum. The growth curve of SFV and the

[*] Present address: Institute of Microbiology, Medical University, Szeged, Hungary.

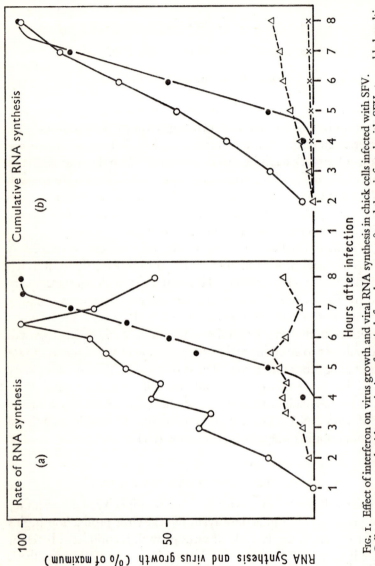

FIG. 1. Effect of interferon on virus growth and viral RNA synthesis in chick cells infected with SFV. Cells were pretreated with 40 units interferon/ml. for 4 hours at 37°, and then infected with SFV at an added multiplicity of 20 p.f.u./cell in the presence of actinomycin D (2 μg./ml.). (a) Rates of RNA synthesis determined by incubating the cells with [³H]adenosine for 15 minutes at each time point. (b) Cumulative RNA synthesis calculated from the areas under the curves for the rates of RNA synthesis. RNA synthesis in control cells: ●—●; in interferon-treated cells: △---△. Virus growth in control cells: ○—○; in interferon treated cells: ×---×.

rate of actinomycin-resistant RNA synthesis in infected cells are shown in Fig. 1.

When RNA is extracted from infected cells which have been labelled with [14C]uridine in the presence of actinomycin D and analysed by sedimentation through a sucrose gradient, the viral RNA can be resolved into

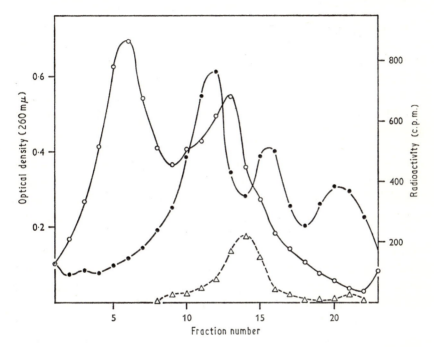

Fig. 2. Sucrose gradient analysis of RNA extracted from chick cells infected with SFV.

Cells were infected with SFV (20 p.f.u./cell) in the presence of actinomycin D (2 μg./ml.) and incubated with [3H]adenosine. Six hours after infection the RNA was extracted from the cytoplasm with phenol and sodium dodecyl sulphate. Chick ribosomal RNA (0·25 mg.) was added to 0·3 ml. of the extract which was then layered on a 5–20 per cent linear sucrose gradient (5 ml. containing tris-HCl 0·01M, pH 7·2; EDTA, 0·001M; KCl, 0·1M) and centrifuged for 2·5 hours at 39,000 rev./min.

Total acid-insoluble radioactivity: ○—○; acid-insoluble radioactivity resistant to 2 μg./ml. ribonuclease: △----△; optical density at 260 mμ: ●—●.

three components (Friedman, Levy and Carter, 1966; Sonnabend, Martin and Mécs, 1967). This is shown in Fig. 2. The optical density peaks are due to 30 S and 18 S ribosomal RNA added as markers. Two peaks of radioactivity are seen. One sediments at 45 S and is infectious; it corresponds to the RNA that can be extracted from the purified virus particle. The second peak of radioactivity, sedimenting at 26 S, is not infectious. After treatment of the gradient fractions with ribonuclease, a third peak of radioactivity is revealed which sediments just ahead of the 18 S, ribosomal RNA. The base compositions of 45 S RNA, 26 S RNA and of the RNA extracted from purified virus are identical (Sonnabend, Martin and Mécs, 1967; Friedman, personal communication).

EFFECTS OF INTERFERON ON VIRAL RNA SYNTHESIS

The rate of viral RNA synthesis in cells pretreated with 40 units interferon/ml. is shown in Fig. 1. The figure also shows the cumulative synthesis of viral RNA, calculated by integration of the values for the rates of RNA synthesis. The results show that interferon causes both a delay in the onset and a decrease in the rate of viral RNA synthesis. It is important to note that interferon causes a considerably greater inhibition of virus production than of viral RNA synthesis.

An obvious question arises from this last observation. Since infected cells contain at least three species of virus-specific RNA, only one of which is infectious, is it only the production of the infectious component that is inhibited? To investigate this, we compared the effect of interferon on virus production, infectious RNA formation, and the accumulation of viral RNA as determined by the incorporation of labelled RNA precursors in the presence of actinomycin. The results (Fig. 3) show that the formation of infectious RNA is less affected by interferon than the production of mature virus, and that the incorporation of a radioactive precursor into viral RNA is less inhibited than the formation of infectious RNA.

Further information on the relative amounts of the various viral RNA species in interferon-treated cells was obtained by extracting the RNA and analysing it on sucrose gradients. The distribution of radioactivity among the different viral RNA species in cells treated with interferon can be directly compared with that in untreated infected cells if the two sets of cells are labelled with different isotopes and the extracted RNA mixed before gradient analysis. The results of such an experiment are shown in Fig. 4. The cells which had been treated with interferon were incubated with [³H]uridine, while control cells were labelled with [¹⁴C]uridine, both in the presence of actinomycin D. The precursors were added at the time of infection, the RNA extracted 6·5 hours later, mixed, and sedimented through a sucrose gradient. The three species of virus-specific RNA previously described can be seen in the [¹⁴C]uridine-labelled RNA: 45 S, 26 S and 20 S. Although these three components are all present in the RNA extracted from interferon-treated cells, their relative amounts differ from that seen in the RNA extracted from untreated infected cells. The most striking difference is that there is relatively more 26 S RNA in the interferon-treated cells, although the absolute amount of this type of RNA that can be detected in these cells is less than that demonstrable in untreated infected cells. The relative effects of interferon on the accumulation of the three species of viral RNA were further investigated. Cells treated with interferon were labelled with the same precursor under identical conditions to untreated infected cells. The proportion of each species of RNA at a

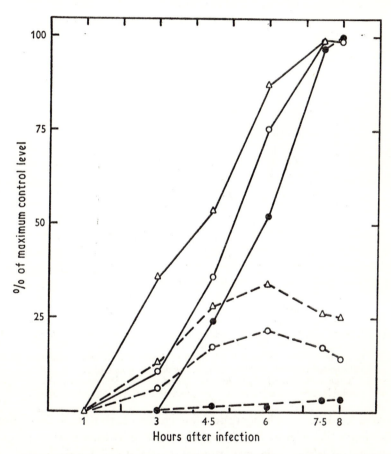

FIG. 3. Effect of interferon on the synthesis of viral RNA and infectious RNA in chick cells infected with SFV.

Cells were infected in the presence of actinomycin D as in Fig. 1, after pre-treatment with 10 units interferon/ml. for 4 hours. [³H]Adenosine was added, and at various times the RNA was extracted with phenol and sodium dodecyl sulphate; it was assayed for infectivity and its specific radioactivity determined.

RNA synthesis (counts/min. per microgram of RNA) in control cells (△—△) and interferon-treated cells (△----△); infectious titre of RNA (p.f.u./ml.) in control (○—○) and interferon-treated (○----○) cells; virus growth (p.f.u./ml.) in control (●—●) and interferon-treated cells (●----●). Results expressed as a percentage of the maximum values of the control series.

given time after infection was determined by measuring the area under each peak of radioactivity and expressing it as a percentage of the total radioactivity on the gradient. This figure, multiplied by the specific activity of the total RNA extracted (counts/min. per microgram of RNA), gives a measure of the relative amounts of each RNA species at each time during the infection cycle. The results, expressed as a percentage of the amount of 45 S RNA present in untreated cells 7·5 hours after infection,

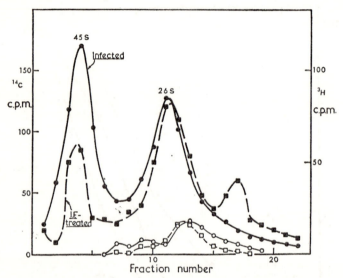

Fig. 4. Sucrose gradient analysis of RNA extracted from control and interferon-treated cells infected with SFV in the presence of actinomycin. Cells were pretreated with interferon and infected as in Fig. 1. [³H]-Uridine and [¹⁴C]uridine were added to interferon-treated and control cells respectively and the RNA extracted 6·5 hours after infection as described in the text. The extracted RNA from both sets of cells was mixed and sedimented through a sucrose gradient as described in Fig. 2.
Total acid-insoluble radioactivity: ³H (■----■); ¹⁴C (●—●). Acid-insoluble radioactivity resistant to ribonuclease: ³H (□----□); ¹⁴C (○—○).

are shown in Fig. 5. The increase in infectivity of the RNA is also shown. It rises in parallel with 45 S RNA, and is inhibited by interferon to a similar extent as 45 S RNA. The greater resistance of both 26 S and ribonuclease-resistant (20 S) RNA is clearly seen.

The effect of interferon therefore is not only to inhibit the overall incorporation of a precursor into viral RNA but also to alter the distribution of radioactivity among the various RNA species, particularly late in infection. It is apparent that 45 S RNA does not accumulate in interferon-treated cells, and that 26 S RNA remains the major component in these cells throughout infection.

It is difficult to account for this observation without some idea of the structure of 26 S RNA and its relevance to the growth of the virus. This is not known. We have suggested that the difference between 26 S and 45 S RNA may be one of configuration—45 S RNA having a more compact structure, required for infectivity and for packaging into the particle

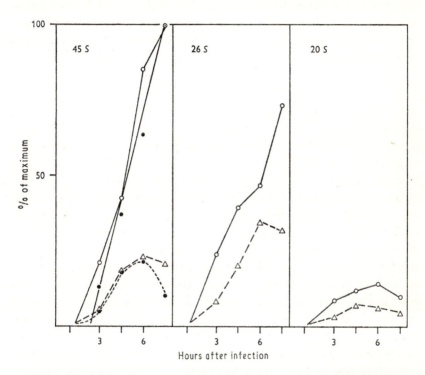

FIG. 5. Effect of interferon on synthesis of 45 S, 26 S, 20 S, and infectious RNA in chick cells infected with SFV.

The amounts of the various RNA components were determined as described in the text, and the results expressed as a percentage of 45 S RNA in control cells 7·5 hours after infection (150 counts/min. per microgram of RNA). RNA synthesis in control (○—○) and interferon-treated (△----△) cells. Infectious RNA titre (p.f.u./μg. RNA) in control (●—●) and interferon-treated cells (●----●).

(Sonnabend, Martin and Mécs, 1967). The base composition of 45 S and 26 S RNA is the same, and in labelling experiments radioactivity appears in 26 S RNA before 45 S RNA (Friedman, Levy and Carter, 1966; Sonnabend, Martin and Mécs, 1967). If 26 S RNA is a precursor of 45 S RNA, its transition to the 45 S form may require the participation of a specific protein—possibly the coat protein of the virus. If this suggestion about the nature of the 26 S RNA is correct, then its relative preponderance

INTER.—6

in interferon-treated cells may be a reflection of a diminished level of virus proteins in these cells.

A specific viral protein is responsible for the replication of viral RNA. The synthesis of this protein—the viral RNA polymerase—is directed by the viral RNA itself. The inhibition of viral RNA synthesis that has been observed in interferon-treated cells could therefore result from a primary action of interferon in blocking the synthesis of the viral RNA polymerase. Alternatively, the action of interferon may be exerted at a point beyond the synthesis of the enzyme, for example inhibiting its activity.

EFFECTS OF INTERFERON ON THE VIRAL RNA POLYMERASE

From the cytoplasm of chick cells infected with SFV we have isolated an enzyme that catalyses the incorporation of ribonucleoside triphosphates into an acid-insoluble product with the properties of the ribonuclease-resistant form of SFV RNA which appears in infected cells (Martin and Sonnabend, 1967). The activity of this RNA polymerase requires the presence of all four ribonucleoside triphosphates and is resistant to actinomycin D and to deoxyribonuclease. The enzyme reaction product, when extracted and examined by sedimentation through a sucrose gradient, gives the result shown in Fig. 6a. The labelled substrate for the enzyme reaction was [^{3}H]GTP. Before gradient analysis, the reaction product was mixed with RNA which had been extracted from infected cells labelled with [^{14}C]uridine. The sedimentation of [^{14}C]uridine-labelled RNA shows the three viral RNA components previously described, the 20 S component being revealed only after treatment with ribonuclease. The enzyme reaction product sediments as a homogeneous component at 20 S and is highly resistant to ribonuclease. It shows a sharp transition to ribonuclease sensitivity as it is heated, and this occurs over the same temperature range as is seen with the 20 S RNA isolated from infected cells. 20 S RNA from infected cells and the enzyme reaction product also have the same buoyant density in caesium sulphate (Martin and Sonnabend, 1967). The enzyme thus catalyses the incorporation of ribonucleoside triphosphates into a specific viral product. We have been unable to detect 45 S and 26 S RNAs in the enzyme reaction product. It is possible that these components are made but degraded by nucleases during incubation.

Pretreatment of cells with interferon before infection inhibits the development of polymerase activity (Fig. 7). The effect is dose-dependent, enzyme levels being lowest in those cells treated with the largest amounts of interferon. Only a small part of the low enzyme activity that can be detected in interferon-treated cells (Fig. 7) is due to the virus-specific

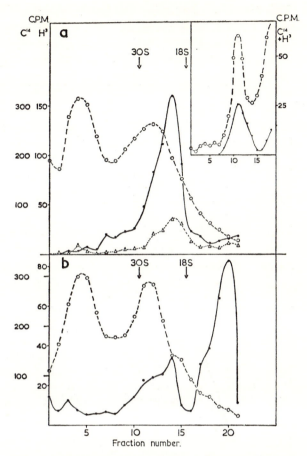

FIG. 6. Sucrose gradient analysis of reaction products of polymerase from control and interferon-treated cells. Polymerase was prepared 6 hours after infection and incubated with [³H]GTP. The product of the reaction was extracted with phenol-sodium dodecyl sulphate and analysed on a sucrose gradient as in Fig. 2, after the addition of ¹⁴C-labelled RNA extracted from untreated cells infected in the presence of actinomycin.

a. Polymerase from untreated cells.

b. Polymerase from interferon-treated cells.

³H radioactivity (reaction product): ●—●; ¹⁴C radioactivity (virus-specific RNA labelled *in vivo*): ○----○; ribonuclease-resistant ¹⁴C-labelled RNA: △----△. Arrows refer to positions of chick ribosomal RNA.

Inset: Distribution of radioactivity after ribonuclease treatment of ¹⁴C-labelled and ³H-labelled RNA before centrifugation.

polymerase. This was shown by the fact that incorporation of GTP by the enzyme prepared from interferon-treated cells was unaffected by the omission of ATP, UTP and CTP. When the reaction product of this enzyme was extracted and analysed on a sucrose gradient, most of the

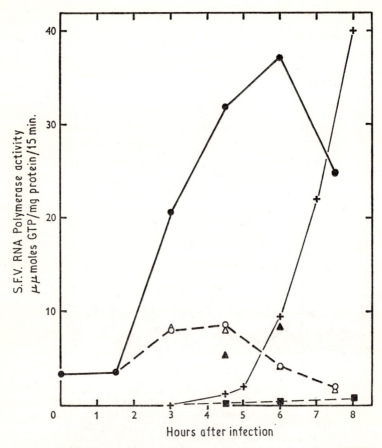

FIG. 7. Polymerase activity in control and interferon-pretreated (5 units/ml.) cells infected with SFV.

RNA polymerase activity of infected untreated cells: ●—●; of interferon-pretreated cells ○----○. Results of assays performed without the addition of three ribonucleoside triphosphates in untreated (▲) and interferon-treated (△) cells. Virus titres in control (+—+) and interferon-treated (■----■) cells.

radioactivity was seen to have been incorporated into low molecular weight material (Fig. 6b).

How does treatment with interferon prevent the development of polymerase activity? Two explanations were considered. The primary action of interferon or of any antiviral agent induced by interferon may be either to inhibit the synthesis of the enzyme or to inhibit its activity. In an attempt to resolve these alternatives we tested the effect of highly purified and partially purified interferon preparations (made by Dr. Karl Fantes) on the activity of the polymerase. As many as 150 units of interferon were without effect. (The amount of polymerase in the assay represented material from 10^7 cells. Ten units of interferon would have been sufficient to inhibit virus growth in this number of cells by 99 per cent.) However, since there is evidence that the action of interferon may be indirect and mediated by a cellular protein (Sonnabend and Friedman, 1966), we also looked for an inhibitor of polymerase activity in extracts from infected and uninfected cells pretreated with interferon. None of these extracts inhibited the *in vitro* activity of the viral polymerase. Essentially similar findings on the effects of interferon on the synthesis and activity of a viral RNA polymerase, but in a different system (Mengo-virus-infected L cells) were reported by Miner, Ray and Simon (1966). Although our results do not prove the absence of a viral polymerase inhibitor in interferon-pretreated cells they do suggest that the low polymerase activity found in these cells more probably reflects a reduced synthesis of the enzyme. These results are consistent with a mechanism of interferon action which is primarily directed towards an inhibition of the synthesis of viral proteins, an interpretation which has received more direct support from the experiments of Marcus and Salb (1966), and of Joklik and Merigan (1966).

We have undertaken some experiments which relate to the development of resistance by the cell on exposure to interferon. The observations that inhibitors of cellular RNA and protein synthesis prevent the development of resistance in response to interferon have led to the proposal that cells treated with interferon synthesize a specific protein possessing antiviral activity (Taylor, 1964; Friedman and Sonnabend, 1964; Lockart, 1964; Sonnabend and Friedman, 1966). However, merely to demonstrate that the effect of any agent on a cell has a requirement for RNA and protein synthesis is very far from demonstrating that the effect depends on the induced synthesis of a specific protein, let alone by a mechanism which involves the derepression of the synthesis of a specific messenger RNA. This is particularly true when, as is the case with interferon action, the evidence is derived from studies with metabolic inhibitors, such as actinomycin, puromycin and fluorophenylalanine. More evidence is needed to show that the sensitivity of interferon action to these inhibitors reflects the need for the synthesis of a specific antiviral protein by the host cell. For example a direct demonstration that interferon-treated cells contain a new protein not present in untreated cells, or present in these cells in reduced amounts, and that this protein has appropriate antiviral activity would strongly support such a mechanism. This is a difficult undertaking. However, the resolving power of acrylamide gel electrophoresis combined with other preliminary fractionation procedures should be sufficient to enable one to identify such a newly synthesized protein. The work of Marcus and Salb (1966) further suggests that the target for the action of this postulated antiviral protein is likely to be the ribosomes and that the cell-free protein-synthesizing system might provide an assay for its activity.

We have embarked on a search for this postulated antiviral protein, and as a beginning have looked for differences in newly synthesized ribosome-associated proteins after exposing cells to interferon. The technique used was to incubate interferon-treated cells with [^{14}C]amino acids, and untreated cells with the same amino acids but labelled in this case with tritium. Ribosomes were prepared from these cells, their proteins dissociated with sodium dodecyl sulphate and urea, and fractionated by electrophoresis on polyacrylamide gels. Ribosomal proteins from interferon-treated and untreated cells were either run separately or mixed and run together. In the latter case, we were looking for differences in the ratio of ^{14}C to tritium, which would indicate differences in the synthesis of any protein component in response to interferon. It is of course just as likely that a protein will be missing as that a new one will be found.

Despite several variations in the conditions of labelling no differences could be detected between the interferon-treated and control series. Labelled ribosomes and their subunits were also compared with regard to their sedimentation in sucrose gradients. No differences were noted, and the proportions of the two ribosomal subunits were the same in both sets of cells.

We have also examined the soluble proteins of the cell. Preliminary fractionation with ammonium sulphate and electrophoresis on acrylamide gels has so far revealed no consistent differences in the proteins synthesized after treatment with interferon. However, in view of the evidence that ribosomes derived from interferon-treated cells have an abnormal function with respect to the translation of viral messenger RNA (Marcus and Salb, 1966) it is important to continue to look for physical, chemical and other functional differences.

Our experiments on the growth of SFV in interferon-treated chick cells indicate that interferon probably inhibits viral RNA synthesis by inhibiting the synthesis of the viral RNA polymerase. In other words, the primary action of interferon is to block viral protein synthesis. We have so far been unable to show that this action depends on a specific cellular protein newly synthesized on exposure to interferon. It may well be that the requirement for cellular RNA and protein synthesis for interferon to demonstrate antiviral activity does not reflect the necessity for the synthesis of a *specific* antiviral protein. Interferon itself may be directly antiviral, and an operation involved in its action—e.g. its entry into the cell or transport to its site of action—may require the continuation of normal cellular RNA and protein synthesis without any qualitative or quantitative differences being necessary.

SUMMARY

The effects of chick interferon on the synthesis of viral RNA and on the RNA polymerase responsible for this synthesis in chick cells infected with Semliki Forest virus are described. It was found that interferon inhibited the rate of total viral RNA synthesis and caused an alteration in the proportions of the three virus-specific RNA components that appear in infected cells. The synthesis of the two poorly-infectious components—26 S RNA and the 20 S ribonuclease-resistant RNA—was less affected than that of the infectious 45 S progeny RNA, and the synthesis of the latter was less inhibited than the formation of mature virus. The levels of virus-specific RNA polymerase were also reduced by interferon treatment. In the absence of any evidence for an inhibitor of polymerase activity in treated cells it was concluded that interferon treatment resulted in the inhibition of polymerase synthesis and that this may reflect a general effect of interferon on viral protein synthesis.

In view of the evidence suggesting that the primary action of interferon is to induce the formation of a protein which is the effective antiviral agent, attempts were made, using polyacrylamide gel electrophoresis, to detect the synthesis of proteins uniquely present in interferon-treated uninfected cells. However, no newly-formed proteins were found in the ribosomes or the cell sap of interferon-treated cells.

ACKNOWLEDGEMENTS

We are grateful to Dr. Ian Kerr and to Dr. Robert Friedman for many helpful discussions during the course of this work.

REFERENCES

FRIEDMAN, R. M., LEVY, H. B., and CARTER, W. B. (1966). *Proc. natn. Acad. Sci. U.S.A.*, **56**, 440.
FRIEDMAN, R. M., and SONNABEND, J. A. (1964). *Nature, Lond.*, **203**, 366.
HELLER, E. (1963). *Virology*, **21**, 652.
JOKLIK, W. K., and MERIGAN, T. C. (1966). *Proc. natn. Acad. Sci. U.S.A.*, **56**, 558.
LOCKART, R. Z. (1964). *Biochem. biophys. Res. Commun.*, **15**, 513.

MARCUS, P. I., and SALB, J. M. (1966). *Virology*, **30**, 502.
MARTIN, E. M., and SONNABEND, J. A. (1967). *J. gen. Virol.*, **1**, 97.
MINER, N., RAY, W. J., and SIMON, E. H. (1966). *Biochem. biophys. Res. Commun.*, **24**, 264.
SONNABEND, J. A., and FRIEDMAN, R. M. (1966). In *Interferons*, pp. 202–231, ed. Finter, N. Amsterdam: North-Holland Publishing Co.
SONNABEND, J. A., MARTIN, E. M., and MÉCS, E. (1967). *Nature, Lond.*, **213**, 365.
TAYLOR, J. (1964). *Biochem. biophys. Res. Commun.*, **14**, 447.
TAYLOR, J. (1965). *Virology*, **25**, 340.

DISCUSSION

Joklik: The polymerase from interferon-treated cells seems to differ in the product it forms. Have you any comments on this?

Sonnabend: Most of the incorporation by the polymerase from interferon-treated cells is into low molecular weight RNA. I think it is likely that a similar amount of low molecular weight RNA is made by the enzyme from untreated cells but is being obscured on the gradient by the much greater incorporation into 20 S RNA. It is of course possible that the material at the top of the gradient represents degradation products rather than a specific enzyme reaction product. The material at the top of the gradient was sensitive to ribonuclease in the case of the product made by the enzyme from untreated cells. Incorporation by the polymerase from interferon-treated cells was so low that we got just enough counts to run on a gradient. There wasn't enough to get anything reliable from treating each fraction with ribonuclease.

Ho: Have you tested for a viral inhibitory protein by a biological test?

Martin: We hope to develop a biological assay for our interferon-induced inhibitory protein by testing the cytoplasmic fractions, and perhaps proteins derived from interferon-treated ribosomes, in a cell-free protein synthetic system using viral messenger RNA. We have no results from this work yet, but we think it is essential that we try to find some test based on its inhibitory activity, and not rely solely on a demonstration of a new band on the gel.

Stoker: You wouldn't necessarily expect any cell specificity in the action of the inhibitory protein. This might be a way of distinguishing it from interferon.

Martin: As soon as we isolate a protein which shows inhibitory activity in a cell-free system we want to test it in a heterologous system, say an inhibitor induced by chick interferon tested in the EMC-RNA-mouse ascites cell system, which we also have going at the moment.

Sonnabend: I think what Dr. Ho was suggesting was simply putting extracts from interferon-treated cells back onto cells. I doubt if this would be very helpful.

Ho: There haven't been many positive results in attempts to detect intracellular interferon. Whatever virus inhibitor you find will be of interest, and you can then attempt to prove subsequently that it is the protein you are looking for.

Martin: Crude chick interferon contains an inhibitor of the polymerase which is not present in highly purified preparations. Some high-titre, mouse-serum interferon which Dr. Baron sent us also inhibited the RNA polymerase from EMC-infected mouse cells. This inhibition was actinomycin-resistant, since actinomycin is present in the polymerase assay. This material may, in fact, be one of the non-interferon factors causing virus interference.

Wagner: Have you characterized the 26 S RNA by base composition?

Sonnabend: It has the same base composition as 45 S RNA. That is really a puzzle to us.

Wagner: Are you guessing it is a minus strand?

Sonnabend: No. I think one would guess that this was a question of secondary structure and that it was perhaps a less compact form of 45 S RNA and just sediments more slowly.

Merigan: We have studied the interesting problem of some of the larger organisms that are interferon-sensitive—the trachoma-inclusion virus agents, which have their own ribosomes (Hanna, L., Merigan, T. C., and Jawetz, E. [1966]. *Proc. Soc. exp. Biol. Med.*, **122**, 421). If the model is as we visualize it, they have a messenger RNA that diffuses out and then they use the host ribosomes as well as their own in becoming mature infective particles. It really is quite complicated to visualize.

Stoker: Are these the largest known organisms that are sensitive to interferon?

Merigan: I think so.

Crick: If you get modified ribosomes, do you think all the ribosomes will be modified?

Sonnabend: Possibly, or the virus uses a special class of ribosomes.

Crick: But is it known whether the virus uses most of the ribosomes?

Sonnabend: No.

Crick: The effect might be due to a new protein giving one new molecule per ribosome, or it might be due to an enzyme which modifies an existing ribosomal protein. If it was an enzyme one should be able to modify ribosomes in a cell-free system.

Joklik: But I disagree that one could pick up one protein molecule per ribosome.

Crick: Are you sure? Of course you may get one which is in a pretty dense band. How many bands did you get?

Martin: Twenty-two or twenty-three.

Joklik: That means there are about 20 species and there may be 100 molecules in each of these species.

Crick: You have to think how much there is per ribosome. If there is one per ribosome, then it is going to make a difference somewhere, and you can work out roughly what sort of difference it would be.

Joklik: One can work out how many ribosomes you apply to the gel and I would be surprised if you put on many more than 10^7 ribosomes.

Martin: Material from roughly 2 to 4×10^7 cells was put onto the gel. We can detect, for instance, 2 µg. of protein as a stained band; with highly radioactive material showing no stained bands we were detecting levels of protein very much lower than this, say at least 0·1 μg. I don't know how many ribosomes per cell there are in the cells we use.★

Crick: It is the number of proteins per ribosome that matters. If it is about 100 and you are detecting one, roughly speaking, then if you have 20 bands, all equally strong, you are looking for roughly a fifth of a band.

Joklik: How long did you label for?

Sonnabend: For periods of five to 21 hours. In some cases we pre-labelled cells with tritiated amino acids and then with [¹⁴C]amino acids for six hours in the presence of interferon. Cells become resistant rapidly and one would think that the rate of synthesis of this protein was at least as rapid as that of the ribosomal proteins.

Levy: Assuming that the virus requires a newly synthesized ribosomal subunit to attach to under ordinary circumstances, if a cell only develops the antiviral state when new interferon-type subunits are in the majority, then when the protein is prepared from the whole ribosomes, the old ribosomes will be diluted to some extent with the new ribosomes. The label of course should only be on the newly synthesized ones. This is a point for conjecture: if the viral RNA has to attach to a ribosomal subunit and if this can only be a newly-synthesized ribosomal subunit, then it will take three to four hours for the pool of newly-synthesized ribosomal subunits to become the majority; this then provides the antiviral state when these are interferon-type subunits.

Joklik: This is simply not so in at least one small RNA virus—polio—nor in vaccinia virus. In neither case do significant numbers of new subunits get into the cytoplasm and form ribosomes: at the most it could be 5 per cent. Certainly the number of ribosomes that are recruited by viral messenger RNA is much larger. This is relevant to the question that Dr. Crick raised, i.e. that in cells infected with Mengo or vaccinia virus, although not all the ribosomes combine with viral messenger RNA, the proportion is between 33 and 50 per cent, that is, a significant proportion.

Crick: I had better ask the question the other way round: what fraction of ribosomes does one need to affect to prevent most of the ribosomes going on? It isn't obvious that you have to affect all of them.

Martin: There is much evidence to suggest that, say, a 50 per cent inhibition in polymerase synthesis produces nearly 90 per cent inhibition of mature virus production (Sonnabend, J. A., Martin, E. M., Mécs, E., and Fantes, K. [1967]. *J. gen. Virol.*, **1**, 41). Presumably this is due to a cascade effect, that is, interferon inhibits first viral protein synthesis and then viral RNA synthesis, and any subsequent process which depends on both RNA and protein is inhibited to a greater extent.

★ Note added in proof:

Dr. Ian Kerr, who is preparing ribosomes from chick embryo fibroblasts for the cell-free protein synthetic work, routinely gets a yield of 250 μg. of ribosomes from 10⁸ cells. This gives a figure of roughly 5,000 ribosomes per cell. It also means I was putting 80 μg. of ribosomes, or 40 μg. of ribosomal protein, onto each gel.

Crick: There may be a number of explanations. If you alter 5 per cent of the ribosomes it might prevent all the others from acting.

Sonnabend: If you give a dose of interferon which is below the amount needed for its maximal effect, then at multiplicities of anything above one it should presumably be possible to overcome the effect. However, our work was at high multiplicities and we never tested for this. Most of the studies on overcoming the effect of interferon were at low multiplicities.

Wagner: It would be interesting to work this out. The argument about a single molecule and changing a single site on the ribosome should hold regardless of the multiplicity of viral RNA going into the cell as challenge. The blocked ribosome shouldn't be usable regardless of multiplicity of viral challenge. My best recollection (and this goes back some years) is that one can overcome the effect by increasing the multiplicity, that is, one gets viral replication and presumably viral RNA synthesis under those conditions. That would weaken the argument for a very specific site on the ribosome for action of the inhibitory protein.

Sonnabend: Surely the outcome will depend on whether one is using a saturating dose of interferon?

Joklik: One need not postulate that this protein completely abolishes the interaction between ribosomes and messenger RNA, but merely that it decreases its probability, so that if the concentration of messenger RNA was increased one might be able partially to overcome its effect.

Ho: Cantell and co-workers (Cantell, K., Skursko, Z., Paucker, K., and Henle, W. [1962]. *Virology*, **17**, 312–323), Dr. Hermodsson (Hermodsson, S., and Phillipson, L. [1963]. *Proc. Soc. exp. Biol. Med.*, **114**, 574–579) and I (Ho, M. [1962]. *Virology*, **17**, 262–275) have investigated whether interferon action is a one-hit phenomenon or an all-or-none phenomenon. Our conclusion was that it was not an all-or-none phenomenon, and that partial inhibition can occur.

THE MECHANISM OF ACTION OF INTERFERON

Hilton B. Levy and William A. Carter

National Institutes of Health, National Institute of Allergy and Infectious Diseases, Laboratory of Biology of Viruses, Bethesda, Maryland

Research on the mechanism of action of interferon has shown that this protein blocks an event in virus replication which occurs very shortly after eclipse of the virus, and before new viral RNA molecules are synthesized. For example, in Semliki Forest virus infection of chicken cells, interferon prevents the formation of the viral RNA polymerase (Sonnabend *et al.*, 1967; for review see Baron and Levy, 1966). With Mengo virus infection of mouse L cells, a rapid cessation of cellular RNA and protein synthesis occurs shortly after infection (Franklin and Baltimore, 1962; McCormick and Penman, 1967). The cell-specific polysomes are disaggregated, and after a latent period of one to $1 \cdot 5$ hours the infected cell undergoes a transition from host to virus-directed RNA and protein synthesis. The virus-induced inhibition of cellular RNA synthesis is postponed by interferon treatment whereas the inhibition of cellular protein synthesis is not (Levy, 1964).

These observations deal with periods very early during the course of virus infection, and indicate that interferon (or more correctly, the product induced by this protein) acts upon the genome of the infecting virus particle. Relatively little is known of the events which immediately follow the uncoating of Mengo virus. The experiments reported here were performed to study the early processing of the RNA of infecting Mengo virus and to determine whether interferon treatment affected this processing.

Mengo virus was grown in suspended cultures of L cells in the presence of actinomycin D and [³H]uridine. The virus was purified by a combination of enzyme treatments (DNase, RNase, and trypsin), differential centrifugation, and isopycnic centrifugation in caesium chloride. The radiopurity of the virus is indicated in Fig. 1, which shows the coincidence of the infectivity and radioactivity of fractions obtained from a caesium chloride gradient. On density gradient sedimentation of the RNA extracted from the virus by phenol (Scherrer and Darnell, 1962) a characteristic 37 *S* peak is revealed (Fig. 2).

Mouse L cells, with or without prior interferon treatment (16 hours, 10 units/ml.), were infected with the purified virus at a multiplicity of infection of 2. This low multiplicity was used to ensure a more efficient uptake of the labelled virus. The fact that a significant proportion of the cells remains uninfected (approximately 15–20 per cent) under these conditions is not relevant since these experiments measured only the radioactivity

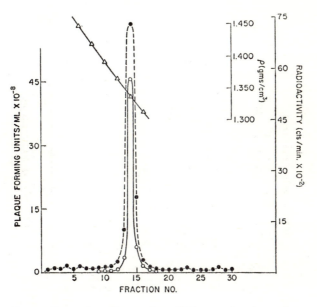

FIG. 1. Isopycnic sedimentation of Mengo virus in caesium chloride. Mengo virus labelled with [³H]uridine was sedimented at 39,000 rev./min. (SW39 swinging bucket rotor, Model L-2 ultracentrifuge, 5°C) for 20 hours. Fractions (0·25 ml.) were collected in tryptose phosphate and the radioactivity determined. Samples were assayed for infectivity in mouse L cells. o—o, plaque-forming units/ml. × 10⁻⁸; ●---●, radioactivity, counts/min. × 10⁻²; △—△, density of CsCl.

of the input virus, and not biochemical changes in the whole cell population. In experiments in which newly synthesized viral RNA or protein molecules were measured, multiplicities of 20 ensured uniform infection. In some early experiments polysomes were prepared from control infected and interferon-treated, infected cultures by disrupting the cells in a hypotonic solution (RSB: 0·01 M-tris at pH 7·4, 0·01 M-KCl, 0·003 M-MgCl₂), using a Dounce homogenizer. The post-mitochondrial supernatant fraction was adjusted to 1 per cent sodium deoxycholate, and polysomes were purified by sedimentation through successive layers of 0·5 and 2·0 M-sucrose

(Wettstein, Staehelin and Noll, 1963). Polysomes were prepared from cells at 30 minutes after infection with the radioactive virus, and were analysed on 10–34 per cent (w/v) sucrose gradients containing RSB, as shown in Fig. 3. At the concentration of Mg²⁺ used in this experiment (0·003 M) the ribosomal subunits are not detectable as discrete optical density peaks. Essentially two peaks of radioactivity, at 150 S and 50 S, are seen in the preparation

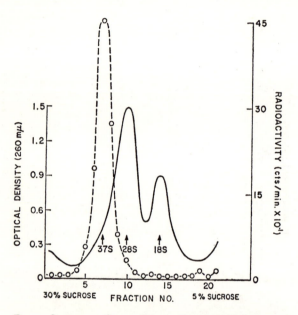

FIG. 2. Sucrose gradient sedimentation of purified Mengo RNA. RNA was extracted from the purified virus in the presence of purified mouse L cell ribosomes (see text). The final product was sedimented on a 5 to 30 per cent sucrose gradient (containing acetate buffer) at 39,000 rev./min. (SW39 swinging bucket rotor, Model L-2 ultracentrifuge, 3°) for 3 hours. The collection of samples is described in the text. ———, optical density; O----O, radioactivity of Mengo virus RNA.

obtained from control infected cells. There is some indication of less resolved heavier sedimenting label. The purified virus sediments at 150 S in this solvent. Infectivity titrations of individual fractions from this gradient confirm that the 150 S fraction represented unmodified virus sedimented with polysomes. The amount of virus at 150 S is also compatible with the known specific activity (counts/min. per p.f.u.) of the virus preparation used. In addition, RNase treatment of the preparation before centrifugation affects neither the radioactivity nor the infectivity of the

150 S product. On the other hand, the 50 S radioactive component is RNase-sensitive and non-infectious. In the polysome gradient from interferon-treated infected cells, the amount of uneclipsed virus at 30 minutes is equal to that in control infected cells, but the 50 S particle is not seen.

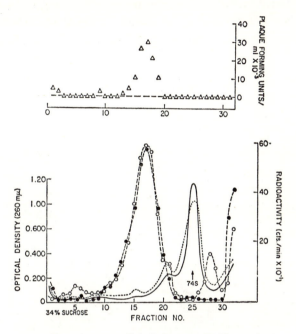

FIG. 3. The processing of labelled Mengo RNA 30 minutes post-infection. Polysomes were isolated by sedimentation through 2·0M-sucrose at 30 minutes after infection. The ribosomal pellet was resuspended in polysome medium, clarified by centrifugation at 10,000 g for 10 minutes, placed on a 10 to 34 per cent linear sucrose gradient (containing polysome buffer) and sedimented at 25,000 rev./min. (SW25.1 swinging bucket rotor, model L-2 ultracentrifuge, 3°) for 3 hours. The collection and assay of samples are described in the text. ———, optical density, control ribosomes; O---O, radioactivity, control ribosomes; ----, optical density, ribosomes from cells exposed to interferon; ●---●, radioactivity, ribosomes from cells exposed to interferon; △---△, plaque-forming units, control ribosome sample.

After longer centrifugation of polysomes prepared at 45 minutes post-infection, the labelled virus is sedimented to the bottom of the centrifuge tube and the 50 S particle is better resolved (Fig. 4). In cells exposed to interferon for 16 hours no evidence for a 50 S particle bearing the input labelled viral RNA is seen.

The 50 S structure is distinguishable from ^{32}P-labelled viral RNA in a gradient where they are compared directly (Fig. 5). The sedimentation behaviour of 37 S Mengo RNA is constant in all solvents studied (RSB, polysome buffer and acetate buffer). Since ribosomes purified from cells exposed to interferon do not form specific complexes with Mengo RNA *in vitro* (Carter and Levy, 1967*a*, *b*), co-sedimentation of viral RNA with these particles should reflect any non-specific interactions which might change

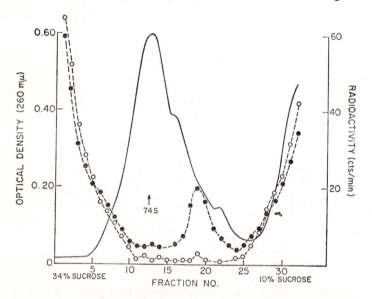

Fig. 4. The 50 S particle bearing viral RNA. Ribosomes were prepared from cells after 45 minutes of infection, as described in Fig. 9 and in the text. The products were sedimented on 10 to 34 per cent sucrose gradients (containing polysome buffer) at 22,000 rev./min. (SW25.1 swinging bucket rotor, model L-2 ultracentrifuge, 3°) for 16 hours. ——, optical density, control ribosomes; ●---●, radioactivity, control ribosomes; ○---○, radioactivity, ribosomes from cells exposed to interferon.

the apparent mass of viral RNA. The 50 S particle is clearly separable from 37 S RNA. However, 37 S RNA can be isolated from the 50 S structure by phenol extraction. The 50 S particle therefore represents an association of viral RNA with a cellular element, probably the 40 S ribosomal subunit.

The method of preparation of ribosomes used in the experiments of Figs. 3 and 4 concentrates the free radioactive virus as well as polysomes, and thereby obscures the examination of possible large viral-specific polysomes. Succeeding experiments were done with Mg^{++}-purified ribosomes (Takanami, 1960; Attardi and Smith, 1962): sodium deoxycholate and BRIJ 58 were added to the post-mitochondrial supernatant fluid to concentrations of 0·5 per cent and Mg++ to a concentration of 0·07 M. The mixture was allowed to stand for one hour at 2°c and the particles were centrifuged at 15,000 *g* for 15 minutes. The resultant pellet was gently washed with RSB and then resuspended in RSB, using a Dounce homogenizer. The sedimentation patterns of the monomer and subunits obtained

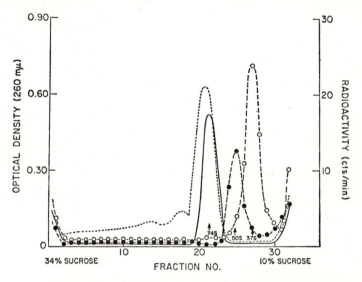

FIG. 5. Sedimentation of the isolated 50 S particle containing viral RNA. The 50 S particle bearing viral RNA was compared directly with the purified monomer (74 S) and ^{32}P-labelled 37 S viral RNA, which has been incubated at 0°c for 30 minutes (Carter and Levy, 1967*b*). The reaction mixture consisted of 0·2 ml. polysome medium, 0·4 mg. ribosomes from cells exposed to interferon, and 100 μg. ^{32}P-labelled viral RNA + ribosomal RNA. In the reaction mixture ribosomes were in excess and viral RNA is the limiting component. The products were sedimented on 10 to 34 per cent linear sucrose gradients (containing polysome buffer) for 4 hours at 25,000 rev./min. (SW25.1 swinging bucket rotor, model L-2 ultracentrifuge, 3°). (1) ——, optical density of the purified monomer (74 S); (2) ●---●, radioactivity of the 50 S particle; (3) ○---○ radioactivity of 37 S RNA after reaction with ribosomes (from cells treated with interferon); (4) ----, optical density, 37 S viral RNA + ribosomes from cells exposed to interferon. (1) and (2) were centrifuged together in one gradient, (3) and (4) in another at the same time as (1) and (2).

from such preparations depend upon the concentration of Mg++ in the buffer used, as shown in Figs. 6 and 7. With a stepwise lowering of the Mg^{2+} concentration, a decrease in the sedimentation value of the monomer occurs, presumably due to swelling of the spherical particle (Tashiro and Siekevitz, 1965). Subsequent experiments were performed in RSB at 1×10^{-3} M-Mg++. Polysome patterns obtained from such preparations are

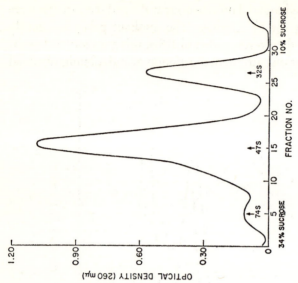

FIG. 7. Sedimentation of the large and small subunit in the presence of EDTA. The transformation of the monomer into 47 *S* and 32 *S* subunits was studied, using EDTA as the chelating agent (see text). When the monomer is finally dissociated, the subunits demonstrate a mass ratio of 2·0:1. The sample was studied on a 10 to 34 per cent sucrose gradient (containing 0·01M-EDTA, 0·01M-tris, 0·2M-NaCl) by centrifugation at 25,000 rev./min. (SW25.1 swinging bucket rotor, model L-2 ultracentrifuge, 3°) for 18 hours. ——, optical density.

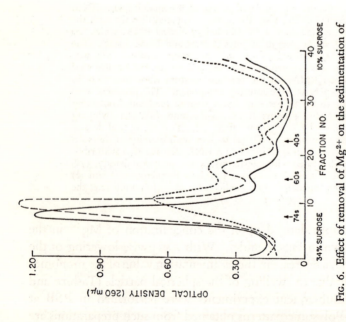

FIG. 6. Effect of removal of Mg²⁺ on the sedimentation of the monomer and its transformation into subunits. Mg²⁺-purified particles were studied in RSB with varying concentrations of Mg²⁺. Samples were sedimented at 22,000 rev./min. (SW25.1 swinging bucket rotor, Model L-2 ultracentrifuge, 3°) on 10 to 34 per cent linear sucrose gradients (with RSB and varying Mg²⁺ concentrations) for 16 hours. The collection of samples is described in the text. ——, 3 × 10⁻³M-Mg²⁺; ——, 1 × 10⁻³M-Mg²⁺; ‥‥, 3 × 10⁻³M-Mg²⁺; ----, 1 × 10⁻⁴M-Mg²⁺.

similar to those of polysomes concentrated by sedimentation through dense sucrose, as seen in Fig. 8. By direct comparison, it was demonstrated that polysomes, as well as monomers and their subunits, were quantitatively recovered by Mg^{++} precipitation.

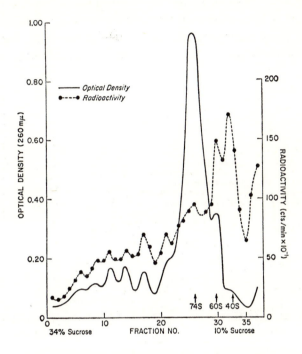

FIG. 8. Polysome profiles after Mg^{2+} purification. Mouse cells were pulsed with [³H]uridine (0·2 μc/ml.) for 30 minutes and rapidly cooled. Polysomes were precipitated from the post-mitochondrial fraction with 0·07M-$MgCl_2$ as described in the text. The product was sedimented on 10 to 34 per cent linear sucrose gradients (containing RSB buffer) for 3 hours at 25,000 rev./min. (SW25.1 swinging bucket rotor, model L-2 ultracentrifuge, 3°). The collection of samples is described in the text.

Mengo virus is not concentrated by Mg^{++} precipitation and under these conditions, 95–98 per cent of the free virus is thus eliminated from the polysome preparation.

Measurements made in the analytical ultracentrifuge indicated that the monomer sediments at 74 S_{20} in 0· 1 M-NaCl, 0·01M-tris (pH 7· 4), and 0· 003M-$MgCl_2$. In the same solvent with the Mg^{2+} concentration adjusted to 0· 0005 M the subunits sediment at 47 S_{20} and 32 S_{20}.

LOCALIZATION OF INPUT MENGO RNA INTO 50 S AND 240 S
STRUCTURES

To determine whether the parental viral RNA was incorporated into a polysome, L cells were exposed to radioactive Mengo virus (as before) and polysomes were prepared by the Mg^{++} precipitation procedure.

Figs. 9 and 10 present data comparing the processing of the labelled input viral RNA in interferon-treated and control mouse cells. Fig. 9 demonstrates a polysome pattern in cells infected for 45 minutes, and Fig. 10 a

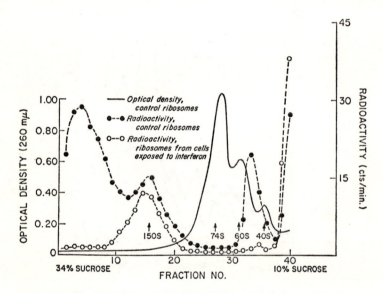

FIG. 9. The assembly of the Mengo-specific polysome. Ribosomes were prepared by Mg^{2+} precipitation at 45 minutes post-infection with radioactive Mengo virus. The ribosomal pellet was resuspended in RSB, clarified by centrifugation at 10,000 g for 10 minutes and analysed on a 10 to 34 per cent linear sucrose gradient (containing RSB) by centrifugation at 25,000 rev./min. for 4 hours (SW25.1 rotor, model L-2 ultracentrifuge, 3°).

pattern in cells infected for 2·5 hours. In the polysome profiles of control infected cells, three peaks of radioactivity are discernible, at 240 S, 150 S, and 50 S. Fig. 10 reveals that the 240 S and the 50 S components are RNase-sensitive, while the 150 S material, the residual free virus, is not. At the earlier time period, in the interferon-treated cells, there is very little incorporation of the radioactive Mengo virus RNA into either the 50 S or 240 S particles (Fig. 9). After 2·5 hours of infection there is still no evidence in the interferon-treated culture of a 50 S particle bearing the viral RNA, but the labelled RNA has entered the 240 S complex to a significant extent. Only a 40–60 per cent inhibition in formation of the 240 S polysome exists at this time (Fig. 10).

Any biochemical mechanism which explains the action of interferon must relate quantitatively to the amount of inhibition of virus growth. The interferon-induced inhibition of viral RNA association with the 50 S particle is of the same magnitude as the inhibition of virus growth (> 99 per

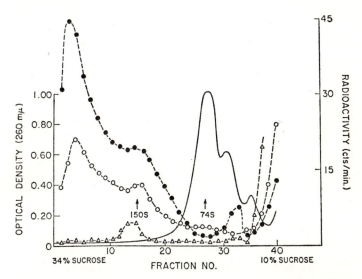

FIG. 10. The Mengo-specific polysome at 2·5 hours after infection. Ribosomes were prepared from cells infected with radioactive virus for 2·5 hours as described under Fig. 9 and in the text. The products were sedimented on 10 to 34 per cent linear sucrose gradients (containing RSB) for 4 hours at 25,000 rev./min. (SW25.1 swinging bucket rotor, model L-2 ultracentrifuge at 3°). ———, optical density of control ribosomes; ●---●, radioactivity of control ribosomes; ○---○, radioactivity of ribosomes from cells exposed to interferon; △---△, control ribosomes incubated with bovine pancreatic RNase (1 μg./ml., 0°c for 15 minutes in RSB).

cent). However, there is no evidence of protein or RNA synthetic activity on this subunit which might be related to the degree of inhibition of virus growth. The reduction in parental RNA incorporation into the 240 S polysome appears insufficient to be the direct and immediate explanation of the inhibition of virus yield. The function of the 240 S complex found in infected cells was then considered.

THE 240 S POLYSOME AS A SITE OF VIRAL PROTEIN SYNTHESIS

Mengo infection of mouse L cells rapidly stops normal protein synthesis (Franklin and Baltimore, 1962). Fig. 11 demonstrates the virus-induced termination of cellular protein synthesis, as well as the fact that by 3·5 hours after infection viral proteins are being rapidly synthesized. These data were obtained by direct use of a post-mitochondrial supernatant fraction of cells pulse-labelled with [³H]valine for one hour. Free (ribosome-dissociated) labelled viral proteins and those incorporated into virus conceal any resolution of the 240 S particle. The data of Fig. 12 were obtained from a similar

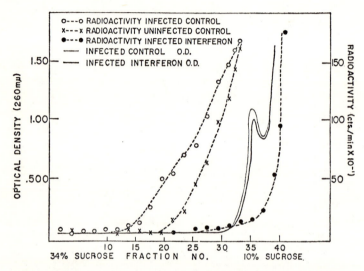

FIG. 11. Effect of interferon on protein synthesis by Mengo-virus-infected cells. L cells were exposed to actinomycin D (2 μg./ml.) for 1 hour, concentrated by centrifugation, exposed to Mengo virus (multiplicity of infection=20) for 30 minutes at room temperature, resuspended in Eagle's Basal Medium (BME) containing actinomycin D (2 μg./ml.) for 2 hours, centrifuged and suspended in valine-free BME for 20 minutes at 37°, and exposed to [³H]valine, (1 μc/ml.) for 1 hour. The cells were centrifuged, washed twice with phosphate-buffered saline, and disrupted in RSB with a Dounce homogenizer. The supernatant fluid after sedimentation at 14,000 g for 10 minutes was applied to a 10 to 34 per cent sucrose gradient in RSB, and sedimented for 60 minutes at 25,000 rev./min. O.D., optical density.

experiment in which infected cells were pulse-labelled with [³H]valine for only ten minutes, and polysomes were purified by Mg⁺⁺ precipitation, which eliminated most of the virus and free proteins. A small but definite peak of radioactive polypeptide on polysomes sediments broadly at about 240 S; no evidence of protein synthesis is detectable in gradients from interferon-treated infected cells. Assays for RNA-dependent RNA polymerase, with the technique of Plagemann and Swim (1966), show in particular that this protein is not made in interferon-treated cells. Addition of EDTA to the polysome preparation completely eliminates the faster-sedimenting radioactivity, probably reflecting the dependence of this complex on Mg^{++} for its stability.

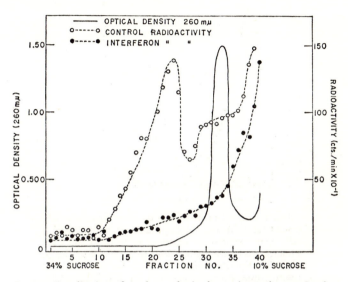

FIG. 12. Localization of newly synthesized protein on the 240 S polysome. Conditions as for Fig. 11 except that cells (2×10^6/ml.) were pulse-labelled for 10 minutes with [³H]valine (5 μc/ml.) in valine-free medium. The ribosomes were precipitated from the post-mitochondrial supernatant fluid by Mg^{2+}, resuspended in RSB, and sedimented through a 10 to 34 per cent sucrose gradient for 90 minutes at 25,000 rev./min.

LOCALIZATION OF PROGENY RNA MOLECULES ON THE 240 S PARTICLE

Newly synthesized RNA molecules are also localized on the 240 S and 50 S particles (Fig. 13). Although the data of Fig. 13 were obtained with cells pulse-labelled for one hour, labelling for as brief a time as five minutes gives comparable results. Therefore, new viral RNA molecules are either synthesized on the 240 S component, or transferred to it very rapidly after synthesis. It should be noted from Fig. 13 that newly made viral RNA also passes through the 50 S particle, presumably during its assembly into a 240 S polysome. RNase treatment (0·1 μg./ml. for 10 minutes at 2°c) of these polysome fractions before gradient analysis removes the 240 S and 50 S radioactive peaks. Also, treatment of the polysomes with EDTA before centrifugation removes the polysome and subunit-bound newly labelled RNA. The effectiveness of the stripping off of Mg^{2+} is reflected in the quantitative conversion of the 74 S monomer into its subunits (Fig. 7).

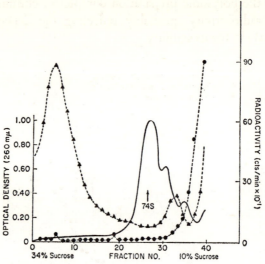

FIG. 13. Effect of interferon on association of newly made viral RNA with the 240 S and 50 S components. L cells were exposed to actinomycin D (2 µg./ml.) for 1 hour, concentrated by centrifugation, exposed to Mengo virus (multiplicity of infection=20) for 30 minutes at room temperature, resuspended in BME containing actinomycin D (2 µg./ml.) for 2·5 hours, and exposed to [³H]uridine for 1 hour. Polysomes were prepared from the post-mitochondrial supernatant fluid by Mg^{2+} precipitation, and sedimented for 4 hours at 25,000 rev./min. on a 10 to 34 per cent sucrose gradient in RSB.
——— optical density; ▲----▲ radioactivity, polysomes from normally infected cells; ●---● radioactivity, polysomes from infected cells that had been pre-exposed to interferon.

THE INTERACTION OF TEMPLATE RNAS WITH RIBOSOMES *in vitro*

Experiments performed with an *in vitro* system confirm and amplify the *in vivo* observations just discussed (Carter and Levy, 1967*a*, *b*). To determine whether the inhibition of the viral RNA-ribosome interaction represents the primary action of interferon, or whether it is a reflection of some earlier alteration, we compared the interaction of viral and cell RNAs with purified ribosomes from control and interferon-treated cells. Interferon does not affect the rate of macromolecular RNA and protein synthesis in uninfected cells (Levy and Merigan, 1966). Ribosomes from interferon-treated cells should therefore be able to make functionally important distinctions between cell and viral messenger molecules if the decreased *in vivo* binding of viral RNA is to be attributed to altered ribosomes.

Rapidly-labelled ^{32}P cell RNA was prepared by exposing L cells in suspension culture (phosphate-free medium) to [^{32}P]phosphate (3 μc/ml.) for 15 minutes. The RNA was extracted with phenol and sodium dodecyl

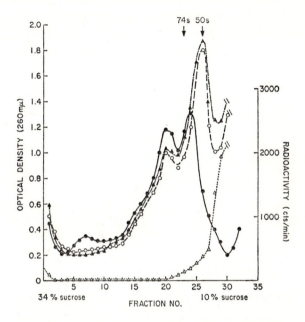

FIG. 14. Association of rapidly labelled RNA with ribosomes from normal cells and those exposed to interferon. Two of the reaction mixtures contained 200 μg. of ^{32}P-labelled RNA and 1·2 mg. of ribosomes; a third tube (control) contained 200 μg. of ^{32}P-labelled RNA but no ribosomes. The mixtures were incubated for 45 minutes at 0°c and layered over linear sucrose gradients (10 to 34 per cent). The tubes were sedimented for 3 hours at 25,000 rev./min. ●----●, optical density of normal ribosomes; ○---○, radioactivity of cellular [^{32}P]RNA and normal ribosomes; ▲---▲, radioactivity of cellular [^{32}P]RNA and ribosomes from cells exposed to interferon; △---△, radioactivity of cellular [^{32}P]RNA sedimented without ribosomes.

sulphate in the presence of polyvinyl sulphate and bentonite (Scherrer and Darnell, 1962). The alcohol-precipitated RNA was passed through Sephadex G25. As shown by sucrose density gradient centrifugation, the radioactivity of this RNA was polydisperse, sedimenting between 4 and 45 S.

Mengo virus RNA, labelled with ^{32}P, was obtained by infecting L cells with Mengo virus in the presence of actinomycin D and ^{32}P. After eight hours of infection, RNA was extracted from the infected cells and the 37 S viral RNA isolated by density gradient centrifugation.

Ribosomes were prepared from control cells, and from cells exposed for 16 hours to 10 units/ml. of mouse interferon. Ribosomes were incubated with the labelled cell or viral RNA for 45 minutes at 0–2° in polysome buffer (0·05 M-tris-HCl at pH 7·8, 0·025 M-KCl, 0·005 M-MgCl$_2$, 0·006 M-mercaptoethanol), adjusted to 0·005 M-NH$_4$Cl and 0·25 M-sucrose (Carter

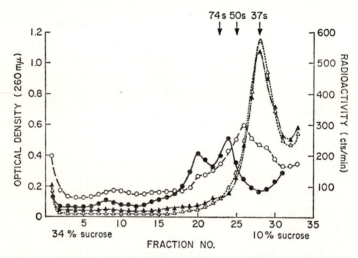

FIG. 15. Interaction of viral RNA with ribosomes from normal cells and those exposed to interferon. Reaction mixtures contained 100 μg. of viral [^{32}P]RNA and unlabelled ribosomal RNA, and 0·6 mg. of ribosomes. Ribosomes from normal cells and those exposed to interferon (10 units/ml. for 16 hours) were reacted with viral RNA at 0°c for 45 minutes. ●---●, optical density of normal ribosomes; ○---○, radioactivity of normal ribosomes and viral [^{32}P]RNA; ▲---▲, radioactivity of ribosomes from cells exposed to interferon and viral [^{32}P]RNA; △---△, radioactivity of viral [^{32}P]RNA sedimented without ribosomes.

and Levy, 1967a, b). The reaction mixture was examined on 10–34 per cent sucrose gradients containing the polysome buffer.

Fig. 14 presents data obtained from the interaction of both types of ribosomes with rapidly labelled cell RNA. Under these conditions of centrifugation, unreacted cell RNA does not descend far into the gradient. Ribosomes from control and interferon-treated cells bind the cell RNA in an indistinguishable way.

However, when labelled viral RNA is incubated with the two types of ribosomes, large differences in the fraction of stable complexes are detectable (Fig. 15). Control ribosomes bind viral RNA, in a quantitatively important way, with peaks of association observed at 100 S and 50 S, while the ribosomes from cells which have been exposed to interferon form no detectable complexes. The optical density profiles do not suggest that many 45 S ribosomal subunits are available for binding; apparently there is a strong preference for binding to this particle even over intact monomers. Steady-state labelled cell RNA, in which virtually all of the label is in the two ribosomal RNA species and transfer RNA, does not interact with ribosomes under these conditions. Thus the ribosome-template RNA complexes formed *in vitro* appear analogous to those assembled during polysome formation *in vivo*.

THE TRANSLATION OF VIRAL RNA MOLECULES *in vitro*

The enzyme fraction obtained at pH 5 (Keller and Zamecnik, 1956) from cells exposed to interferon supports the translation of Mengo RNA with normal ribosomes (Carter and Levy, unpublished). Combinations of these enzyme fractions and ribosome preparations from normal cells and those exposed to interferon demonstrate that the restriction in translation of Mengo RNA is a property of the ribosomal particle only. These critical functional tests, by comparing simultaneously the translation of homopolymers, endogenous messenger and viral RNA templates, thus confirm the ability of the ribosomes to be selective in the formation of functional complexes with different types of RNA molecules.

Thus, *in vitro* as well as *in vivo*, ribosomes from interferon-treated cells, while able to interact with and translate normal cellular templates, are greatly restricted in their ability to form functional complexes with animal viral RNA.

DISCUSSION

The 40 S particle may be utilized by both DNA and RNA animal viruses, as well as mammalian cells, in the assembly of polysomes. Nascent vaccinia messenger RNA (Joklik and Becker, 1965) and rapidly-labelled RNA of rat liver (Henshaw, Revel and Hiatt, 1965) interact with sub-ribosomal particles during polysome assembly. The present data suggest that the *input* viral RNA in the Mengo-L cell system attaches to a similar particle before assembly into a viral specific structure. Godson and Sinsheimer (1967) have recently demonstrated that the RNA of ^{32}P-labelled bacteriophage MS 2 forms an association with the smaller of the ribosomal subunits as one of the earliest interactions of the viral genome with the host cell. The kinetics and the conversion process of the input phage RNA into a polysome-bound form are similar to those reported here with an animal virus. For instance, with time the input Mengo virus RNA is converted from the 50 S particle to the 240 S polysome (Figs. 9 and 10). After 45 minutes of infection, 25 per cent of the ribosome-bound viral RNA sediments at 50 S, while at two hours only 10 per cent of the ribosome-associated RNA is attached to the 50 S particle. At 45 minutes post-infection, 70 to 75 per cent of the input virus remains uneclipsed, as previously noted by Homma and Graham (1964).

The 240 S complex appears to be a polysome, perhaps with an additional function. It is present in post-mitochondrial fractions, precipitates with Mg^{++}, and is sensitive to the action of RNase and EDTA, thus depending upon RNA and Mg^{2+} ion for its stability. In addition this complex may also be the site of synthesis of progeny viral RNA, although the possibility that viral RNA is synthesized elsewhere and rapidly transferred to the polysome has not been rigorously excluded. We have not observed any other virus-specific structure in L cells infected with Mengo virus. In a previous study of this system (Tobey, 1964) the labelled input virus was all found broadly distributed in polysome gradients, but examination of the patterns presented suggest that the bulk of the radioactivity observed represented free uneclipsed virus, sedimenting at about 150 S.

A poliovirus RNA replication complex has recently been described (Girard, Baltimore and Darnell, 1967). This is a complex similar in size (250 S) to the polysome seen in the Mengo system, but ribosomes are not responsible for its rapid sedimentation, since the complex is EDTA- and puromycin-insensitive. Both the polio and Mengo RNA polymerase activities are on membraneous structures sedimentable at 20,000 g for 30 minutes in the absence of detergent (DOC). Treatment with detergent may artificially partition the polio polysome from the replication complex. Late in infection the polio polysome is transformed from a 380 S to a 220 S structure which is still capable of making the same spectrum of protein molecules (Summers and Maizel, 1967).

Interferon blocks the *in vivo* and *in vitro* translation of messenger RNA of several other animal viruses. Messenger RNA transcribed from vaccinia virus DNA does not enter the polysome in HeLa cells exposed to this protein (Joklik and Merigan, 1966). In an *in vitro* protein-synthesizing system requiring Sindbis virus RNA and chicken ribosomes, translation of the viral genome is also inhibited, although stable viral RNA-ribosome complexes are formed (Marcus and Salb, 1966). This latter *in vitro* system resembles to some extent the results reported here *in vivo* (Fig. 9).

The molecular nature of the recognition of viral RNA by the ribosome, as well as the nature of the non-functional and functional bonds between template RNA and ribosomes, remain to be determined. Although other possibilities are not excluded, attachment of viral RNA to the 40 S ribosomal subunit may be an obligatory step for the formation of a functional polysome. Whether animal viral and mammalian cell messages differ in their initiating codons (Noll, 1966; Summers and Maizel, 1967) or possess distinguishable differences in secondary structure is as yet unknown.

SUMMARY

Previous work from this and other laboratories demonstrated that the locus of antiviral action of interferon is an event that occurs very early during virus replication—so early as to suggest that the infecting virus particle may be involved. Radioactive Mengo virus was used to study the early intracellular processing of the RNA of infecting virus particles, and the effect of interferon on such processing. In normally infected L cells, the Mengo RNA attaches rapidly to the smaller ribosomal subunit, just prior to the RNA being incorporated into a functional viral polysome. The polysome is the site of synthesis of viral proteins, including the viral RNA polymerase. Progeny viral RNA molecules are also found on this polysome, probably having been made there. In cells that had been rendered resistant to Mengo virus by exposure to interferon, the parental viral RNA never attaches to the ribosomal subunit. A pseudo-polysome is formed slowly and to a lesser extent than in normally infected cells. The polysome-like structure formed in interferon-treated cells is non-functional in that it is severely restricted in its ability to synthesize viral RNA and viral proteins, including the viral RNA polymerase. It is suggested that passage of the viral RNA through the 40 S ribosome subunit may be a necessary step for the formation of a functional polysome.

These data are supported by studies *in vitro*. Ribosomes and their subunits from normal cells bind and translate cellular messenger RNA as well as Mengo viral RNA. Ribosomes from interferon-treated cells, on the other hand, while reacting normally with cellular messenger RNA, neither bind to nor translate Mengo viral RNA.

It follows, then, that the action of interferon is to lead to the formation of altered ribosomes and subunits which selectively reject viral RNA, though continuing to accept cellular messenger RNAs.

REFERENCES

ATTARDI, G., and SMITH, J. (1962). *Cold Spring Harb. Symp. quant. Biol.*, **27**, 271.
BARON, S., and LEVY, H. B. (1966). *A. Rev. Microbiol.*, **20**, 291.
CARTER, W. A., and LEVY, H. B. (1967a). *Science*, **155**, 1254.
CARTER, W. A., and LEVY, H. B. (1967b). *Archs Biochem. Biophys.*, **120**, 563–570.
FRANKLIN, R., and BALTIMORE, D. (1962). *Cold Spring Harb. Symp. quant. Biol.*, **27**, 175.
GIRARD, M., BALTIMORE, D., and DARNELL, J. E. (1967). *J. molec. Biol.*, **24**, 59.

GODSON, G. N., and SINSHEIMER, R. L. (1967). *J. molec. Biol.*, **23**, 495.
HENSHAW, E., REVEL, M., and HIATT, H. (1965). *J. molec. Biol.*, **14**, 241.
HOMMA, M., and GRAHAM, A. F. (1964). *J. Bact.*, **89**, 64.
JOKLIK, W. K., and BECKER, Y. (1965). *J. molec. Biol.*, **13**, 511.
JOKLIK, W. K., and MERIGAN, T. C. (1966). *Proc. natn. Acad. Sci. U.S.A.*, **56**, 558.
KELLER, E. B., and ZAMECNIK, P. C. (1956). *J. biol. Chem*, **221**, 45.
LEVY, H. B. (1964). *Virology*, **22**, 575.
LEVY, H. B., and MERIGAN, T. C. (1966). *Proc. Soc. exp. Biol. Med.*, **121**, 53.
MARCUS, P. I., and SALB, J. M. (1966). *Virology*, **30**, 502.
McCORMICK, W., and PENMAN, S. (1967). *Virology*, **31**, 135.
NOLL, H. (1966). *Science*, **151**, 1241.
PLAGEMANN, P. G. W., and SWIM, H. E. (1966). *J. Bact.*, **91**, 2327.
SCHERRER, K., and DARNELL, J. E. (1962). *Biochem. biophys. Res. Commun.*, **7**, 486.
SONNABEND, J., MARTIN, E., MÉCS, E., and FANTES, K. (1967). *J. gen. Virol.*, **1**, 41.
SUMMERS, D., and MAIZEL, J. (1967). *Virology*, **31**, 550.
TAKANAMI, M. (1960). *Biochim. biophys. Acta*, **39**, 318.
TASHIRO, Y., and SIEKEVITZ, P. (1965). *J. molec. Biol.*, **11**, 149.
TOBEY, R. A. (1964). *Virology*, **23**, 23.
WETTSTEIN, D. F., STAEHELIN, T., and NOLL, H. (1963). *Nature, Lond.*, **197**, 430.

DISCUSSION

Mécs: Do you get breakdown of Mengo RNA during binding in the *in vitro* system?

Levy: Not much in the *in vitro* system but some breakdown occurs *in vivo*. The ribosomes we use *in vitro* have been purified. There is still some RNase there but a lot of the free RNase has been eliminated.

Martin: You mentioned the 50 S particle in the polysome gradients of infected cells and said that it was possibly a 40 S ribosomal subunit plus the virus RNA. Could it be equally well explained by the effect that M. Girard and D. Baltimore have described (1966. *Proc. natn. Acad. Sci. U.S.A.*, **56**, 999), of the cell sap containing a protein which increases the sedimentation of viral RNA to values of this order?

Levy: Mengo RNA sediments the same in all the buffers we studied—at 37 S. This was true for RSB, tris, and some other buffers. It still sediments at 37 S in the presence of interferon-type ribosomes. Baltimore's effect dealt with cell sap. In our experiments no cell sap is present: we are using precipitated purified preparations. The polysomes were recovered by magnesium precipitation. ^{32}P-labelled Mengo RNA and the 50 S particles were sedimented in the same gradient; they separated from each other by several fractions.

Fantes: What concentration of magnesium do you use?

Levy: We ended up adding 1×10^{-3} M, but the actual concentration might be as high as $1 \cdot 5 \times 10^{-3}$ M. The RSB that we use contains 1×10^{-3} M-magnesium, but our ribosomes are prepared by precipitation with $0 \cdot 07$ M-magnesium, so there may still be some magnesium present in the pellet which would bring the concentration up a little.

Joklik: I am heartened by your conviction that this association with the 40 S particle is real. We first saw this with vaccinia messenger RNA (Joklik, W. K., and Becker, Y. [1965]. *J. molec. Biol.*, **13**, 511). Then David Baltimore fully confirmed in our laboratory his finding that the sedimentation rate of polio RNA or vaccinia messenger RNA is increased by the addition of cell sap which contains no particles. You seem to have ruled this out by your experiments and you still find the association with 40 S particles.

Levy: The only cell sap in these preparations is any that may be wetting the ribosomes. When the ribosomes from the interferon-treated cells are incubated, we don't see the 37 S material sedimenting at 50 S. Of course we haven't rigidly demonstrated that this is an association of the RNA with a ribosomal subunit.

Joklik: Early in your one-hour experiments you had nothing heavier than whole virus particles in interferon-treated cells—the peak was at 150 S. The radioactivity only went up right at the top of the gradient. Was there free messenger RNA up there or only soluble material? It seemed to me that there could almost have been a marked delay in uncoating of the virus.

Levy: We are worried about that too. If one looks carefully at the curves in the heavy part of the gradient, one can see some viral RNA heavier than 150 S in the normally infected cultures, but it is masked by the large 150 S peak. I can't really rule out a delay in uncoating, although we have done some book-keeping experiments where we followed the radioactivity in all the various subcellular fractions that one gets before this point. About the same amount of acid-precipitable radioactivity is present in the post-mitochondrial fluid in both interferon-treated and control cells. The difference comes in the amount of viral RNA that is ribosomal-bound. This is a fairly small portion, and of the total material that winds up in the post-mitochondrial fluid, possibly only 15 per cent is ribosomal-bound. So it would really be very difficult to see if there is any difference in the amount of uncoating. We are not able to pick up free 37 S RNA in these gradient studies.

Stoker: Which RNAs do not combine with ribosomes from interferon-treated cells?

Levy: We tried TMV in a translating system, not in a binding system. Ribosomes from interferon-treated cells translate the TMV RNA as well or as poorly as the control ribosomes did. Polyuridylic acid is also translated equally well by both types of ribosomes.

Stoker: Are there any interferon-resistant variants of the sensitive viruses?

Levy: Some strains of Mengo are fairly resistant to interferon, but the Mengo strain we use is extremely sensitive. We get 99·9 per cent inhibition of virus growth.

Chany: Lwoff (personal communication) tried to select out interferon-resistant mutants from poliovirus populations, but as far as I know it has not been possible to demonstrate such a variant.

GENERAL DISCUSSION

Baron: Early viral messenger RNA is apparently prevented from functioning in the interferon-treated cell. What happens with the late viral messenger RNA?

Joklik: There isn't any, because there is no progeny DNA.

Baron: But in virus-infected cells two things are going on: the virus is being replicated and the cell gets ready to make interferon and the antiviral protein. In those viruses which grow slowly it is possible that there is sufficient time for the antiviral protein to be made late in the virus growth cycle. Would the antiviral protein then interfere with the functioning of a late viral messenger RNA?

Joklik: It might be possible, with adenovirus in particular, to add interferon to an infected cell in a system which does not cause inhibition of host-cell RNA synthesis. The trouble is that in most systems host-cell RNA synthesis is also stopped at about the time viral DNA replication starts. There might be a short period in which host-cell messenger RNA as well as late viral messenger RNA could be transcribed, but it would probably not be much more than an hour or so. These conditions would be necessary to answer your question, Dr. Baron.

Wagner: In some old experiments we infected cells with eastern equine encephalomyelitis virus and then added interferon in large amounts to the infected cell cultures (Wagner, R. R. [1961]. *Virology*, **13**, 323). The cells were infected at a multiplicity which gave a one-step growth curve. The interferon had a partial effect for three to four hours after infection of the cells. In other words some virus had actually been formed inside the cell before treatment with interferon. We added interferon and got a reduction in final virus yields of some 80–90 per cent, which was probably real. I suppose that some late product made in the cycle of viral replication, presumably protein, might have been inhibited.

Joklik: If large amounts of interferon were used and these were relatively impure preparations, one could not be sure the effect was not caused by something other than interferon.

Tyrrell: Another problem here is that you can't be sure that you have got truly synchronous infection—some of the particles may have been starting to multiply an hour or so after you started your incubation.

Wagner: We were certainly beginning to get a rising titre which tapered off after interferon was added. Lockart did virtually the same experiment with exactly the same results (Lockart, R. Z., Sreevalsan, T., and Horn, B. [1962]. *Virology*, **18**, 493).

Tyrrell: What about one of these viruses like SV5 which goes on pouring out of monkey kidney cells for days? The virus doesn't seem to damage the cells seriously because they remain intact.

Wagner: They don't make any interferon.

Tyrrell: But they might be susceptible to interferon.

Chany: They might even block the action of interferon.

Baron: Perhaps another reason for being concerned with the late viral messenger is the cascade effect which was mentioned. It has been pointed out that the infectivity is decreased more than some of the viral synthetic functions. Perhaps a contributing factor to the disproportionately large inhibition of infectivity is that not only is the early viral messenger RNA depressed but also the later messenger RNAs which are also essential for viral replication.

Merigan: With the TRIC agents interferon sensitivity extends to late in the cycle, apparently to 18 to 24 hours after the agent has infected the cell. If they do have a messenger RNA species that uses the host ribosomes instead of their own, it is one that apparently acts late in their cycle, which lasts anywhere from 48 to 72 hours.

Wagner: Is this species-specific?

Merigan: Yes, it is. We also used interferon purified by column chromatography to confirm that the anti-TRIC action was due to interferon, although it is 100-fold less active than against VSV. TRIC agents are an interesting tool for the study of interferon action. One can follow their replication within the cell with fluorescent antibody and electron microscopy. In contrast to viruses, you can really see the agent most of the time during its replicative cycle.

Chany: Does the TRIC agent multiply only in the cell?

Merigan: Yes, it is an obligate intracellular parasite.

Stoker: The rickettsiae have thick walls and it would be very difficult to see how messenger could get onto the cell ribosomes.

Levy: There may be some antiviral protein not bound to ribosomes which somehow gets into the TRIC agent and works there.

Chany: I don't quite understand the species specificity. The TRIC agent itself is not of the same species as the cell in which it multiplies.

Merigan: The action of interferon against these agents is species specific in the sense that the cells in which the replication is to be blocked must be treated by interferon prepared in the same cell species.

Joklik: Impure preparations of interferon contain a fair amount of carbohydrate. Is it possible to inactivate purified interferon by some sort of enzyme acting on carbohydrate?

Fantes: We have not tried any carbohydrate enzymes. All the interferons are inactivated by proteolytic enzymes, according to the literature. Crude chick interferon, according to Isaacs and colleagues, is not inactivated by periodate, which is supposed to be fairly specific for carbohydrates, but other interferons, including mouse and possibly human, are inactivated by periodate. I am not sure whether periodate can be considered to be absolutely specific for carbohydrates. For instance, performic acid breaks disulphide bonds, and possibly periodate does something similar; the moment disulphide bonds are broken, by oxidation or reduction, all interferon activity disappears.

Joklik: At the moment there are a number of interferons of different sizes, but these do not fall into any regular molecular weight series. If interferon is adsorbed onto some sort of carrier molecule, this might explain its heterogeneous electrophoretic behaviour, its odd behaviour on Sephadex chromatography, where the bands seem to be much broader than for pure proteins, and so on.

Fantes: Nagano postulates that interferon is an active polysaccharide that can associate with quite a number of proteins, thus explaining the different specificities (Nagano, Y., Kojima, Y., and Kanashiro, R. S. [1966]. *Jap. J. exp. Med.*, **36**, 477–480). Even if one doesn't accept this, one could perhaps more readily accept that it associates with proteins of different molecular weights, giving rise to a series of interferons of different molecular weights (Nagano, Y., Kojima, Y., Shirasaka, M., and Haneishi, T. [1965]. *Jap. J. exp. Med.*, **35**, 133–140), though I myself am doubtful even about this.

Wagner: These presumably different molecular species of interferon in rabbit cell systems could certainly be attributable to carrier proteins or other biologically inactive molecules. If so, however, they do seem to associate in a reasonably regular way, because the results of Sephadex diffusion are relatively reproducible. It is certainly a possibility that we are dealing with aggregates; this would explain the varieties of presumably different molecular species. Dr. Merigan has mentioned this several times in his papers.

Burke: One still needs new protein synthesis to make interferon, and puromycin and *p*-fluorophenylalanine block its formation. So if you are going to talk about carrier proteins then you have to say that you make a new carrier protein at the time when interferon is formed, and this becomes a semantic difference from saying that interferon is partially protein.

Ho: The essential protein synthesized or required might be either a carrier or a molecule associated with interferon itself; or maybe something else is required to obtain the final product.

Martin: Perhaps you might be able to resolve some of these problems with the preparations that you showed us, Dr. Fantes—particularly the one where you had two major bands of protein and a diffuse region of biological activity. If this is due to multimolecular forms, or to the presence of proteins of the same molecular weight but with varying charges, you might be able to eliminate these effects by treating the interferon with sodium dodecyl sulphate. Alternatively, if you have dimers or trimers then it should be possible to dissociate it into monomers with urea. You might then find that all this material, which you now find spread over a large region, runs as a single band. Of course it would no longer have biological activity but may appear as a third sharp band.

Burke: We have done that and the biological activity is lost.

Fantes: Chick interferon is reported as being relatively stable to urea; mouse and others are not.

Merigan: We have done some electrophoresis of highly purified chick interferon in urea. Unfortunately it increases the number of protein bands observed—probably through dissociation of contaminant proteins into their subunits.

Levy: Urea wouldn't solve the unifying of the charge, would it?

Martin: Sodium dodecyl sulphate may do this, as the charge on the treated proteins is mostly due to the bound SDS. In theory, SDS-treated proteins should separate on the basis of molecular weight only.

Stoker: Dr. Wagner, why do you call your interferon constitutive? Do you get it when the macrophages are put in culture?

Wagner: The term is used as an analogy to inducible enzyme systems and bacteria mutants that synthesize enzymes without induction. Some of them may have a defect in the regulator gene that controls synthesis of the specific enzyme. In other words no repressor would operate in the cell. We harvest the cells from the peritoneal cavity in a fairly large volume of fluid, so that any interferon will be diluted, possibly below the levels of detection. But on a number of occasions we have found that we can get some interferon in the peritoneal fluid before we put the cells into culture; it is present at very low levels but it is there. The presumption, therefore, is that it is made continuously in the animal at these inflammatory sites, and that the cells will continue to make it when they are explanted into cultures, provided of course that they are given proper conditions, including a temperature of 37°. There may be contaminating bacterial endotoxin in the system which we used, but we are not aware that any inducing agent is present.

Stoker: But it is known in other tissue culture systems that as soon as cells are taken out of the body and placed in culture they change very rapidly—they produce new antigens, they lose pre-existing antigens and they alter in viral sensitivity. Even without any obvious inducing agent the change is very marked.

Wagner: This is certainly possible—in other words the inducer could be the process of removing the cells to a different environment, in which case we would not be entitled to say that they are in the constitutive state *in vivo*. Incidentally, as far as I can recall, we have not put the cells on siliconized surfaces so that they wouldn't attach; some interaction with glass might be producing this effect.

Baron: In one of your experiments you explanted cells from the peritoneum, treated them with actinomycin and showed that interferon was not produced. This finding suggests that the messenger RNA for interferon is produced after explantation.

Wagner: Messenger RNA might be produced all the time—but if we presume that it is stable, it must be stable for a few hours at any rate. When we explant the cells, hold the culture at 4° for a period of time, then add the actinomycin and bring the temperature up to 37°, no interferon is produced; but if we wait 30–60 minutes after bringing the culture to 37° and then add the actinomycin, the full amount of interferon is produced. I am not sure how to explain this or what went on before we took the cells out of the peritoneal cavity.

Finter: It seems a very attractive idea that macrophages may form interferon very readily, perhaps even continuously. After all, the macrophage is an important element in the body's defence against viruses—this is the cell that is mobilized in virus infections.

Wagner: The theory we hold at present is that there must be some function of these cells that can localize in areas of virus inflammatory responses. They might develop this function, e.g. interferon production, particularly if they are mobilized and then mature in some way so that the capacity to synthes izeinter-feron "spontaneously" comes about over a period of some days. This may be relevant to host defence mechanisms, but this is pure speculation.

Finter: There are now contradictions in the literature as to whether poly-morphonuclear cells form interferon or not. S. H. S. Lee and R. L. Ozere (1965. *Proc. Soc. exp. Biol. Med.*, **118**, 190) originally reported that polymorphs did form interferon on stimulation with Sendai virus, though in fact they tested production by preparations of mononuclear cells, and by mixed preparations of mononuclear cells and polymorphs. In your paper, Dr. Wagner, you said that your polymorph preparations also contained macrophages. Do you think that the macrophages present were probably responsible for the interferon production?

Wagner: The polymorphs form no interferon spontaneously. With viral induction there seems no question that the polymorphonuclear leucocytes make interferon less well. The acute exudates have many more cells, yet one gets lower yields of virus-induced interferon. The yields appear to be determined, in the counts that we have done, by the relative number of macrophages that we can count in these preparations. We cannot rule out polymorphs as inter-feron-synthesizing cells, but they are certainly far less efficient than macrophages. I think E. F. Wheelock (1966. *J. Bact.*, **92**, 1415) found that mononuclear cells (? lymphocytes) were the interferon-producing cells in cultures prepared from circulating human leucocytes.

Chany: Four or five years ago with Dr. Gresser we did some model experiments (Falcoff, E., Gresser, J., and Chany, C. [1964]. *C. r. hebd Séanc. Acad. Sci., Paris*, **258**, 1096–1098; Chany, C. [1964]. *Ciba Fdn Symp. Cellular Biology of Myxovirus Infections*, pp. 310–313, London: Churchill), using human white blood cells, and we tested their ability to protect a cell culture against poliovirus in a mixed culture system. We found that if we preinfected the leucocytes with a myxo-virus, then the leucocytes protected the tissue culture underneath against polio-virus, while uninfected leucocytes did not provide any protection. Poliovirus penetrates into the white cells only when leucocytes are kept for two to three days in a tissue culture medium. Consequently, in this experiment the challenge virus could not produce interferon. Since in this very sensitive test the uninfected WBC did not protect the cells, it seems likely that macrophages have to be infected before they can play a protective role.

Wagner: That is possible.

De Maeyer: We must realize that if we test for the induction of interferon *in vitro*, almost any cell will produce interferon under the right conditions. But however interesting *in vitro* studies may be, a more important problem in the physiopathology of virus infections is to know which cell produces interferon after intravenous injection of the virus. I suspect that this is a matter of clearance and depends on which cells first take up the virus particles. I think there is a basic difference *in vitro* and *in vivo*; *in vitro* it seems that one can safely say that any cell will produce interferon.

Baron: To my knowledge there is no evidence that the white cell and macrophages can produce interferon more rapidly or to a higher titre than many other cells. But leucocytes are mobile and perhaps they can, at the site of the virus infection, pick up the stimulus to produce interferon and migrate to other parts of the body. Production of interferon may then occur at distant sites, thereby disseminating the resistance from the local site of infection to the rest of the body.

Ho: This brings out the two possible mechanisms by which macrophages in the reticuloendothelial system may act. On the one hand, the macrophage itself may produce interferon and on the other, it may perform some function over and above that of producing interferon. This may be migration, as Dr. Baron says, but it may also be transmission of inducing information. There is actually some evidence on the role of the macrophages with respect to the first point. Y. Kono (1967. *Proc. Soc. exp. Biol. Med.*, **124**, 155) showed that leucocytes from bovine blood which turned into macrophages after 12 days of incubation produced, on a per cell basis, more interferon faster than other types of cells. This fits in very well with Professor Wagner's hypotheses.

Actually Kono's work is a little at variance with Wheelock's studies. Wheelock (in work not yet published) found that to get peripheral leucocytes to produce interferon optimally, it was very important to induce them as soon as possible after collecting them from blood.

Baron: Interferon may be produced as rapidly in some tissue culture systems as in white cell systems; for example in Chikungunya-infected chick embryo cells in culture, interferon will be produced within two hours of virus infection.

SOME DETERMINANTS OF THE INTERFERON-INDUCED ANTIVIRAL STATE

S. BARON, C. E. BUCKLER AND F. DIANZANI[*]

Laboratory of Biology of Viruses, National Institutes of Health, Bethesda, Maryland

SEVERAL factors have been observed to affect the cellular resistance to viruses which is associated with the interferon system. The interferon system may be composed of two distinct cellular proteins. The first is the interferon protein which is induced by viral infection (Isaacs, 1963) and which has been interpreted to react with cells to induce a second substance —the proposed intracellular, antiviral protein (Taylor, 1964). The present communication will consider some of the factors which influence the interferon-induced, second component of the interferon system—the proposed antiviral protein.

Interferon was produced in the serum of NIH-strain mice by intravenous injection of Newcastle disease virus (NDV), as previously described (Baron and Buckler, 1963). It was desirable to measure interferon-induced antiviral activity at a time close to experimental manipulations. For this purpose antiviral activity was determined by inhibition of yield of vesicular stomatitis virus, Indiana strain (VSV), in a single growth cycle as detailed below. Since interferon-induced inhibition of virus multiplication is thought to occur within one hour of infection (Levy, 1964), it is likely that this method determines antiviral activity close to the time of VSV infection. The plaque reduction assay was not used because multiple cycles of virus growth occur over an interval of several days between the time of virus challenge and the development of plaques. The unit of interferon is the highest dilution of the sample which decreases the yield of VSV by $0 \cdot 5$ $\log_{10}$ in a one-step growth cycle. The dose-response curve is shown in Fig. 1. For this assay of mouse interferon and for determination of the level of antiviral activity, primary mouse embryo cells were cultured in unstoppered 16×150 mm. tubes in $1 \cdot 0$ ml. of medium in a vertical position in a CO_2 incubator at $37°c$ until a confluent and non-dividing cell popula-

* Institute of Microbiology, University of Siena, Italy. At present a guest worker at the NIH under a fellowship from the Italian National Research Council, Group of Experimental Medicine.

tion developed. Thereafter cultures were maintained at 33° in Eagle's medium containing 10 per cent skim milk for three to five days. For the experiments three cultures per point were maintained in Eagle's medium containing 2 per cent foetal bovine serum and incubated at 37°. Dilutions of interferon were applied, and at the intervals described for each experiment the cultures were washed three times and challenged with 0·2 ml. of a VSV preparation containing an input of 20 plaque-forming units (p.f.u.) of VSV per cell. After one hour at 37° the cultures were rinsed four times, re-fed with maintenance medium and reincubated for 14 to 24 hours. Culture fluids were then harvested for virus plaque assay on

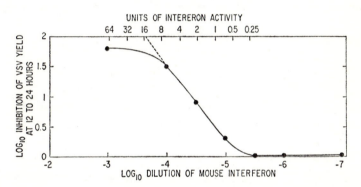

FIG. 1. Effect of concentration of mouse interferon on yield of VSV in a one-step growth cycle in primary cultures of mouse embryo cells. The curve was similar when cells were exposed to interferon for 8 to 30 hours before virus infection.

mouse L-cell cultures. Control experiments demonstrated that VSV yield was maximal at 12 hours, and virus titres remained constant through 30 hours. Fluids from the three replicate cultures were pooled before assay. Inhibition of 0·5 $\log_{10}$ yield of virus was found to be significant.

Rates of cellular protein or RNA synthesis were determined as follows. [^{14}C]Phenylalanine in phenylalanine-free medium or [^{3}H]uridine (New England Nuclear Corporation) were added to triplicate cultures of cells, to a concentration of 0·1 μc/ml. The cells were incubated at 37° for 45 minutes, the medium poured off, the cells washed three times with phosphate-buffered saline, and scraped into 1 ml. of 10 per cent trichloroacetic acid. The cells were washed twice with 10 per cent trichloroacetic acid, and dissolved in 1 ml. of 1 N-NaOH; 0·4 ml. was acidified, filtered onto a Schleicher and Schuell membrane filter and counted in a Packard Tricarb scintillation counter. Protein contents were determined on 0·2 ml. of the NaOH solution by the method of Lowry and co-workers (1951).

EFFECT OF TIME ON THE INDUCTION BY INTERFERON OF INTRACELLULAR ANTIVIRAL ACTIVITY

The time course of development of antiviral activity by cultured mouse embryo cells exposed to varying amounts of interferon is shown in Fig. 2. The level of antiviral activity is expressed as $\log_{10}$ inhibition of VSV yield. It may be seen that the time of onset of antiviral activity is directly correlated with units of interferon applied per millilitre. The rate of increase of antiviral activity at each dose level began to diminish at seven hours. These findings are similar to those reported for mouse L cells exposed to interferon (Lockart, 1963). After seven hours the level of antiviral activity at each dose level tended to remain more stable for the duration of the experi-

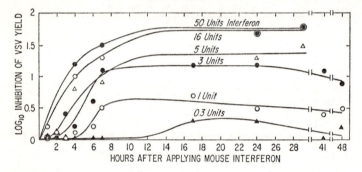

FIG. 2. Time course of development of resistance to multiplication of VSV, by cultures of mouse embryo cells treated with varying amounts of interferon.

ment. Previous studies have shown that in this experimental system the extracellular concentration of interferon does not detectably decrease during the development and maintenance of the antiviral state (Buckler, Baron and Levy, 1966; Youngner, Taube and Stinebring, 1966).

EFFECT OF DOSE OF INTERFERON ON ANTIVIRAL ACTIVITY

As may be seen in Figs. 1 and 2, the final level of resistance to virus was directly related to the dose of interferon up to 16 units of interferon/ml. The apparent lack of increased inhibition of VSV by doses greater than about 16 units/ml. was subsequently shown to be an artifact of the experimental procedure. As described earlier, interferon-treated cell cultures were challenged with a large virus inoculum, incubated for one hour and then washed four times. With this procedure the amount of virus residual from the inoculum was greater than the subsequent virus yield from cells treated with more than 16 units of interferon/ml. This leads to a levelling off of the upper portion of the curve in Fig. 1. With increased washing to remove more of the unadsorbed virus inoculum, inhibition of VSV was progressive through at least 100 units/ml. and is indicated by the dashed line in Fig. 1. These findings indicate that the degree of resistance to viruses by mouse embryo cells was directly proportional to the dose of interferon.

To help to determine whether resistance was dependent on the concentration or total amount of interferon, cultures were exposed to different volumes of interferon (0·1 ml. to 1·0 ml.) at a fixed concentration of

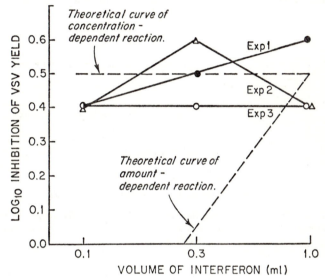

FIG. 3. Relationship of concentration of interferon and total amount of interferon to the degree of antiviral activity.

1 unit/ml. As may be seen in Fig. 3, the degree of antiviral activity was dependent on the concentration applied and was largely independent of the total amount of interferon. Similar concentration dependency has been observed independently by Youngner and Hallum (1966). However, the finding that the degree of antiviral activity is independent of amount has not been observed under all experimental conditions and will be considered later.

EFFECT OF CHANGING CONCENTRATION OF INTERFERON IN THE
EXTRACELLULAR FLUID ON ESTABLISHED ANTIVIRAL ACTIVITY

Experiments were done to determine whether the continued presence of the same concentration of interferon in the fluid was required for the maintenance of antiviral activity.

7*

Mouse embryo cells were treated with five units of interferon/ml. (enough to inhibit VSV yield $1 \cdot 2 \log_{10}$) for 24 hours at 37° so that their antiviral activity had reached a steady level (Fig. 4). A group of cultures was then washed five times with Earle's balanced salt solution to remove interferon and re-fed with Eagle's medium containing 2 per cent foetal bovine serum (maintenance medium). Fig. 4 shows that after removal of extracellular interferon there was no significant loss of antiviral activity during the first seven hours of continued incubation at 37° in the absence of interferon. Thereafter the level of antiviral activity decreased but at a

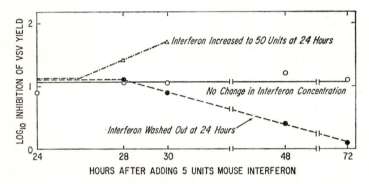

FIG. 4. Effect of changing the concentration of interferon on the pre-existing level of resistance to VSV by mouse embryo cultures pretreated with interferon.

slower rate than the initial rise in antiviral activity, as shown in Fig. 2. This rate of decline is comparable with previous reports of decline of antiviral activity after removal of interferon (Isaacs and Westwood, 1959; Lockart, 1963; Paucker and Cantell, 1963).

In the same experiment another group of cultures was also pretreated with five units of interferon for 24 hours. The interferon was then replaced by a tenfold higher concentration of interferon (50 units/ml.), and the level of antiviral activity was determined four and six hours later. It may be seen that the degree of antiviral activity increased at four and six hours (Fig. 4). The degree of activity at six hours was equal to that of cultures which had not been pretreated with interferon but were exposed to 50 units of interferon/ml. for six hours.

The findings demonstrate that prolonged maintenance of relatively stable antiviral activity required the continued presence of the same concentration of interferon in the extracellular fluid of mouse embryo cells.

EFFECT OF INHIBITION OF CELLULAR PROTEIN SYNTHESIS ON ESTABLISHED ANTIVIRAL ACTIVITY

To help to determine whether protein synthesis was required for maintenance of established antiviral activity, mouse embryo cells were treated with interferon (100 units/ml.) overnight at 37° so that antiviral activity had reached a constant level. Inhibitors of protein synthesis were added to the cultures, and at the intervals shown in Tables I and II the cultures were

TABLE I

EFFECT OF INHIBITION OF FUNCTIONAL CELLULAR PROTEIN SYNTHESIS BY FPA*
ON ESTABLISHED ANTIVIRAL ACTIVITY

Pretreatment for 24 hours	Second treatment	Time of 2nd treatment before wash + VSV challenge (hours)	Yield of VSV (log_{10})	Reduction of VSV yield (log_{10})	Percentage reduction of VSV yield
Medium	None	0	6·7	—	—
Interferon	None	0	5·1	1·6	97·5
Medium	Medium	2	6·7	—	—
Interferon	Interferon	2	5·1	1·6	97·5
Medium	FPA*	2	6·6	—	—
Interferon	Interferon+FPA	2	4·8	1·8	98·3
Medium	Medium	4	6·7	—	—
Interferon	Interferon	4	5·2	1·5	97·0
Medium	FPA	4	6·7	—	—
Interteron	Interferon+FPA	4	4·7	2·0	99·0
Medium	Medium	6	6·8	—	—
Interferon	Interferon	6	4·9	1·9	98·7
Medium	FPA	6	6·5	—	—
Interferon	Interferon+FPA	6	4·6	1·9	98·7
Medium	Medium	24	7·0	—	—
Interferon	Interferon	24	4·8	2·2	99·4
Medium	FPA	24	6·4	—	—
Interferon	Interferon+FPA	24	5·8	0·6	75·0

* FPA = 60 µg. fluorophenylalanine/ml. in phenylalanine-free medium.

washed three times to remove the inhibitor and interferon and then challenged with a high multiplicity of VSV. The results demonstrate that inhibition of (functional) protein synthesis by DL-p-fluorophenylalanine (FPA) (in the presence of phenylalanine-free medium) or cycloheximide for 16 or more hours decreased the degree of established resistance to virus in the continued presence of interferon. Multiplication of VSV after removal of the inhibitors indicated that the effect of inhibitors could be fully reversed for virus multiplication up to seven hours after application. At later times reversal of inhibitors was not complete although the yield of VSV was still high.

The effectiveness of the inhibition of protein synthesis was shown in two ways. Incorporation of [^{14}C]phenylalanine showed 60 per cent inhibition of specific activity at four hours, 61 per cent inhibition at six hours, and 74 per cent inhibition at 24 hours in cultures treated with 60 μg. FPA/ml. At the same time there was no inhibition and sometimes there was

TABLE II

EFFECT OF INHIBITION OF CELLULAR PROTEIN SYNTHESIS BY CYCLOHEXIMIDE
ON ESTABLISHED ANTIVIRAL ACTIVITY

Pretreatment for 24 hours	Second treatment	Time of 2nd treatment before wash + VSV challenge (hours)	Yield of VSV ($\log_{10}$)	Reduction of VSV yield ($\log_{10}$)	Percentage reduction of VSV yield
Medium	None	0	7·0	—	—
Interferon	None	0	4·8	2·2	99·4
Medium	Medium	4	6·6	—	—
Interferon	Interferon	4	4·4	2·2	99·4
Medium	Cycloheximide	4	6·6	—	—
Interferon	Interferon + cycloheximide	4	4·4	2·2	99·4
Medium	Medium	7	6·8	—	—
Interferon	Interferon	7	4·4	2·4	99·6
Medium	Cycloheximide	7	6·4	—	—
Interferon	Interferon + cycloheximide	7	4·4	2·0	99·0
Medium	Medium	16	6·4	—	—
Interferon	Interferon	16	4·6	1·8	98·3
Medium	Cycloheximide	16	6·0	—	—
Interferon	Interferon + cycloheximide	16	5·0	1·0	90·0
Medium	Medium	24	6·2	—	—
Interferon	Interferon	24	4·5	1·7	98·0
Medium	Cycloheximide	24	5·9	—	—
Interferon	Interferon + cycloheximide	24	5·0	0·9	87·0

enhancement of incorporation of [^{3}H]uridine. Similarly 10 μg. of cycloheximide/ml. was followed by 93 per cent inhibition of incorporation of [^{14}C]phenylalanine at one hour. Also both inhibitors suppressed multiplication of VSV more than 1,000-fold in a single growth cycle.

Similar FPA experiments with chicken interferon in chick embryo cultures have given similar results (Baron and Friedman, 1966).

EFFECT OF INHIBITION OF CELLULAR PROTEIN SYNTHESIS ON THE
DEVELOPMENT OF ANTIVIRAL ACTIVITY

A comparison was made of the ability of FPA and cycloheximide to inhibit the development of antiviral activity. Mouse embryo cells were treated with a mixture of interferon and inhibitor for five hours and challenged with VSV after removal of inhibitor, as shown by the representative experiment outlined in Table III. Inhibition of protein synthesis by FPA resulted in marked inhibition of development of antiviral activity, as has been reported (Taylor, 1964; Friedman and Sonnabend, 1964; Lockart, 1964, Levine, 1964). Surprisingly, cycloheximide caused only slight inhibition of development of antiviral activity. Mouse embryo cells

TABLE III

EFFECT OF COMBINED FPA AND CYCLOHEXIMIDE ON DEVELOPMENT OF INTERFERON-
INDUCED ANTIVIRAL ACTIVITY

Treatment for 5 hours before wash + VSV challenge	Yield of VSV (log_{10})	Reduction of VSV yield (log_{10})	Percentage reduction of VSV yield
Medium*	6·4	—	—
Interferon	5·6	0·8	84
Interferon + FPA†	6·6	0·0	0
Interferon + cycloheximide‡	5·4	1·0	90
Interferon + FPA + cycloheximide	5·6	0·8	84
Medium + FPA + cycloheximide	6·4	—	—

* Phenylalanine-free medium.
† FPA = 80 μg./ml. in phenylalanine-free medium.
‡ 10 μg./ml.

treated simultaneously with interferon, cycloheximide and FPA also showed only slight inhibition of development of resistance after removal of inhibition and challenge with VSV (Table III). Possible reasons for this finding will be considered later.

EFFECT OF INHIBITION OF CELLULAR RNA SYNTHESIS ON
ESTABLISHED ANTIVIRAL ACTIVITY

To help to determine whether RNA synthesis was required for maintenance of antiviral activity, mouse embryo cells were treated with 100 units interferon/ml. overnight at 37° so that resistance to virus had reached a constant level. Actinomycin D (0·1 μg./ml.) was added to the cultures, and at the intervals shown in Table IV the cultures were washed three times to remove both unbound inhibitor and interferon, and then they were challenged with a high multiplicity of VSV. Treatment with actinomycin D up to eight hours did not measurably decrease resistance to VSV. Treatment for 21 to 24 hours did significantly decrease resistance to VSV, as shown in Table IV.

Challenge of mouse embryo cells with VSV at intervals after the addition of actinomycin D indicated that the cells lost the ability fully to support multiplication of VSV after 21 hours of treatment with actinomycin D (Table IV), although treatment for up to five hours did not inhibit multiplication. Biochemical controls incorporating labelled uridine or phenylalanine showed that by eight hours and 24 hours after treatment with actinomycin D, RNA synthesis was inhibited more than 95 per cent. Protein synthesis was inhibited 46 per cent eight hours after actinomycin D,

TABLE IV

EFFECT OF INHIBITION OF CELLULAR RNA SYNTHESIS BY ACTINOMYCIN D ON ESTABLISHED ANTIVIRAL ACTIVITY

Pretreatment for 24 hours	Second treatment	Time of 2nd treatment before wash + VSV challenge (hours)	Yield of VSV (log_{10})	Reduction of VSV yield (log_{10})	Percentage reduction of VSV yield
EXPERIMENT 1					
Medium	Medium	24	7·5	—	—
Interferon	Interferon	24	5·4	2·1	99·2
Medium	Actinomycin D*	24	5·3	—	—
Interferon	Interferon + actinomycin D	24	4·7	0·6	75·0
EXPERIMENT 2					
Medium	Medium	21	7·4	—	—
Interferon	Interferon	21	5·3	2·1	99·2
Medium	Actinomycin D	21	5·8	—	—
Interferon	Interferon + actinomycin D	21	4·8	1·0	90·0
Medium	Medium	24	7·4	—	—
Interferon	Interferon	24	5·4	2·0	99·0
Medium	Actinomycin D	24	5·6	—	—
Interferon	Interferon + actinomycin D	24	4·4	1·2	93·7

* 0·1 µg./ml.

and 87 per cent 24 hours afterwards. These results are consistent with the current viewpoint that actinomycin D acts primarily to inhibit the synthesis of DNA-primed RNA, including messenger RNA, and that as a consequence of decay of pre-existing messenger RNA a secondary inhibition of protein synthesis occurs (Reich, 1963), The assumption is made that the decay of ribosomes during this period would not be sufficient to account for the observed decrease in protein synthesis. Therefore, a decrease in antiviral protein after treatment of resistant cells with actinomycin D would probably reflect a decreased production due to decreased availability of its messenger RNA.

TREATMENT OF MOUSE EMBRYO CELL CULTURES WITH A MIXTURE OF INTER-
FERON AND AN INHIBITOR OF PROTEIN SYNTHESIS FOLLOWED BY REPLACEMENT
WITH ACTINOMYCIN D

If interferon-induced resistance is actually due to induction of an antiviral protein (Taylor, 1964), then reaction of cells with interferon and a
specific inhibitor of protein synthesis should result in formation of the
messenger RNA but should not result in formation of the proposed antiviral protein (resistance). Subsequent removal of the inhibitor and addition
of actinomycin D would be expected to result in translation of the formed
messenger RNA into antiviral protein (resistance) if the message were
sufficiently stable.

TABLE V

EFFECT OF TREATMENT OF MOUSE EMBRYO CELLS WITH INTERFERON AND CYCLOHEXIMIDE
FOLLOWED BY REPLACEMENT WITH ACTINOMYCIN D

Treatment for 5 hours before addition of actinomycin D*	Yield of VSV (log_{10}) after wash, re-feeding with actinomycin D, incubation for 3 hours + challenge with VSV	Reduction of VSV yield (log_{10})	Percentage reduction of VSV yield
EXPERIMENT 1			
None	6·2	—	—
Interferon†	3·9	2·3	99·5
Interferon + cycloheximide	4·2	1·8	98·4
EXPERIMENT 2			
None	6·3	—	—
Interferon	4·2	2·1	99·2
Interferon + cycloheximide	4·4	1·9	98·7
EXPERIMENT 3			
None	6·4	—	—
Interferon	4·2	2·2	99·4
Interferon + cycloheximide	4·7	1·7	98·0

* 0·2 ml. of 5 μg./ml. added to 1 ml. volume in each tube.
† 100 units/ml.

For this purpose mouse embryo cell cultures were treated simultaneously
with 100 units interferon/ml. (enough to inhibit the yield of VSV by 2·5
log_{10}) and with 10 μg. cycloheximide/ml. in a total volume of 1 ml. After
five hours at 37°, 0·2 ml. of actinomycin D was added to give a final concentration of 5 μg./ml. After an additional 30 minutes at 37° the cultures
were washed three times to remove interferon and cycloheximide, and then
reincubated for three more hours in the presence of 1 μg. actinomycin D/ml.
before challenge with a high multiplicity of VSV.

The results are presented in Table V. Resistance to VSV developed in
mouse embryo cells after removal of interferon and cycloheximide and

replacement with actinomycin D. Control experiments demonstrated that this dose of actinomycin D was capable of completely inhibiting the development of interferon-induced resistance. Cycloheximide permits full virus yield after it is removed at 5·5 hours.

DISCUSSION

Any interpretation of the mechanism of induction and maintenance of antiviral activity by interferon must account for the observed variables. Some factors which affect interferon-induced resistance to viruses in mouse embryo cells may be considered under the following headings:

(1) *Time after application of interferon.* Exposure of mouse embryo cells to interferon results in increasing antiviral activity over about seven hours. Thereafter antiviral activity does not continue to increase, and the level of resistance tends to remain relatively stable through at least 72 hours (Fig. 2).

(2) *Interferon in the extracellular fluid.* Previous studies have shown that there was no detectable disappearance of interferon from culture fluids under the conditions of the present experiment (Buckler, Baron and Levy, 1966). Thus the initial rise of antiviral activity and the subsequent levelling off of resistance occurs in the presence of an undetectable change in the quantity of interferon.

(3) *Concentration of interferon.* The dose of interferon was directly related to the time of onset of detectable antiviral activity and to the final stable level of resistance (Fig. 1). The effect of dosage was determined by the concentration of interferon rather than by the amount applied under the present experimental conditions (Fig. 3).

(4) *Continued presence of interferon.* Continued presence of the same concentration of interferon was required to maintain the final, established level of resistance. Removal of interferon resulted in gradual loss of antiviral activity after a significant lag period. Addition of an increased concentration of interferon resulted in a further rise of resistance (Fig. 4).

(5) *Protein synthesis.* Development of resistance by cells exposed to interferon is prevented by inhibitors of protein synthesis (FPA and puromycin) (Taylor, 1964; Friedman and Sonnabend, 1964; Lockart, 1964; Levine, 1964). The effect of FPA was confirmed in the present study, but brief inhibition of protein synthesis by cycloheximide did not prevent the induction by interferon of a high degree of antiviral activity (Table III). Resistance of cells continually exposed to interferon was decreased by prolonged treatment with inhibitors of protein synthesis (FPA and cyclo-

heximide) (Tables I and II). Any interpretation must allow for the inability to reverse fully the virus-inhibitory effects of prolonged treatment with FPA and cycloheximide.

(6) *RNA synthesis.* Development of resistance by cells exposed to interferon is prevented by inhibition of RNA synthesis by actinomycin D (Taylor, 1964; Lockart, 1964; Levine, 1964). We have been able to confirm this finding in several unpublished experiments. Resistance of cells continually exposed to interferon was also decreased by inhibition of RNA synthesis by actinomycin D in the present study (Table IV). The latter effect of actinomycin D must be interpreted with caution since a toxic action of actinomycin D to retard RNA virus occurred after prolonged treatment of mouse embryo cells with actinomycin D (Table IV).

(7) *Different effects of FPA and cycloheximide.* The development of antiviral activity was inhibited more completely by FPA than by cycloheximide. In some experiments cycloheximide did not inhibit development of resistance at all (Tables III and V). Combined FPA and cycloheximide permitted substantial development of resistance (Table III). Moderate resistance did develop in mouse embryo cells treated with interferon and cycloheximide and then challenged with VSV in the presence of actinomycin D after removal of interferon and cycloheximide (Table V) (Dianzani, Buckler and Baron, 1967).

The main question is whether these findings can lead to an understanding of some of the mechanisms which govern the development and maintenance of antiviral activity in cells exposed to interferon. Development of resistance seems most simply explained by the previous suggestion that interferon induces the production of an antiviral substance (protein) which accumulates intracellularly and accounts for the increasing resistance (Taylor, 1964). Maintenance of a relatively stable level of antiviral activity after development of resistance in cells exposed to interferon can be interpreted in several ways. The possibility that antiviral activity is maintained because cells acquire refractoriness to responding further to interferon is not supported by the observations: (a) that resistant cells respond appropriately to an increased concentration of interferon, and (b) that maintenance of antiviral activity requires the continued presence of interferon in the extracellular fluid. The possibility that the resistance level is maintained by continual induction of the antiviral protein is supported by (a) the requirement for the continued presence of interferon in the extracellular fluids, and (b) the requirement for continued protein synthesis and the probable requirement for continued RNA synthesis. If the resistance level is maintained by continued induction of the antiviral protein, it may be further deduced that antiviral activity could remain relatively stable only if the hypothesized production were offset by an equal rate of degradation.

Certain of the present findings bear on the question: how much uptake of interferon by cells is required to induce antiviral activity? Several laboratories have now contributed information on the disappearance or lack of disappearance of interferon from culture fluids during the induction of antiviral activity. Several laboratories (Lindenmann, Burke and Isaacs, 1957; Wagner, 1961; Sellers and Fitzpatrick, 1962; Gifford, 1963) observe substantial losses of interferon from culture fluids. Consistent with this loss is their finding that induction of antiviral activity is dependent on the total amount (volume) as well as the concentration of interferon applied (Lockart, 1966; Ke, Armstrong and Ho, 1966). However, loss from the medium could be due to either specific or non-specific causes.

In other laboratories (see references in Buckler, Baron and Levy, 1966; Youngner, Taube and Stinebring, 1966) no disappearance of interferon from culture fluids could be detected during the development of antiviral activity. Consistent with undetectable loss in these laboratories is the finding that the level of antiviral activity of mouse embryo or mouse L cells is dependent upon the concentration of interferon and independent of the total amount (Fig. 3) (Youngner and Hallum, 1966). If interferon is largely adsorbed and the amount taken up determines the degree of antiviral activity, then the addition of large volumes of the same concentration of interferon would result in the availability of more total interferon, which in turn would induce more antiviral activity. Since this is not the case in the latter laboratories, the results support the finding of undetectable loss of interferon. Further evidence comes from the finding that the antiviral state of cultures of mouse embryo cells remains constant as long as the applied interferon is left in contact with the cells (Figs. 2 and 4). If large amounts of interferon were irreversibly taken up by cells, the level of antiviral activity would fall because experimental removal of the applied interferon is followed by gradual loss of the antiviral state (Isaacs, 1963). Whereas the observed level of antiviral activity did not decrease during exposure to interferon, the major portion of the interferon could not have been bound to the cells under the present experimental conditions.

It seems reasonable to assume that all the experimental observations are correct. Since under certain experimental conditions, antiviral activity can develop in the absence of detectable loss of interferon, it necessarily follows that disappearance of measurable quantities of interferon is not a prerequisite for development of antiviral activity. This conclusion would be invalid only if antiviral activity is induced by different mechanisms under the differing experimental conditions.

The relative inefficiency of cycloheximide, as compared with FPA, in inhibiting development of interferon-induced resistance (Table III) raises some interesting possibilities. Cycloheximide is a potent inhibitor of protein synthesis, as reported in the literature (Colombo, Felicetti and Baglioni, 1965) and confirmed for the present system. One possibility is that cycloheximide may inhibit protein synthesis and permit the accumulation of messenger RNA. Thus when interferon and cycloheximide are removed from mouse embryo cells, the formed messenger RNA for the antiviral protein could be rapidly translated and thereby inhibit the challenge VSV. FPA may inhibit protein synthesis but somehow prevent accumulation of messenger RNA and thereby prevent the development of resistance to VSV. An alternative possibility, that the antiviral protein is produced before the removal of cycloheximide and interferon, seems less likely because resistance to VSV developed in mouse embryo cells after treatment with cycloheximide combined with FPA and interferon. In this case FPA would be expected to prevent the formation of functional antiviral protein until FPA was removed. The possibility that the messenger RNA for the antiviral protein is produced after removal of cycloheximide and interferon is ruled out by the development of resistance after removal of cycloheximide and interferon and replacement with actinomycin D. The apparent formation of messenger RNA for the antiviral protein in mouse embryo cells treated with both cycloheximide and interferon also suggests that the production of the messenger RNA does not require induction of intermediary proteins. This working model of the action of cycloheximide is currently being tested (Dianzani, Buckler and Baron, 1967), including the observation that prolonged treatment of mouse embryo cells with cycloheximide may inhibit maintenance of resistance, perhaps by eventually inhibiting cellular RNA synthesis or by eventual decay of messenger RNA for the antiviral protein (Tobey, Anderson and Petersen, 1966).

SUMMARY

Several factors which affect the interferon-induced antiviral activity of mouse embryo cultures have been considered. These include interferon concentration, time of interferon reaction with cells, change of interferon concentration, and cellular protein and RNA synthesis. A proposed working model which accounts for most of these observations follows. Development of antiviral activity by mouse embryo cells exposed to interferon could be due to the production of the hypothesized intracellular antiviral protein (Taylor, 1964). Maintenance of stable antiviral activity in the presence of interferon could be the result of continued production of enough antiviral protein to offset decay.

Evidence is considered which supports the interpretation that, under certain conditions, interferon may induce full antiviral activity without detectable loss of interferon from the extracellular fluid.

Finally the possibility is considered that in the presence of interferon and cycloheximide, mouse embryo cells produce the messenger RNA for the antiviral protein.

REFERENCES

BARON, S., and BUCKLER, C. E. (1963). *Science*, **141**, 1061.
BARON, S., and FRIEDMAN, R. M. (1966). Unpublished results.
BUCKLER, C. E., BARON, S., and LEVY, H. B. (1966). *Science*, **152**, 80.
COLOMBO, B., FELICETTI, L., and BAGLIONI, C. (1965). *Biochem. biophys. Res. Commun.*, **18**, 389.
DIANZANI, F., BUCKLER, C. E., and BARON, S. (1967). *Bact. Proc.*, 157.
FRIEDMAN, R. M., and SONNABEND, J. A. (1964). *Nature, Lond.*, **203**, 366.
GIFFORD, F. E. (1963). *J. gen. Microbiol.*, **33**, 437.
ISAACS, A. (1963). *Adv. Virus Res.*, **10**, 1.
ISAACS, A., and WESTWOOD, M. A. (1959). *Nature, Lond.*, **184**, 1232.
KE, Y., ARMSTRONG, J., and HO, M. (1966). Personal communication.
LEVINE, S. (1964). *Virology*, **24**, 229.
LEVY, H. B. (1964). *Virology*, **22**, 575.
LINDENMANN, J., BURKE, A., and ISAACS, A. (1957). *Br. J. exp. Path.*, **38**, 551.
LOCKART, R. Z. (1963). *J. Bact.*, **85**, 996.
LOCKART, R. Z. (1964). *Biochem biophys. Res. Commun.*, **15**, 513.
LOCKART, R. Z. (1966). Personal communication.
LOWRY, O. J., ROSEBROUGH, N. J., FARR, A. L., and RANDALL, R. J. (1951). *J. biol. Chem.*, **193**, 265.
PAUCKER, K., and CANTELL, K. (1963). *Virology*, **21**, 22.
REICH, E. (1963). *Cancer Res.*, **23**, 1428.
SELLERS, R. F., and FITZPATRICK, M. (1962). *Br. J. exp. Path.*, **43**, 674.
TAYLOR, J. (1964). *Biochem. biophys. Res. Commun.*, **14**, 447.
TOBEY, R. A., ANDERSON, E. C., and PETERSEN, D. F. (1966). *Proc. natn. Acad. Sci. U.S.A.*, **56**, 1520.
WAGNER, R. R. (1961). *Virology*, **13**, 323.
YOUNGNER, J. S., and HALLUM, J. V. (1966). Personal communication.
YOUNGNER, J. S., TAUBE, S. E., and STINEBRING, W. R. (1966). Personal communication.

DISCUSSION

Tyrrell: Why should you get a different result with FPA and cycloheximide?

Baron: We do not really understand that. FPA apparently allows the translation of the messenger RNA to occur, but the resulting polypeptide is fallacious because it incorporates FPA. Cycloheximide is reported to delay the progression of messenger RNA on the ribosomes, and to hold it on polysomes; after removal of the cycloheximide, there is a rapid translation. We know from our experiments that in the presence of cycloheximide messenger RNA is conserved in mouse embryo cells. In the presence of FPA perhaps the translation results in natural degradation of the messenger RNA. The messenger RNA may be unstable in use.

Martin: Did you check that you could recover protein synthetic activity when you removed the cycloheximide?

Baron: Protein synthesis was rapidly restored after removal of inhibitors.

Joklik: In the presence of FPA a faulty protein may be made, which could then compete successfully with good protein made later on.

Baron: We tested the idea that an FPA-containing fallacious antiviral protein might compete with the functional protein. There was no competition. We would have liked to have seen such a competing protein.

Chany: The observation that interferon must be present in the medium to maintain the antiviral activity is very interesting. It reminds me of an observation many people have made: in a chronically infected cell system, if one trypsinizes the cells or changes the medium, an outburst of viral multiplication and cell destruction occurs very soon afterwards (Daniel, P., and Chany, C. [1962]. *Can. J. Microbiol.*, **8**, 709–718). This is probably related to the fact that antiviral activity is lost when interferon is removed.

Ho: When did you collect the VSV?

Baron: Usually between 14 and 20 hours after challenge, because in control experiments we have shown that the virus yield levels off after about 12 hours and remains stable up to about 30 hours.

Ho: Did you remove interferon at times other than at 24 hours?

Baron: Yes, at 4 hours, and 48 hours, with the same result.

Stoker: Could the reduction in yield be due either to a reduced yield per cell, or to a reduced number of cells yielding?

Baron: Yes, either explanation is possible. The first to occur is a reduced yield per cell and as the yield per cell decreases the number of yielding cells becomes smaller.

Stoker: When you add more interferon and get an increase in resistance, could you then be blocking more cells?

Baron: We have not checked whether this is the explanation in the cell system we used, but Lockart (Lockart, R. Z., and Horn, B. [1963]. *J. Bact.*, **85**, 996) has shown that the application of interferon to cells will determine the yield from individual cells and the number of yielders, in his system.

Crick: Could the active protein be a combination of the antiviral protein and interferon?

Baron: That cannot be ruled out, but if Dr. Merigan's rough calculation is right and only about one interferon molecule per cell is required for antiviral activity, it seems unlikely.

Wagner: The optimum virus yields we get with VSV at a multiplicity of infection of about 20 to 30 plaque-forming units per cell occur six to eight hours after infection, and in our experience replication tapers off after this time. This is in the mouse-cell system, or in any other kind of cells that we have tested. At 14 to 24 hours we see a considerable amount of variation in the final yields although they seem to be more constant at six hours than later.

Baron: We have a maximum yield at ten hours, and before that the yield is variable. The reliability of this system is greatest after the maximum yield occurs: at from 12 to 30 hours after infection there is an essentially constant amount of virus.

Wagner: Are all the cells infected early in your experiments?

Baron: The multiplicity is between 20 and 30 p.f.u./cell, which should infect almost all the cells. This is calculated on the mouse infectivity titre, and it would be close to 100 p.f.u./cell on a chick infectivity titre. CPE occurs synchronously, that is, by 12 to 14 hours all the cells are becoming involved and showing CPE.

Wagner: Another point is that only a $0 \cdot 6 \log_{10}$ difference is shown between the top and bottom levels in your experiments on concentration versus amount. In the interpretation of the validity of your experiment is that amount of difference significant?

Baron: In our system $0 \cdot 5 \log_{10}$ inhibition of yield is highly significant. Dr. J. S. Youngner and Dr. J. Hallum (personal communication) also found a concentration dependency in their system, which also shows no detectable loss of interferon from the fluid.

Joklik: For how long do you adsorb before you remove the VSV inoculum?

Baron: One hour.

Joklik: When you remove it, what is your yield per cell?

Baron: Sixty per cell if we assay in the mouse system. It is more like 130 plaque-forming units per cell if we assay in a chick system.

Pereira: What is the ratio of particles per infective dose?

Wagner: It depends on how you prepare the virus. Preparations that we have looked at have lots of non-infective virus which can be separated on sucrose gradients. The best possible preparation has a ratio very close to 1, such as in a good vaccinia preparation. Do you still believe in a 10:1 ratio, Dr. Joklik?

Joklik: The best ratio that has been recorded with vaccinia is 3 to 4:1.

What is the purity of interferon now? What is the dilution factor of your preparation with the highest interferon concentration, Dr. Baron?

Baron: This is crude mouse-serum interferon, with the two further features that the titre is very high, up to 100,000 units/ml. In many of these experiments we used less than 10 units/ml. and therefore diluted at least 10,000-fold. Also we have been very careful to characterize the interferon preparation biologically and biochemically. We are working with a resistance which has all the characteristics of being interferon-induced, and not due to extraneous materials.

Stoker: I do not quite see how one reconciles the calculation that it may take only one molecule of interferon per cell to be effective, with the fact that when one varies the amount of interferon one varies the yield of virus per individual cell, rather than the numbers of cells infected. If you lower the amount of interferon, you ought to lower the number of cells infected, surely?

Baron: There is no evidence that it goes in irreversibly. It may go in, but it may come out again.

Tyrrell: How does the relationship between dose and the speed of the detectable response fit in with this theory?

Wagner: With the very low dose one could not detect what happened before six hours.

Tyrrell: But the titres had levelled off by six hours, and if you expressed those early values as percentages of the final yield, the curves would still have been different, I think—that is, if you think that those with 0·3 of a unit would be reliable.

Baron: You are correct in that resistance develops earlier and more rapidly in cells exposed to higher concentrations of interferon. I believe that this effect may be most closely related to the derepression mechanism for production of the antiviral protein.

OF MICE AND MEN: STUDIES WITH INTERFERON

N. B. FINTER

*Research Department, Imperial Chemical Industries Limited, Pharmaceuticals Division,
Mereside, Alderley Park, Macclesfield, Cheshire*

SEVERAL investigators have now shown that interferon can protect animals against local or systemic virus infections (see review by Finter, 1966a). In man, interferon has been found to be locally effective in the skin (Scientific Committee, 1962) and probably also in the eye (Jones, Galbraith and Al-Hussaini, 1962), and it is reasonable to suppose that it will also be active against systemic virus infections, as it is in animals. Thus presumptively interferon may be of value in clinical medicine.

There appear to be two ways in which it might be used. One might inject interferon prepared from human cells *in vitro*, or one might inject some substance which leads to the formation of interferon in the patient's body. On the face of it, this second possibility seems much the more attractive. Many substances are now known which stimulate formation of interferon in animals, and some of these, namely viruses and the mould products statolon and helenine (reviewed by Finter, 1966a), and certain synthetic polyanions (Regelson, 1967), have been shown to protect animals against virus infections. Ho and Postic (1967a), however, have recently pointed out that, because of their toxicity or for other reasons, none of these inducers could at present be used clinically, except perhaps under very special circumstances. Thus, in spite of the obvious problems involved, one must still seriously consider the possibility of making interferon for injection into man for therapeutic purposes. There is also the point that the injection of interferon could under certain circumstances have a decisive advantage over the injection of an inducer of interferon. With the latter, several hours may elapse before the formation of significant amounts of interferon, which may then be too late to influence the course of the infection. Results of an experiment illustrating this point are shown in Table I. Injection of mouse brain interferon into mice 24 hours after they had been infected with Semliki Forest virus (SFV) led to a significant increase in the number of survivors, whereas injection at this same time of a large amount of Newcastle disease virus (NDV), an efficient inducer of interferon, was ineffective; statolon, another inducer of interferon, was ineffective when injected 17 hours after the virus. All three substances in the doses used were found to be highly effective when injected 18 hours before the virus, leading to the survival of all or nearly all of the mice treated. Comparable results have been obtained in other experiments, though injection of NDV 17 hours after virus infection sometimes led to significant protection of mice. By analogy, injection of a relatively small amount of interferon into a child promptly at the onset of the prodromal symptoms of measles might abort the clinical disease, whereas injection of an inducer might be ineffective, despite the ultimate formation of much larger amounts of interferon.

TABLE I

MICE INFECTED WITH SFV

Inoculum	Route	Time after infection (hours)	Survivors (out of 30)	P (%)
Diluent	i.v.	17	5	
NMB	i.v.		5	
Statolon	i.p.		2	
Interferon	i.v.		17	$\ll 0.5$
NMB	i.v.	24	2	
NDV	i.v.		8	> 10
Statolon	i.p.		5	
Interferon	i.v.		12	2.5
Mean control			4	

Groups of 30 mice were infected intraperitoneally with SFV, and inoculated 17 or 24 hours later by the intravenous (i.v.) or intraperitoneal (i.p.) route with the substances shown.

NMB, normal mouse brain; NDV, $10^{8.7}$ EID_{50} of NDV; statolon, 143 µg. of active material; interferon, 1,600 units; diluent, Hanks saline (used to dilute the other substances).

If the use of preformed interferon in clinical practice is to be considered, there are three relevant questions:

First, how could interferon suitable for injection into man be obtained?

Second, in what viral infections might interferon be particularly useful?

Third, how much interferon would be needed to produce beneficial effects?

The first question will only be considered briefly here. Interferon has been obtained from tissue cultures of many different human cells, including primary cells, diploid cell strains, and continuous cell lines. Relatively potent preparations have been obtained from cultures of human leucocytes, e.g. by Strander and Cantell (1966) and by Falcoff and co-workers (1966), and these and preparations made from human amnion cultures have already been used in therapeutic experiments in man (Falcoff et al., 1966). To produce and purify large amounts of interferon from cell cultures would certainly pose many practical problems, but probably none of these is ultimately insuperable, if there should be the need.

The second question may seem academic at the present time, when little interferon is available even for clinical trials. Nevertheless, suitable preparations of interferon will doubtless become available one day, and there are certain virus infections of man where, potentially, the use of interferon has particular attractions. It thus seems worth testing the effects of interferon in appropriate animal models resembling such human infections. We have therefore studied interferon in mice infected with rabies virus, a life-endangering infection, and in mice infected with influenza virus, a particular instance of a respiratory virus infection.

Groups of mice weighing 12 to 14 g. were treated locally with 250 units of interferon 24 hours and again five hours before infection with one median lethal dose (LD_{50}) of the CVS strain of rabies virus, injected subcutaneously into the footpad. Other mice received 2,500 units of interferon, one-third injected intramuscularly and the rest intraperitoneally, 24 hours before they were infected. In two experiments there was no evidence that the treated mice were protected. This result does not necessarily mean that interferon cannot influence the course of rabies virus infections in man or other animals. The relative sensitivity to interferon of the CVS and of field strains of rabies is unknown, and there are important differences in the course of the infection with CVS virus in mice and with street virus in mice, dogs and bats (Johnson, 1965). Possibly a much larger dose of interferon injected locally might have had some effect, although, as Johnson (1965) has pointed out, CVS virus does not necessarily multiply at the site of inoculation before it spreads centripetally. The failure of a total of 2,500 units of interferon to protect the mice is disappointing, since this amount is approximately 20 times more than that required to protect mice against infection with a comparable dose of SFV (Finter, 1967). Possibly, however, only a little of the injected interferon penetrated into the cerebrospinal fluid, so that the cells of the central nervous system were inadequately protected: by fluorescent antibody techniques, Johnson (1965) could detect multiplication of CVS virus only in the cells of the spinal cord and brain, when mice were infected by footpad inoculation. Further experiments will be required, perhaps in other species, to evaluate the place of interferon in the prophylaxis of rabies virus infections.

Many different viruses can infect the human respiratory tract, and such infections are an important and frequent cause of disease in man. Interferon seems potentially to have particular advantages for their prevention or treatment, because of its broad antiviral spectrum. As a model of a respiratory virus infection, influenza virus in the mouse has been much studied, and several groups of workers have claimed beneficial effects from interferon in this system: whether the observed effects were in fact due to the interferon in the preparations used seems, however, conjectural, for reasons given elsewhere (Finter, 1966a). We have therefore further investigated the effects of interferon in mice which were infected by exposure to aerosols of the DSP strain of influenza A virus, under the conditions described by Bowers, Davies and Hurst (1952). Delivery of the virus as an aerosol led to a more uniform infection than resulted from intranasal instillation of virus to anaesthetized mice.

As a preliminary, the infectivity of the virus, when delivered as an aerosol, was determined. In subsequent experiments, mice were exposed to a calculated 100 aerosol ID_{50} (median infectious dose) of virus. The animals were killed 27 hours later and the titre of infectious virus in the lungs of each mouse was determined by subculture. In a number of experiments, interferon was inoculated into mice by the intravenous or intramuscular or intraperitoneal route, or by a combination of these routes. When the mice were exposed to an influenza virus aerosol 18 to 24 hours later, the virus grew in their lungs at the same rate as in the controls, even though total amounts of interferon of up to 29,000 units were administered.

One possible explanation for such results could be that influenza virus growing in the cells of the respiratory tract of mice is relatively or very insensitive to the antiviral action of interferon. We have investigated this, using organ cultures of mouse trachea prepared according to the general procedure described by Hoorn (1966). The trachea of a mouse was exposed by blunt dissection, and cut across just below the thyroid cartilage. The cut end was gripped with two pairs of very fine forceps, and the trachea was cut longitudinally into two halves down to the level of the sternum. Each half was placed in a separate plastic Petri dish with 1 ml. of medium 199, and incubated in an atmosphere containing 5 per cent CO_2. After 24 hours, the medium was drained off, and half of each trachea was treated with mouse brain interferon diluted in medium 199; the other half received an equivalent dilution of a control preparation of normal mouse brain and thus served as a direct control. After incubation for a further 24 hours, the medium was again exchanged, and now 100 ID_{50} (as measured in trachea organ cultures) of DSP influenza virus were added. Each 24 hours for the next three days the medium was collected and fresh medium was added. All the harvested media were assayed for infectious virus. Four or five replicate cultures were used to test each interferon dilution, and the amounts of virus found in these at a given time were generally in good agreement.

Results of an experiment in which cultures were treated with 250 units or 62 units of interferon are shown in Fig. 1. Virus titres were high in the first harvest from the control cultures, 24 hours after challenge, and slightly higher in the second harvest. In the third harvest, they were very much lower: at this time the ciliated epithelium had largely been destroyed, due to the considerable growth of virus in the previous 48 hours. Similar findings in organ cultures of human respiratory epithelium infected with

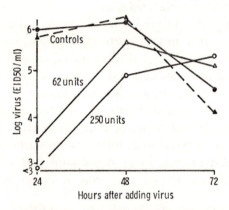

FIG. 1. Effect of interferon on the growth of influenza virus in mouse trachea organ cultures. Cultures were treated for 24 hours with interferon or an equivalent dilution of control material, and then challenged with $100 \: ID_{50}$ of virus.

influenza viruses have been reported by Tyrrell, Bynoe and Hoorn (1965). The cultures treated with interferon formed very much less virus than the controls in the first 24-hour period after infection, but there were larger amounts in the media collected at the end of the next two periods. In the third harvest, 72 hours after infection, there was actually more virus in the interferon-treated cultures than in the controls, in which at this time virus growth was declining. The maximum amounts formed in a 24-hour period in the treated cultures never reached those found in the control cultures. Histologically, the respiratory epithelium was better preserved in the interferon-treated cultures than in the controls, 24 hours after they had been infected with the virus.

In a similar experiment, cultures were treated with eight units of interferon, and six times less virus was formed in the first 24 hours after infection than in control cultures; with 32 units, there was 80 times less virus. These results suggest that the growth of influenza virus in the respiratory tract of a mouse is quite sensitive to interferon.

Another possible reason why injected interferon failed to inhibit the growth of influenza virus in mice is that it does not readily come in contact with the cells of the respiratory epithelium. If it did, it should presumably be found in the respiratory mucus, and might then be detected in bronchial washings. Mice were therefore injected intravenously with 1,800 units of interferon, or with an inducer of interferon (10^8 EID_{50} of NDV). At intervals, a mouse was killed by injection of Nembutal, and blood was collected. Bronchial washings were obtained by aspirating and expelling in succession two volumes of 0·5 ml. of Hanks saline into the bronchial tree, using the technique described by Fazekas de St. Groth (1948). The washings from individual mice were assayed from a 1/4 dilution. No interferon was detected in any, even when the serum collected at the same time contained as much as 800 units of interferon/ml. This failure could, however, simply reflect excessive dilution of a small volume of bronchial mucus in the wash fluid and assay diluent, and the use of an insufficiently sensitive assay method. Further studies are needed.

Even if little or no interferon passes from the blood into the respiratory mucus of a mouse, nevertheless interferon given by intranasal instillation or as an aerosol, and thus brought more directly into contact with the respiratory cells, might be effective against a respiratory virus infection. Unfortunately, administration of substances to anaesthetized mice by intranasal instillation is an erratic procedure, as pointed out by Bowers, Davies and Hurst (1952) and confirmed in our own experience. The amount of administered material which is inhaled depends on the depth of anaesthesia, and much of it is in fact swallowed. If several mice are infected intranasally with the same virus inoculum, their lungs at a given time thereafter may sometimes contain widely differing amounts of virus. After intranasal administration, there may presumably be similar differences in the amounts of interferon retained in the lungs of individual mice, and correspondingly the mice may be protected to differing extents against a subsequent virus challenge. Experiments have confirmed this prediction. For example ten mice were dosed intranasally with 250 units of interferon, and 18 with comparable control material. They were challenged 24 hours later with an aerosol of influenza virus. After 26 hours, their lungs were harvested and assayed for infectious virus. In four of the treated mice, the amounts of virus in the lungs were very significantly (at least 20 times) less than in the control mice, but in the other six treated mice, the differences were smaller: the mean titre of virus in the lungs of all the treated mice was eight times less than in the controls, a statistically highly significant effect.

A more satisfactory method of protecting mice might be to administer interferon also as an aerosol. Experiments to determine the feasibility of this are currently in progress. So far the aerosols have for various reasons contained inadequate concentrations of interferon, in part due to inactivation of the interferon in the nebulizer, and in part due to the design of the particular apparatus used. It should be possible to overcome these difficulties.

The third topic to be considered concerns the amounts of interferon that might be needed to produce clinically useful effects in man. Eventually this point may be settled from direct clinical experience, but although interferon has already been used on a few occasions in volunteers and patients with virus infections, the published data from these studies give no guide. At the present time, it would be very helpful to those planning clinical trials to have estimates of probable dose requirements: the failure of interferon to protect volunteers against viruses causing colds (Scientific Committee, 1965) may have resulted merely from the use of inadequate amounts, and other trials in the future may similarly fail in the absence of guidance on dosage.

Some estimates of amounts of interferon which might be needed in man have already been published, and as an example of one type of calculation, the following data may be considered. It has been found that as little as 100 units of mouse interferon can protect a 20 g. mouse against the lethal effects of an intraperitoneal injection of approximately 1 LD_{50} of SFV (Finter, 1967). Scaled up directly on a weight-to-weight basis, this figure might suggest that $3 \cdot 5 \times 10^6$ units of interferon would protect a 70 kg. man against a comparable infection. Unfortunately, however, there is at present no direct way of translating an amount of mouse interferon, measured in arbitrary units, into an equivalent amount of human interferon, so that this calculation is probably meaningless. Hilleman (1965) and Ho and Postic (1967a) have given estimates of the amounts of interferon which might be required for use in man: unfortunately, in their calculations similar assumptions of the equivalence of units of mouse or chick interferon and human interferon are involved.

The following consideration may provide an alternative basis for calculation. It may be a reasonable assumption to suppose that the relation between the amount of interferon needed to protect against a particular type of virus infection, and the total amount of interferon which is formed in the species concerned in response to a virus infection, is roughly constant from species to species. If so, we have the equation:

$$\frac{\text{Species } A}{\underset{\text{Amount of interferon formed}}{\text{Amount of interferon needed to protect}}} = \frac{\text{Species } B}{\underset{\text{Amount of interferon formed}}{\text{Amount of interferon needed to protect}}}$$

(Obviously the amount required and the amount formed in species A must be measured in the same units, and similarly for species B, but equivalence of the units for the two species is not assumed.)

Some data relevant to this equation are available from studies with mice. Firstly, 100 units of interferon will protect a mouse against 1 LD_{50} of SFV (Finter, 1967). Secondly, if mice are infected intracerebrally with West Nile virus, much more interferon is subsequently found in the brain than in any other organ (Subrahmanyan and Mims, 1966): when the brain interferon is at its highest level, the total content is approximately 17,000 units/brain (Finter, 1964). However, since the interferon found in an organ at any one time represents the balance between its production and its destruction or loss to other parts of the body, this figure must considerably underestimate the total amount formed in such mice.

Another estimate has been given by Baron and co-workers (1966). From the amounts of interferon found in the blood of mice at different times after intravenous injection of 10^8 or more p.f.u. of NDV, and the rate at which injected interferon disappeared from the blood of mice, they suggested that such mice formed in total very large amounts of interferon (100,000 units in their unitage, which is known to be equivalent to 750,000 of the units used in my laboratory).

A sudden rise of virus in the blood to a level of 10^8 p.f.u./ml. or more is of course a highly unnatural occurrence, and when 1/10 or 1/100 as much NDV was inoculated intravenously into mice, very much lower titres of circulating interferon were subsequently found (Baron and Buckler, 1963; Youngner et al., 1966). Baron and co-workers (1966) also found lower titres of interferon in sera from mice with viraemias developing naturally during various virus infections. Thus the total amount of interferon formed in a mouse during a natural virus infection may be considerably less than the estimate of 750,000 units given above. These two figures, 17,000 units and 750,000 units, may however set lower and upper limits, respectively, to the amounts of interferon formed in a mouse during a virus infection, and it may be reasonable to take as a working figure the geometric mean value of approximately 100,000 units.

If these figures, 100 units of interferon to protect a mouse and 100,000 units formed in a mouse, are substituted in the equation above, and if the basic assumption is correct, then the amount of human interferon required to protect a man against an LD_{50} of a virulent arbovirus, e.g. one of the equine encephalitis viruses, will be of the order of (100/100,000) × the amount formed in man during a systemic virus infection.

Some data on the amounts of interferon formed in man during various virus infections are available (reviewed by Wheelock, 1967). In a few studies in which volunteers were inoculated with virus vaccines, interferon was found in sera obtained on successive days from the same individuals (Petralli, Merigan and Wilbur, 1965; Wheelock and Sibley, 1965). From these and similar data, it might be possible to calculate the total amounts of interferon formed in these volunteers, if the rate at which interferon is cleared from the blood in man was known. Data on the rate of clearance of injected interferon from the blood of mice and rabbits are available (Baron et al., 1966; Finter, 1966b and unpublished; Gresser et al., 1967; Ho and Postic, 1967a), but unfortunately different laboratories have obtained rates for mouse interferon which differ quite considerably. In view of this divergency within a single species, it seems unwise to assume a rate of clearance of injected interferon from the blood of man. Also, results discussed below suggest that the distribution and excretion of interferon in man may differ from that in the rabbit and mouse. Thus at present no estimates of the total interferon formed in man can be made from the data on blood interferon levels.

Another way of estimating what total amounts of interferon are formed was suggested by Ho and Postic (1967b). They found that 0·2 to 2 per cent of a dose of interferon injected into rabbits appeared in the urine. They then induced a viraemia in rabbits by injecting NDV, collected the urine, and determined the total interferon present. On the assumption that the fraction of the serum interferon excreted was similarly 0·2 to 2 per cent, they calculated that the rabbits formed between 5 and 150 million units of interferon. However, it seems likely that the amount of interferon cleared from the blood into the urine will depend to a considerable extent on the concentration of interferon in the blood. Thus the proportion appearing in the urine of rabbits during a viraemia could be considerably greater than 0·2 to 2 per cent, and the estimates obtained for total interferon formed may be on the high side.

In view of the data of Ho and Postic (1967b), we have looked for interferon in urine collected from children with measles, chickenpox or mumps. Between ten and twelve children with each disease were studied.

All urine passed in each period of eight to ten hours was collected from the first onset of symptoms for four to five days, except that from three family contacts who later developed measles, urine was collected from five days before appearance of the rash until two days after. Samples from the first ten children were treated at pH 2 for 48 hours, then dialysed against Hanks saline, and tested for interferon at 1/4 dilution. Since no interferon was detected in any of the samples, the remaining samples were merely dialysed against Hanks saline before testing, lest the pH treatment destroyed any interferon present. A few samples, including all those from one of the measles contact cases, were concentrated five to ten times by pressure dialysis before assay. No interferon was detected in any of the approximately 400 individual urine samples tested. Since no blood samples were obtained, we do not know whether there was any interferon in the blood of any of the children. Nevertheless, Petralli, Merigan and Wilbur (1965) found interferon in the blood of children after subcutaneous injection of measles virus vaccines, with peak titres on the tenth day, and it seems likely that in the natural disease there will be circulating interferon at least at the comparable times. The absence of interferon in any of the urine samples tested suggests that interferon is not readily excreted into the urine of man, apparently in contrast to the rabbit and mouse. Thus this approach to the problem of the amounts of interferon formed in man has not yet been fruitful.

At the present time, then, no reliable estimates of the total amounts of interferon formed in man during natural virus infections can be given. Nevertheless, from further studies, it should be possible to make such estimates, and hence to calculate the probable amounts of interferon required for prophylaxis against virus infections. However, some quite different approach to the problem may perhaps prove more rewarding: for example, experimental studies with monkeys and monkey interferon may give the necessary information, and this line is also being followed.

SUMMARY

Potentially, interferon could be useful in human virus infections. Injections of preformed interferon may be needed, since as yet no suitable inducers of interferon are available. Also, interferon might be effective when injected later in the course of a virus infection than an inducer, as has been shown in mice.

Interferon has been used in mice with experimental virus infections. It had no apparent effect against the CVS strain of rabies virus, though, for reasons discussed, this does not necessarily mean that interferon could not be of value in human rabies.

As a model respiratory virus infection, mice were infected with aerosols of influenza virus. Interferon injected intravenously or by other routes did not reduce virus growth. Nevertheless, in mouse trachea organ cultures, influenza virus was found to be quite sensitive to interferon. Interferon could not be detected in bronchial washings from mice after intravenous injection of interferon, suggesting that little injected interferon comes in contact with the respiratory cells. When interferon was brought into direct contact with the respiratory cells by intranasal administration, the growth of influenza virus was inhibited.

It would be very useful to know how much interferon would produce useful effects in man. The data for the amounts needed in mice do not help directly, since amounts of interferon, measured in arbitrary units, cannot be equated from one species to another. An indirect way of estimating human requirements of interferon is suggested, but for this the total interferon formed in man during a virus infection must be known. Ways of measuring this are considered; since urine samples from children with measles, mumps and chickenpox contained no detectable interferon, no estimates of total interferon formed could be made from these.

REFERENCES

BARON, S., and BUCKLER, C. E. (1963). *Science*, **141**, 1061–1063.

BARON, S., BUCKLER, C. E., McCLOSKEY, R. V., and KIRSCHSTEIN, R. L. (1966). *J. Immun.*, **96**, 12–16.

BOWERS, R. H., DAVIES, O. L., and HURST, E. W. (1952). *Br. J. exp. Path.*, **33**, 601–609.

FALCOFF, E., FALCOFF, R., FOURNIER, F., and CHANY, C. (1966). *Annls Inst. Pasteur, Paris*, **III**, 562–584.

FAZEKAS DE ST. GROTH, S. (1948). *Aust. J. exp. Biol. med. Sci.*, **26**, 29–36.

FINTER, N. B. (1964). *Nature, Lond.*, **204**, 1114–1115.

FINTER, N. B. (1966a). In *Interferons*, pp. 232–267, ed. Finter, N. B. Amsterdam: North-Holland Publishing Co.

FINTER, N. B. (1966b). *Br. J. exp. Path.*, **47**, 361–371.

FINTER, N. B. (1967). *J. gen. Virol.*, **1**, 395–397.

GRESSER, I., FONTAINE, D., COPPEY, J., FALCOFF, R., and FALCOFF, E. (1967). *Proc. Soc. exp. Biol. Med.*, **124**, 91–94.

HILLEMAN, M. R. (1965). *Am. J. Med.*, **38**, 751–766.

HO, M., and POSTIC, B. (1967a). In *First International Conference on Vaccines against Viral and Rickettsial Diseases of Man*, pp. 632–639. Washington, D.C.: PAHO/WHO Scientific Publication 147.

HO, M., and POSTIC, B. (1967b). *Nature, Lond.*, **214**, 1230–1231.

HOORN, B. (1966). *Acta path. microbiol. scand.*, **66**, suppl. 183.

JOHNSON, R. T. (1965). *J. Neuropath. exp. Neurol.*, **24**, 662–674.

JONES, B. R., GALBRAITH, J. E. K., and AL-HUSSAINI, M. K. (1962). *Lancet*, **1**, 875–879.

PETRALLI, J., MERIGAN, T. C., and WILBUR, J. (1965). *New Engl. J. Med.*, **273**, 198–201.

REGELSON, W. (1967). In *Atherosclerosis and the Reticuloendothelial System*. In press.
SCIENTIFIC COMMITTEE ON INTERFERON (1962). *Lancet*, **1**, 873–875.
SCIENTIFIC COMMITTEE ON INTERFERON (1965). *Lancet*, **1**, 505–506.
STRANDER, H., and CANTELL, K. (1966). *Annls Med. exp. Biol. Fenn.*, **44**, 265–273.
SUBRAHMANYAN, T. P., and MIMS, C. A. (1966). *Br. J. exp. Path.*, **47**, 168–176.
TYRRELL, D. A. J., BYNOE, M. L., and HOORN, B. (1965). *Br. J. exp. Path.*, **46**, 370–375.
WHEELOCK, E. F. (1967). *First International Conference on Vaccines against Viral and Rickettsial Diseases of Man*. Washington, D.C.: PAHO/WHO Scientific Publication 147.
WHEELOCK, E. F., and SIBLEY, W. A. (1965). *New Engl. J. Med.*, **273**, 194–198.
YOUNGNER, J., SCOTT, A., HALLUM, J., and STINEBRING, W. (1966). *J. Bact.*, **92**, 862–868.

DISCUSSION

Baron: Using interferon, NDV and statolon, Dr. K. Habel and I were unable to protect mice in experiments similar to those done by Dr. O. Soave and Dr. T. C. Merigan with rabies virus. Even with the very large interferon levels we were able to generate in the mice there was no observable protection. A corollary of what you have said occurred to us. There is time to treat before the rabies virus gets to the target organ. What we did not consider was that the rabies virus enters the axon to travel up to the nervous system. In order to get any resistance to develop within the cytoplasm of that axon we would therefore have to reach the cell nucleus with interferon stimulation. The nucleus however is not where the axon and the cytoplasm are but is often within the central nervous system. So your finding that the neurones themselves have to be treated is reinforced by the fact that the main site of transport of the virus is in the cytoplasmic extension of the far-removed neurone body where the induction of the antiviral protein will have to occur.

Finter: I think this is right, and that interferon is probably not taken into the nerve cell through the axon; perhaps one ought to inject interferon into the cerebrospinal fluid to get an effect, but the technical difficulties of doing lumbar punctures on mice have deterred us from trying this.

Tyrrell: These are two illustrations of a basic principle. In animals or man, we have to consider the anatomical distribution of both the virus and the thing we are trying to treat the virus with. You remarked that the distribution of interferon is probably limited by a barrier which prevents it getting to the bronchial secretion. Fucidic acid, an antibiotic with a relatively small molecule, is capable of inhibiting the multiplication of coxsackie virus A21 very effectively *in vitro*, in concentrations much less than those found in the blood. My colleagues have found that it is quite inactive when given to volunteers infected with this virus, and they cannot find more than small amounts of the drug in the nasal secretions (Acornley, J. E., Bessell, C. J., Bynoe, M. L., Godtfredson, W. O., and Knoyle, J. M. [1967]. *Br. J. Pharmac. Chemother.*, in press). This therefore suggests that a virus infection is taking place in a compartment of the body which the drug does not reach. This may apply to all sorts of antiviral drugs, and interferon may not be exempt from this.

Gresser: Dr. Atanasiu (unpublished observations) at the Pasteur Institute has shown, using an immunofluorescent plaque assay, that fixed rabies virus was inhibited by interferon *in vitro*.

Ho: Do the amounts of interferon calculated to protect man apply to a single type of virus?

Finter: We know the amount needed to protect a mouse against an arbovirus infection, and using this figure, the calculation would give the amount to protect man also against an arbovirus infection. The amounts required to protect a mouse against arbovirus infection and mouse organ cultures against influenza virus seem to be pretty comparable, but I do not think one could generalize to other viruses.

Levy: That formula could perhaps be tested by comparing mouse with rabbit or hamster instead of man.

Finter: We are hoping to compare the amounts needed in the mouse and the monkey.

Merigan: We thought a direct approach to this would be to test endogenous interferon against a challenge virus in humans, simultaneously measuring the serum interferon levels achieved. If we could determine the intravascular disappearance rate of human interferon and combine that with the amount we saw was an effective protective serum level, we could then extrapolate to find what dose of exogenous interferon would protect. The results of the measles–vaccinia protection study in human infants give us knowledge of what serum levels are protective in man, but we are awaiting studies with exogenous interferon to determine its intravascular disappearance rate, which is the crucial missing factor.

Chany: We have done many experiments on the intravenous injection of interferon into patients. The injected interferon was cleared from the blood in a few minutes and we could not recover it in the urine or elsewhere. This might be due to quantitative aspects of the problem. Twice we injected interferon into the spinal fluid of the monkey. We were then able to recover some interferon in the blood four hours after the injection.

Merigan: By a calculation of the blood volume into which you injected your unitage, would you have expected to have seen it?

Chany: The amount of interferon we injected into the human subjects was probably too low. We expected some excretion when we injected interferon in babies but we did not find any.

Merigan: This disappearance rate is still a missing factor.

Finter: Another complication is that the clearance rate in mice varies quite a lot from animal to animal, which may account for discrepancies between findings in different laboratories.

Tyrrell: Even if the clearance rate in a normal person given exogenous interferon was known, this would not necessarily be the same as that in the subject with virus-infected cells.

Baron: Do the calculations you made of the amount of interferon necessary for protection apply mainly for prophylaxis?

Finter: Yes.

Baron: In natural infection, most of the interferon is made locally at the site where the virus is multiplying; therefore the concentration of interferon at that site must be very much higher than can be achieved by passive administration of interferon, and this concentration, at least under conditions in our laboratory, is the determining factor in the level of resistance. So in therapeutic use we would have to think of a much higher concentration at the site of infection than you have calculated for.

Finter: I think the amount needed may depend very much on the sort of infection involved. A hundred units of interferon will protect mice when injected 18 hours before the animals are infected with Semliki Forest virus, but a dose 50 times bigger is needed if it is administered 24 hours after the virus. At this time, this virus is spreading through the blood stream, and it probably gains access to the central nervous system by infecting the vascular endothelium of brain capillaries. One should be able to achieve an effect very much later if one could get the interferon in contact with the target cells. In the mouse the difficulty is that intracerebral injection ruptures the subarachnoid villi, and then the interferon goes out into the blood stream. But I can see no theoretical reason why one should not give interferon very much later after infection, and get protection.

Baron: You are quite right. What I had in mind was the height of the virus infection, which tends to coincide with the greatest production of interferon. The concentration required at the local site is probably very much higher than we can achieve at present with passive administration.

Chany: When we talk about the diffusion of interferon, we must take into consideration the size of the molecule. A small molecule of 25,000 or 30,000 would probably get into the spinal cord and stay there, while one of 160,000 would probably not get in.

Finter: The molecular weight of mouse brain interferon is of the order of 30,000, according to my colleague, Mr. A. Davies.

Stoker: Obviously Dr. Baron's experiments on the concentration effect, which also show how rapidly the protection is lost when interferon is removed, must be relevant to this question of protection *in vivo*.

Finter: A single injection of only 5,000 units will protect mice for up to five days, which is quite a reasonable length of time. I do not know what would happen if a very much bigger dose of interferon was administered.

EFFECT OF DIFFERENT CARCINOGENIC AGENTS ON THE PRODUCTION OF INTERFERON IN TISSUE CULTURE AND IN THE ANIMAL

EDWARD DE MAEYER AND JAQUELINE DE MAEYER-GUIGNARD

Institut du Radium, Orsay (Essonne)

OUR research has been mainly focused on the effect of chemical and physical carcinogens on the interferon defence mechanism. The principal reason for this study is the hope that it may contribute to a better understanding of those forms of carcinogenesis where chemicals or X-irradiation enhance the activity of either a latent oncogenic virus or of a tumour virus administered by the investigator. The intervention of a latent virus in the induction of lymphatic leukaemia in mice by X-irradiation has become increasingly evident, especially from the work of Gross (1959) and of Lieberman and Kaplan (1959). Recently, leukaemia agents have also been isolated from lymphomas induced with dimethylbenz(a)anthracene (DMBA) (Toth, 1963), 4-nitroquinoline-*N*-oxide (4NQO) (Kinosita and Tanaka, 1963), and 3-methylcholanthrene (3-MCA) (Irino *et al.*, 1963), although in these cases more unsuccessful attempts have been made than successful ones (Toth and Shubik, 1966). The aetiological role of a lymphatic leukaemia virus in lymphomas induced by X-irradiation or carcinogens in mice has become well-documented from these studies; the role of a virus in certain other forms of chemical carcinogenesis is suggested by the recent isolation of a filterable agent from DMBA-induced mammary carcinomas in Sprague-Dawley rats (Scholler, Bergs and Groupé, 1964).

The activation of latent viruses by carcinogens is, in our opinion, but one particular aspect of the capacity of these carcinogens to change the host-virus equilibrium in favour of the latter. This capacity has been well documented for a number of host-virus systems, beginning with the work of Rous and Kidd (1936), who demonstrated that previous treatment of rabbit skin with tar rendered this skin much more susceptible to the action of the rabbit papilloma (Shope) virus. Comparable results have been obtained in mice with urethane and leukaemia viruses: induction of leukaemia by Graffi virus in adult C57BL mice is greatly enhanced if the animals receive urethane after injection of the virus (Fiore-Donati, Chieco-Bianchi and De Benedictis, 1964); urethane also increases the susceptibility of C57BL mice to radiation lymphoma virus (Lieberman, Haran-Ghera and Kaplan, 1964). Chemical carcinogens furthermore are capable of increasing the susceptibility of animals to non-oncogenic viruses (see review by Duran-Reynals, 1963).

Little is known about the mechanism by which carcinogens activate or stimulate virus infection in the animal. The great variety of experimental conditions renders an analysis of the phenomenon difficult, and it seems very possible that a combination of different factors is involved, since some carcinogens are known to upset the hormonal balance of the host, for instance, and also to depress certain immune reactions (Malmgren, Bennison and McKinley, 1952; Stjernswärd, 1966). The increasing evidence for the role played by interferon in limiting the spread of viral infection, together with the observation that cortisol could inhibit interferon synthesis (Kilbourne, Smart and Pokorny, 1961), suggested a new approach to this problem. It had been known for some time that under certain conditions cortisol could enhance the severity of viral infection *in vivo*, and the observation of Kilbourne, Smart and Pokorny (1961) provided a clue as to how such an enhancement could take place. The striking steric resemblance between steroid hormones and aromatic carcinogens, as emphasized by Yang and co-workers (1961), suggested the possibility that the latter compounds also inhibit interferon synthesis. This was investigated and, as a result of these experiments, we were able to show that polycyclic carcinogens can inhibit interferon synthesis. These observations have now been extended to carcinogens of widely different chemical structures. Experiments were first carried out under the relatively simple conditions of the tissue culture system; more recently we have studied the effect of carcinogenic chemicals and X-irradiation *in vivo*. The salient features of our previously published results will be reviewed in this paper and new data will be presented.

TISSUE CULTURE EXPERIMENTS

Polycyclic aromatic hydrocarbons

Previous experiments were carried out in rat embryo fibroblast tissue culture; pretreatment of these cells with any one of three carcinogenic hydrocarbons—3-MCA, benzo(a)pyrene (BaP), and DMBA—significantly decreased interferon synthesis induced with live Sindbis virus. Four structurally related but non-carcinogenic compounds had no effect (De Maeyer and De Maeyer-Guignard, 1964; De Maeyer-Guignard and

De Maeyer, 1965). Comparable results have been obtained in L cell or C3H mouse embryo cultures infected with Semliki Forest virus (SFV) (Table I) or Newcastle disease virus (NDV).

In cultures of rat embryo and mouse embryo fibroblasts and in L-cell cultures, plaque size of Sindbis or SFV is increased after pretreatment of the

TABLE I

EFFECT OF CARCINOGENIC AND NON-CARCINOGENIC HYDROCARBONS ON INTERFERON
INDUCTION BY SFV IN C3H EMBRYO FIBROBLASTS

Pretreatment of culture (μg./ml.)	Interferon titre (units/1·6 ml.)	Average
Control	140	
	200	190
	200	
	220	
Non-carcinogenic		
Pyrene, 1·0	210	
	260	243
	260	
BeP, 1·0	200	
	250	233
	250	
Anthracene, 1·0	120	
	200	173
	200	
BA, 1·0	200	
	200	220
	260	
Carcinogenic		
BaP, 1·0	50	
	50	53
	60	
0·1	60	
	80	103
	170	
DMBA, 0·1	0	
	0	0
	0	
0·01	50	
	50	70
	110	

Cultures of C3H embryo fibroblasts were exposed to the compound-containing media for 24 hours. The media were then removed, and the cells were infected with SFV at an input multiplicity of 0·01. Forty-eight hours later the culture media were removed and samples were dialysed against Sörensen buffer at pH 2. Interferon titres were determined in C3H embryo fibroblast cultures against vaccinia virus. Interferon yields of replicate cultures are given in the table. Virus yields were comparable in all instances.

BeP=Benzo(e)pyrene; BA=Benz(a)anthracene; BaP=Benzo(a)pyrene; DMBA=7, 12-Dimethyl-benz(a)anthracene.

cells with carcinogenic hydrocarbons; no effect is obtained with non-carcinogenic compounds (Fig. 1). The increase of plaque size, as compared to untreated cultures, is a result of the inhibition of interferon synthesis in the carcinogen-treated cultures. It is due to the greater influence of endogenous interferon in checking the spread of infection under a solid overlay as opposed to fluid culture medium. Indeed, under either an agar or a starch gel, interferon, because of its smaller molecular size, diffuses more readily than virus particles, and this way it reaches surrounding cells much sooner than the virus, which is an important prerequisite for establishing its protective effect. The enhancement of plaque size by carcinogens is

TABLE II

PROTECTION OF L-CELL CULTURES AGAINST THE INTERFERON INHIBITORY
EFFECT OF BaP BY PRETREATMENT WITH BeP

Treatment of cultures before inoculation of virus		Interferon titre (units/1·6 ml.)
0–24 hours	24–48 hours	
—	—	40
—	BaP, 1 μg./ml.	8
BeP, 10 μg./ml.	—	50
BeP, 10 μg./ml.	BaP, 1 μg./ml.	35

Cultures of L-cell fibroblasts were treated with the compounds as indicated in the table. Thereafter, the chemical-containing culture media were removed, and NDV (Kumarov strain) was added to the cultures. The fluids were harvested 33 hours later, pooled and dialysed against Sörensen buffer at pH 2 for 96 hours. Each pool was derived from three replicate cultures. Interferon titrations were carried out in L-cell fibroblasts against VSV.

not observed in cells unsusceptible to the viral inhibitory activity of interferon (De Maeyer-Guignard and De Maeyer, 1965). Conversely, it is not observed in cells susceptible to interferon but infected with a virus that induces little or no interferon formation. For example, pretreatment of L-cell cultures with BaP is followed by a marked increase of SFV plaque size, but it has no enhancing effect on plaque size of vesicular stomatitis virus (VSV); this virus, in contrast to SFV, does not induce measurable interferon formation in these cultures.

The lack of effect on interferon synthesis and on plaque size of the non-carcinogenic hydrocarbons is not due to lack of uptake by the cells, since we have noticed that cells exposed to these hydrocarbons develop the same pattern of intracellular fluorescence as those exposed to carcinogenic compounds. Furthermore, pretreatment of fibroblast cultures with non-carcinogenic aromatic hydrocarbons renders these cultures resistant to the interferon inhibitory effect of the carcinogenic ones (Table II). This pretreatment not only provided protection against the interferon inhibitory

8*

effect of carcinogenic hydrocarbons, but also against their enhancing effect on plaque size, as was to be expected (Fig. 2). The mechanism of the protective effect is not clear; the non-carcinogenic compound could conceivably impair the penetration of the carcinogen into the cell, or it could, inside the cell, prevent the action of the carcinogen by blocking some site on the target molecules.

The foregoing experiments were carried out in rat or mouse cell cultures, since the carcinogenic activity of aromatic hydrocarbons has been mostly documented in these species. We have done a few comparable experiments in tissue cultures of primate origin (monkey kidney or human foetal lung). In these cells, neither 3-MCA nor BaP, at concentrations up to 50 µg./ml., had any effect on interferon synthesis induced with Sindbis virus.

The lack of effect of carcinogenic hydrocarbons in primate cells cannot be due to a lack of uptake by the cells since it has been shown by Allison and Mallucci (1964) and by Diamond (1965) that these compounds are readily taken up by monkey and human cells. This lack of activity in cells derived from the monkey, a species known to be very refractory to the carcinogenic power of these hydrocarbons (Pfeiffer and Allen, 1948), raised the problem of the relationship between carcinogenic activity and inhibition of interferon synthesis. In addition, the inhibitory effect of carcinogenic hydrocarbons on interferon synthesis in murine cells, as opposed to the lack of effect of their non-carcinogenic counterparts, also suggested a correlation between carcinogenicity and inhibition of interferon production. However, in view of the inhibitory action of cortisol on interferon synthesis, the possibility remained that the comparable effect obtained with carcinogenic hydrocarbons was only related to the steroid-like structure of the latter. Therefore the effect of carcinogens without a steroid-like structure was examined.

4-Nitroquinoline-N-Oxide and Triethylenemelamine

Two compounds, very different chemically but sharing carcinogenic properties, were studied. The bicyclic compound, 4NQO, is a very potent carcinogen (Nakahara, Fukuoka and Sugimura, 1957): it induces lymphomas in BALB/c mice, from which a filterable agent has been isolated (Kinosita and Tanaka, 1963; Ribacchi and Giraldo, 1966). Triethylenemelamine (TEM) on the other hand is a weakly carcinogenic alkylating agent (Walpole, 1958).

Pretreatment of rat embryo cell cultures for 24 hours with 4NQO at 0·1 and 0·01 µg./ml. completely inhibited interferon production upon infection of these cultures with SFV. Furthermore, an increase of SFV

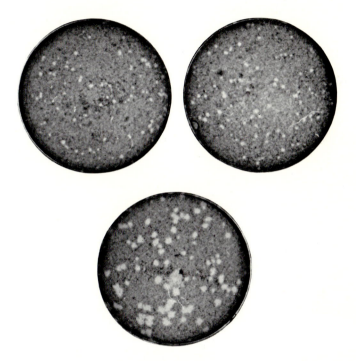

Fig. 1. Semliki Forest virus plaques in C3H embryo cultures pre-treated with either the non-carcinogenic benzo(e)pyrene (BeP) or the carcinogenic benzo(a)pyrene (BaP).

The cultures were exposed for 24 hours to the hydrocarbon-containing culture media (concentration: 1 μg./ml. for both compounds). The hydrocarbon-containing medium was then removed and SFV was plated under a starch overlay. The picture was taken three days after virus inoculation.

Top left: control culture; top right: BeP 1 μg./ml.; bottom: BaP 1 μg./ml. Scale: 2/3.

[*To face page 222*

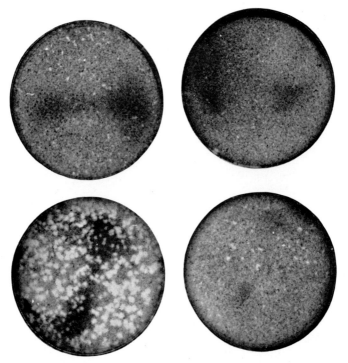

FIG. 2. Protection by a non-carcinogenic hydrocarbon (benzo(e)-pyrene) against the interferon-inhibiting effect of a carcinogenic hydrocarbon (7,12-dimethylbenz(a)anthracene).

C3H mouse embryo cultures were incubated with medium containing BeP at 10 μg./ml. or with control medium for 48 hours. These media were then removed and the cultures were further incubated with medium containing DMBA at 0·1 μg./ml. or with control medium for 24 hours. The media were then removed and SFV was plated under a starch overlay.

	First incubation (48 hrs.)	*Second incubation (24 hrs.)*
Top left:	Control medium	Control medium
right:	BeP 10 μg./ml.	Control medium
Bottom left:	Control medium	DMBA 0·1 μg./ml.
right:	BeP 10 μg./ml.	DMBA 0·1 μg./ml.

Scale: 2/3.

plaque size in rat embryo cell cultures was noticed in carcinogen-treated cultures. The structurally related but non-carcinogenic 4-nitropyridine-N-oxide had no effect (De Maeyer and De Maeyer-Guignard, 1967). Similar results were obtained with TEM, at concentrations of 1 and 0·1 μg./ml., in rat embryo cell cultures infected with Sindbis virus (De Maeyer and De Maeyer-Guignard, 1967).

The results obtained with 4NQO and TEM indicated that a steroid-like structure was not a prerequisite for a carcinogen to be able to inhibit interferon synthesis. Furthermore, it became clear that the correlation with carcinogenic activity was qualitative but not quantitative, since both a weak carcinogen (TEM) and a very strong one (4NQO) had about the same interferon-inhibiting activity when tested in tissue culture.

2-Acetylaminofluorene and N-hydroxy-acetylaminofluorene

Results obtained with the carcinogen 2-acetylaminofluorene (AAF) provided additional evidence for the existence of a correlation between carcinogenicity and inhibition of interferon synthesis. AAF is an aromatic amine with potent carcinogenic activity in rats or mice. Its effect on interferon synthesis was studied in rat and mouse embryo cell cultures infected with Sindbis or SFV. No inhibitory activity was found with concentrations up to 100 μg./ml. However, AAF is not the actual carcinogen, but requires metabolic activation in the animal where, as a result of hydroxylation a more proximate carcinogenic metabolite, N-OH-AAF, is formed (Miller, Miller and Hartmann, 1961). Dr. E. Bisagni of our institute synthesized for us some N-OH-AAF which was then tested for its effect on interferon formation in C3H mouse embryo cells. The cultures were exposed for 48 hours to either AAF or N-OH-AAF at concentrations of 10 μg. and 1 μg./ml. After removal of the culture media the cells were infected with SFV at an input multiplicity of 0·01. The production of infectious virus and of interferon was measured. Interferon

TABLE III

EFFECT OF ACETYLAMINOFLUORENE AND N-HYDROXY-ACETYLAMINOFLUORENE ON INTERFERON SYNTHESIS IN C3H EMBRYO CELLS INFECTED WITH SFV

	Control	AAF (10 μg.)	AAF (1 μg.)	N-OH-AAF (10 μg.)	N-OH-AAF (1 μg.)
Interferon* (units/1·6 ml.)	310	250	200	0	280
Virus† (p.f.u./0·5 ml.)	$4·9 \times 10^3$	$4·6 \times 10^3$	—	$3·3 \times 10^5$	—

* Interferon titrations were carried out in L cells against VSV.
† Virus titrations were carried out in primary cultures of chick embryo fibroblasts.

synthesis was completely blocked by N-OH-AAF at 10 μg./ml., while about 100 times more virus was produced than in control cultures (Table III). In C3H embryo cell cultures, SFV plaque size was enhanced by N-OH-AAF but not by AAF.

EXPERIMENTS *in vivo*

The experiments carried out in rat or mouse embryo fibroblasts indicated that in these cultures carcinogenic agents of a widely different nature significantly reduced the amount of interferon appearing upon infection with Sindbis virus, SFV or NDV. However, the possible implication of these findings for certain forms of carcinogenesis could not be fully assessed until similar experiments had been performed *in vivo*. Our first studies *in vivo* were concerned with the effect of urethane and of X-irradiation on the production of circulating interferon in either BALB/c or C3H mice.

Urethane

Urethane was chosen because of its already well-documented enhancing effect upon infection in mice with several viruses (Braunsteiner and Friend, 1954; Mirick *et al.*, 1952) and especially with leukaemia viruses (see above). Furthermore, in contrast to most carcinogens urethane is very rapidly metabolized and eliminated by the animal (Berenblum *et al.*, 1958), so that a dose-response effect can be established more readily.

The effect of urethane on the production of interferon was studied primarily in BALB/c mice. In these animals circulating interferon was induced by intravenous injection of either NDV or Sindbis virus. Urethane, dissolved in phosphate-buffered saline, was injected intraperitoneally, at a dose of 1 to 1·5 mg./g. body weight. This corresponds to the usual amounts given in order to enhance viral leukaemia. Initial experiments were carried out in BALB/c mice of about two months of age, and a preliminary account of these experiments has been published (De Maeyer-

TABLE IV

EFFECT OF METHYLCARBAMATE ON NDV INTERFERON INDUCTION IN BALB/c MICE

Group	Interferon titre (units/1·6 ml.)
Control	430
Methylcarbamate (1·5 mg./g.)	350

A group of six 8-week-old male BALB/c mice received an intraperitoneal injection of methylcarbamate dissolved in phosphate-buffered saline. Another group received only phosphate-buffered saline. Twenty-three hours later all animals were injected with NDV; blood was drawn 6½ hours after virus injection. Interferon titrations of the pooled sera were carried out in L cell fibroblasts against VSV.

Guignard and De Maeyer, 1967). Intraperitoneal administration of urethane to two-month-old BALB/c mice impaired the capacity of these
animals to produce circulating interferon. The effect appeared rapidly after a
single injection, and was of short duration (Fig. 3). The structurally related

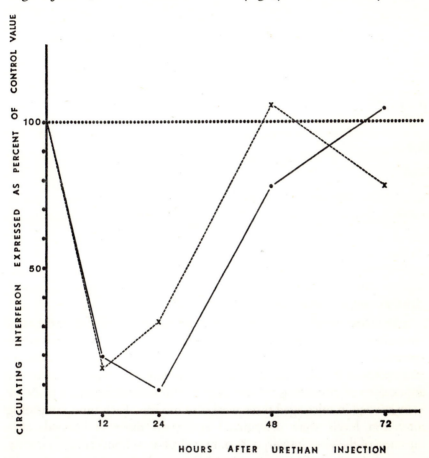

FIG. 3. Effect of urethane on NDV-induced circulating interferon in female BALB/c
mice. The circulating interferon levels were measured six hours after injection of the virus.
Interferon titrations were carried out in L cells against VSV.

●—● 1·5 mg./g.
×---× 1·0 mg./g.

but non-carcinogenic methylcarbamate (Larsen, 1947) had no effect on
interferon synthesis (Table IV). The higher sensitivity of newborn or
suckling mice to the carcinogenic action of urethane is well documented
(Pietra, Rappaport and Shubik, 1961; Fiore-Donati *et al.*, 1961; Trainin,
Precerutti and Law, 1964); we therefore examined the effect of urethane

on interferon formation in BALB/c, C3H and C57BL mice of different ages. It was found that the effect of urethane on circulating interferon was age-dependent, being very striking in weanling animals, and gradually decreasing with increasing age. Some results are summarized in Table V.

TABLE V

EFFECT OF URETHANE ON NDV-INDUCED CIRCULATING INTERFERON IN FEMALE
MICE OF DIFFERENT AGES

Mouse strain BALB/c	Treatment	Interferon titres of control and urethane-treated mice in different age groups		
		2 months	4 months	6 months
Exp. 1	Control	480*	380	275
	Urethane (1·25 mg./g.)	115 (24%)†	145 (38%)	158 (57%)
Exp. 2	Control	380		120
	Urethane (1·25 mg./g.)	72 (19%)		105 (87%)
C3H		1 month	8·5 months	
	Control	4,925	800	
	Urethane (1·25 mg./g.)	2,275 (46%)	575 (72%)	
C57BL		1 month	19 months	
	Control	25,000	3,300	
	Urethane (1·50 mg./g.)	2,000 (8%)	1,320 (40%)	

* Units/1·6 ml.
† Percentage of control value.

Age dependency of circulating interferon response

In the course of the experiments with urethane in mice of different ages, we noticed that the amounts of circulating interferon appearing in the control animals were also age-dependent. A systematic study was therefore undertaken in BALB/c and C3H mice of varying ages; the kinetics of the appearance of circulating interferon after intravenous injection of NDV were studied in mice aged three weeks–19 months. Each time, circulating interferon levels were determined at several different intervals after injection of the virus (usually 2, 6, 9, 12 and 18 or 24 hours later). This was necessary because after a few experiments it became obvious that the maximum levels of circulating interferon did not always appear at the same time after virus injection. Whereas in C3H mice the maximum interferon levels were obtained for all age groups six hours after injection of the virus, in BALB/c mice maximum interferon levels appeared generally in the younger animals (up to two months) at about six hours after injection of the virus, and for the older animals nine to 12 hours after injection of the virus. With due regard for the different kinetics of interferon induction in animals of different ages, our findings can be summarized as follows. The amounts of circulating interferon appearing after intravenous injection of

NDV increase with the age of the animal, reaching a maximum in mice aged two months. From then on the circulating interferon-producing capacity very slowly decreases; for example it was repeatedly observed that 10-month-old C3H or BALB/c mice produced about half as much interferon as animals of two to three months old. Fig. 4 summarizes two representative experiments where the kinetics of induction of circulating interferon were followed in C3H and BALB/c mice of different ages.

X-irradiation

The study of interferon production in X-irradiated mice was undertaken because of the well-known enhancing effect of X-irradiation on virus infection. In addition, we hoped that this study would provide some basic information about certain aspects of interferon synthesis *in vivo*. These experiments were carried out in collaboration with Dr. P. Jullien; some of the results have been published (Jullien and De Maeyer, 1966), and the remainder will be published in greater detail elsewhere.

All experiments discussed in this section were performed in C3H mice, and all irradiation was carried out under conditions of total body exposure. The production of circulating interferon after intravenous injection of Sindbis virus or NDV is significantly reduced after exposure of the mice to a dose of 1,000 r. Different kinetics of the onset of the inhibitory effect suggested that different cells were involved in interferon formation in response to NDV as opposed to Sindbis virus. This suggestion has now received additional support from studies carried out with different irradiation doses. Eight-week-old C3H mice received either 125, 250, 500 or 1,000 r., and four days after irradiation the interferon production upon intravenous injection of either Sindbis virus or NDV was measured. From these experiments it appears that the circulating interferon-producing system is fairly radioresistant if Sindbis virus is used as inducer, since a significant reduction only occurs after 1,000 r.; in contradistinction, circulating interferon production with NDV as inducer is more radiosensitive, since at 125 r. a marked effect is already obtained, and after 250 r. the production is as much reduced as with 1,000 r. (Table VI). The nature of the interferon-producing cells cannot be inferred with absolute certainty from these results, but a plausible guess would be that with Sindbis virus macrophages are involved (Kono and Ho, 1965) and with NDV lymphocytes or granulocytes (Wheelock, 1966). This is borne out by our observation that restoration of the haemopoietic system after 1,000 r. is very closely followed by restoration of the interferon-producing capacity of these animals, the speed of restoration being dependent on the number of

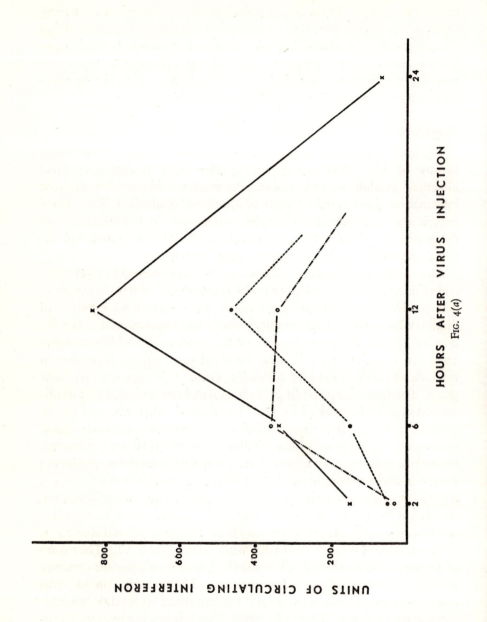

FIG. 4(a)

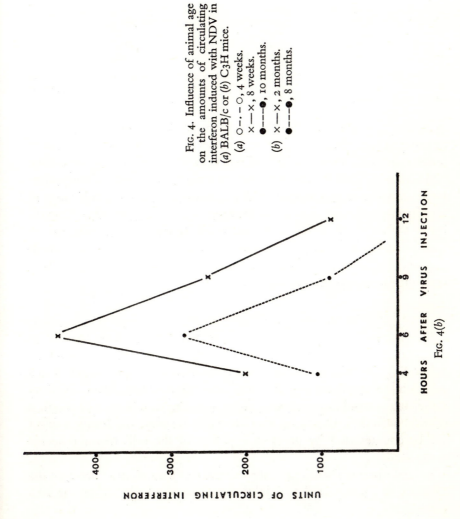

FIG. 4. Influence of animal age on the amounts of circulating interferon induced with NDV in (a) BALB/c or (b) C3H mice.

(a) ○–·–○, 4 weeks.
×—×, 8 weeks.
●———●, 10 months.

(b) ×—×, 2 months.
●––––●, 8 months.

FIG. 4(b)

HOURS AFTER VIRUS INJECTION

UNITS OF CIRCULATING INTERFERON

TABLE VI

EFFECT OF INCREASING DOSES OF X-IRRADIATION ON CIRCULATING INTERFERON
INDUCTION WITH NDV AND SINDBIS VIRUS IN 8-WEEK-OLD C3H MICE

Exposure (r.)	NDV-induced interferon	Sindbis-induced interferon
0	5,000 —	11,000 —
125	1,400 (28%)	14,500 (131%)
250	500 (10%)	7,600 (69%)
500	440 (9%)	4,800 (43%)
1,000	550 (11%)	2,600 (23%)

The circulating interferon production was measured four days after irradiation. Animals were bled six hours after injection of NDV and eight hours after injection of Sindbis. Interferon titrations were carried out in L cells against VSV. Titres are given in units/1·6 ml.

isologous bone marrow cells injected after irradiation. Similar studies with other viruses are planned to find out whether the very radiosensitive type of interferon induction observed with NDV, and the fairly radioresistant one observed with Sindbis, represent the two main systems of circulating interferon induction or just happen to be the two extremes of a whole range of interferon-producing systems of intermediate radiosensitivities. Regardless of the outcome of this study, our results to date indicate that, on the basis of an effect on interferon synthesis, one could expect that animals exposed to relatively low doses of irradiation would be more susceptible to some viruses, but by no means to all.

DISCUSSION

Our *in vitro* experiments show that chemical carcinogens are able to decrease the normal amounts of interferon appearing in virus-infected cell cultures. This effect is obtained with concentrations of carcinogen which do not inhibit replication of the virus used to induce interferon. Furthermore, under conditions where endogenous interferon limits the progress of viral infection, i.e. under agar or starch overlay, the limiting effect can be counteracted by previous exposure of the cells to carcinogenic compounds.

Several observations suggest the existence of a correlation between the capacity of a compound to inhibit interferon synthesis and its carcinogenicity:

(a) The lack of effect on interferon production of structurally related but non-carcinogenic derivates;

(b) The activity of the proximate carcinogen N-OH-AAF as opposed to its non-hydroxylated precursor AAF;

(c) The absence, in monkey cell cultures, of the phenomenon of inhibition of interferon synthesis by hydrocarbons, known to be very carcinogenic for murine species but without demonstrable carcinogenicity in primates.

What is the extent and the meaning of this apparent correlation? It is not an absolute one, since actinomycin D and some steroid hormones can also inhibit interferon synthesis without inhibiting virus replication (Heller, 1963; De Maeyer and De Maeyer-Guignard, 1963). Such compounds can certainly not be considered as carcinogens in the strict sense, even though it has been shown in mice that actinomycin may induce sarcomas (Kawamata et al., 1959) and oestrogens may induce lymphomas from which a filterable leukaemogenic agent can be isolated (Kunii, Takemoto and Furth, 1965).

At present, we have no information concerning the mechanism of inhibition of interferon synthesis by carcinogens. This problem should be approached with due regard for the well-known properties various chemical carcinogens have of interacting with biologically important macromolecules (see review by Miller and Miller, 1966). The interaction could take place with the genomal DNA, as a result of which the transcription of messenger RNA necessary for interferon synthesis would be impaired. Interaction with DNA has been described for polycyclic aromatic carcinogens (Brookes and Lawley, 1964a) and for alkylating agents (Brookes and Lawley, 1964b). Another possible explanation for the action of the carcinogens on interferon formation would be their equally well documented capacity for interacting with proteins (see review by Heidelberger, 1964), and one can imagine an interaction either with enzymes involved in interferon synthesis, or with interferon itself. The possibility of a direct interaction of carcinogens with interferon is now being examined and first results indicate that some inactivation of interferon occurs, but at concentrations of carcinogen more elevated than those required for the effect on interferon formation.

Is the inhibition of interferon synthesis by chemical carcinogens related to their carcinogenic activity? A distinction should be made between "direct" induction of tumour formation by chemicals, where the tumour is the immediate result of an interaction carcinogen-cell, and "indirect" induction of tumour formation, where the carcinogen acts by way of a latent tumour virus. The latter form of carcinogenesis is involved in the induction of murine leukaemia, and possibly also in the origin of mammary tumours. As far as direct tumour induction is concerned, it would appear that the inhibition of interferon synthesis is not directly relevant to the process of carcinogenesis, but is merely a reflection of the capacity of these carcinogens to interact with vital macromolecules, as discussed in the previous paragraph. At the most, the inhibition of interferon formation by chemical carcinogens may serve as an example of how these compounds can interfere with cellular control mechanisms by inhibiting the formation of biologically very active derepressor molecules. The inhibition of interferon synthesis, however, is of immediate relevance to the second type of carcinogenesis by chemicals, the "indirect" form, where the carcinogen acts by way of a virus. Our *in vitro* study of the interaction between the components of the triad, chemical carcinogen-cell-virus, has revealed the existence of a direct mechanism by which the carcinogen alters the cell-virus relationship in favour of the latter. Such a situation was predicted by Lwoff (1960) "... When tumor viruses are involved, and when malignancy is due to the concerted action of a virus and a carcinogen, the role of carcinogens could be the same as when inducers act on lysogenic bacteria: they would upset the balance of the cell virus system by interfering with the synthesis of repressors." Such a mechanism may reveal itself to be an important step in the activation of certain leukaemia and mammary tumour viruses, which are vertically transmitted or acquired neonatally through the milk, and towards which the animal is immunologically tolerant. Equally in favour of this hypothesis are our *in vivo* results, since both urethane and X-irradiation, which are good inducers or enhancers of leukaemia, were very effective in depressing interferon production. However, at least in the case of X-irradiation, the decreased interferon formation *in vivo* seemed not to be due to a direct effect on the synthesis of the interferon, but rather to a depression of bone marrow function resulting in a decrease of interferon-producing cells. The importance of leucocytes and macrophages in the synthesis of interferon during viraemia is becoming increasingly manifest (Gresser, 1961; Glasgow and Habel, 1963; Kono and Ho, 1965) and it would therefore appear that, if interferon synthesis by these cells plays a role in restricting the replication of certain leukaemia viruses, one could expect that most marrow-depressing agents would have an enhancing effect on these forms of leukaemia.

The validity of our hypothesis that oncogenic viruses can be stimulated by carcinogens because the latter depress interferon formation depends upon two assumptions for which the experimental evidence is at present incomplete. The first assumption is that oncogenic viruses are susceptible to interferon; this has been demonstrated *in vivo* for polyoma (Atanasiu and Chany, 1960), and Rous sarcoma virus (Lampson *et al.*, 1963) and *in vitro* for SV40 (Todaro and Baron, 1965). The evidence for leukaemia viruses is less abundant, but studies by Gresser and co-workers (1967) with Friend leukaemia virus indicate that they will prove to be no exception to other oncogenic agents. In addition, as a result of a small pilot experiment we have noticed that the appearance of lymphoma in AK mice can be delayed by giving large amounts of interferon during the neonatal period. The second assumption is that formation of endogenous interferon is part of the mechanism by which an animal can keep its latent virus infections under control. This remains to be proved.

Direct stimulation of virus replication by interference with the synthesis of inhibitors such as interferon may turn out to be an important part of the mechanism by which carcinogens exert their enhancing effect on tumours of viral origin; the immunodepressive effect of these carcinogens (Prehn, 1963; Stjernswärd, 1966; Doell, De Vaux St. Cyr and Grabar, 1967) could then facilitate the acceptance of virus-transformed antigenic cells. To assess the relative importance of virus stimulation in oncogenesis by carcinogens, we plan to give interferon to carcinogen-treated or irradiated animals. This treatment, as far as we know, would not interfere with the immunodepressive effect of the carcinogen, nor is it likely to decrease the number of immature target cells, which, according to Kaplan (1960) and Duplan and Latarjet (1966) may favour development of viral leukaemia. Purified interferon of high potency seems in this respect a promising tool with which to obtain more information about the role of virus stimulation in the origin of some chemically or radiation-induced tumours.

SUMMARY

Polycyclic aromatic carcinogenic hydrocarbons decrease interferon formation in tissue cultures of murine cells, but not of primate cells.

Structurally related but non-carcinogenic hydrocarbons have no effect on interferon synthesis. However, cells preincubated with these compounds become resistant to the interferon inhibitory effect of the carcinogens.

The weakly carcinogenic triethylenemelamine and the potent carcinogen 4-nitroquinoline-N-oxide both inhibit interferon synthesis in tissue cultures of murine cells. The non-carcinogenic 4-nitropyridine-N-oxide has no effect.

The carcinogenic aromatic amine, acetylaminofluorene, has no effect on interferon synthesis in tissue culture, but its more proximate carcinogenic metabolite, N-hydroxy-acetylaminofluorene, inhibits interferon formation in tissue cultures of murine cells.

After intravenous injection of Newcastle disease virus into mice, circulating interferon levels are significantly reduced if the carcinogen urethane (ethylcarbamate) has previously been administered to the animals. The effect of urethane decreases with increasing age of the animal.

very old ??

Interferon formation is reduced in X-irradiated mice; interferon induction with Newcastle disease virus is very radiosensitive, whereas induction with Sindbis virus is much more radioresistant.

The amounts of circulating interferon appearing in BALB/c mice after intravenous injection of Newcastle disease virus are age-dependent. They reach maximum levels in animals of two to three months old, and slowly decrease from then on.

Acknowledgements

This work was supported by the Jane Coffin Childs Memorial Fund for Medical Research (New Haven, U.S.A.); in addition, J. De Maeyer-Guignard was until recently a fellow of the Lady Tata Foundation.

We are greatly indebted to Dr. R. Latarjet for encouragement and help, and to our colleagues, Drs. E. Bisagni, P. Jullien and F. Zajdela, for stimulating discussions and collaboration.

REFERENCES

ALLISON, A. C., and MALLUCCI, L. (1964). *Nature, Lond.,* **203**, 1024–1027.

ATANASIU, P., and CHANY, C. (1960). *C. r. hebd. Séanc. Acad. Sci., Paris,* **251**, 1687–1689.

BERENBLUM, I., HARAN-GHERA, N., WINNICK, R., and WINNICK, T. (1958). *Cancer Res.,* **18**, 181–185.

BRAUNSTEINER, H., and FRIEND, C. (1954). *J. exp. Med.,* **100**, 665–673.

BROOKES, P., and LAWLEY, P. D. (1964a). *Nature, Lond.,* **202**, 781–784.

BROOKES, P., and LAWLEY, P. D. (1964b). *J. cell. comp. Physiol.,* **64**, Suppl. 1, 111–128.

DE MAEYER, E., and DE MAEYER-GUIGNARD, J. (1963). *Nature, Lond.,* **197**, 724–725.

DE MAEYER, E., and DE MAEYER-GUIGNARD, J. (1964). *J. natn. Cancer Inst.,* **32**, 1317–1331.

DE MAEYER, E., and DE MAEYER-GUIGNARD, J. (1967). *Arch. ges. Virusforsch,* in press.

DE MAEYER-GUIGNARD, J., and DE MAEYER, E. (1965). *J. natn. Cancer Inst.,* **34**, 265–276.

DE MAEYER-GUIGNARD, J., and DE MAEYER, E. (1967). *Science,* **155**, 482–484.

DIAMOND, L. (1965). *J. cell. comp. Physiol.,* **66**, 183–198.

DOELL, R. G., DE VAUX ST. CYR, C., and GRABAR, P. (1967). *Int. J. Cancer,* **2**, 103–108.

DUPLAN, J. F., and LATARJET, R. (1966). *Cancer Res.,* **26**, 395–399.

DURAN-REYNALS, M. L. (1963). *Prog. exp. Tumor Res.,* **3**, 148–185.

FIORE-DONATI, L., CHIECO-BIANCHI, L., and DE BENEDICTIS, G. (1964). In *Cellular Control Mechanisms and Cancer,* pp. 268–271, ed. Emmelot, P., and Mühlbock, O. Amsterdam: Elsevier Publishing Co.

FIORE-DONATI, L., CHIECO-BIANCHI, L., DE BENEDICTIS, G., and MAIORANO, G. (1961). *Nature, Lond.,* **190**, 278.

GLASGOW, L. A., and HABEL, K. (1963). *J. exp. Med.,* **117**, 149–160.

GRESSER, I. (1961). *Proc. Soc. exp. Biol. Med.,* **108**, 799–803.

GRESSER, I., COPPEY, J., FALCOFF, E., and FONTAINE, D. (1967). *Proc. Soc. exp. Biol. Med.,* **124**, 84–91.

GROSS, L. (1959). *Proc. Soc. exp. Biol. Med.,* **100**, 102–105.

HEIDELBERGER, C. (1964). *J. cell. comp. Physiol.,* **64**, 129–148.

HELLER, E. (1963). *Virology,* **21**, 652–656.

IRINO, S., OTA, Z., SEZAKI, T., SUZAKI, M., and HIRAKI, K. (1963). *Gann,* **54**, 225–237.

JULLIEN, P., and DE MAEYER, E. (1966). *Int. J. Radiat. Biol.,* **11**, 567–576.

KAPLAN, H. S. (1960). *Natn. Cancer Inst. Monogr.,* no. 4, 141–146.

KAWAMATA, J., NAKABAYASHI, N., KAWAI, A., FUJITA, H., IMANISHI, M., and IKEGAMI, R. (1959). *Biken's J.*, **2**, 105–112.

KILBOURNE, E. D., SMART, K. M., and POKORNY, B. A. (1961). *Nature, Lond.*, **190**, 650–651.

KINOSITA, R., and TANAKA, T. (1963). In *Viruses, Nucleic Acids, and Cancer*, ed. University of Texas. Baltimore: Williams and Wilkins.

KONO, Y., and HO, M. (1965). *Virology*, **25**, 162–166.

KUNII, A., TAKEMOTO, H., and FURTH, J. (1965). *Proc. Soc. exp. Biol. Med.*, **119**, 1211–1215.

LAMPSON, G. P., TYTELL, A. A., NEMES, M. M., and HILLEMAN, M. R. (1963). *Proc. Soc. exp. Biol. Med.*, **112**, 468–478.

LARSEN, C. D. (1947). *J. natn. Cancer Inst.*, **8**, 99–101.

LIEBERMAN, M., HARAN-GHERA, N., and KAPLAN, H. S. (1964). *Nature, Lond.*, **203**, 420–422.

LIEBERMAN, M., and KAPLAN, H. S. (1959). *Science*, **130**, 387–388.

LWOFF, A. (1960). *Cancer Res.*, **20**, 820–829.

MALMGREN, R. A., BENNISON, B. E., and McKINLEY, T. W., JR. (1952). *Proc. Soc. exp. Biol. Med.*, **79**, 484–488.

MILLER, E. C., and MILLER, J. A. (1966). *Pharmac. Rev.*, **18**, 805–838.

MILLER, E. C., MILLER, J. A., and HARTMANN, H. A. (1961). *Cancer Res.*, **21**, 815–824.

MIRICK, G. S., SMITH, J. M., LEFTWICH, C. I., JR., and LEFTWICH, W. B. (1952). *J. exp. Med.*, **95**, 147–160.

NAKAHARA, W., FUKUOKA, F., and SUGIMURA, T. (1957). *Gann*, **48**, 129–137.

PFEIFFER, C. A., and ALLEN, E. (1948). *Cancer Res.*, **8**, 97–127.

PIETRA, G., RAPPAPORT, H., and SHUBIK, P. (1961). *Cancer, N.Y.*, **14**, 308–317.

PREHN, R. T. (1963). *J. natn. Cancer Inst.*, **31**, 791–805.

RIBACCHI, R., and GIRALDO, G. (1966). *Natn. Cancer Inst. Monogr.*, **22**, 701–711.

ROUS, P., and KIDD, J. G. (1936). *Science*, **83**, 468–469.

SCHOLLER, J., BERGS, V. V., and GROUPÉ, V. (1964). *Proc. Am. Ass. Cancer Res.*, **5**, 56.

STJERNSWÄRD, J. (1966). *J. natn. Cancer Inst.*, **36**, 1189–1195.

TODARO, G. J., and BARON, S. (1965). *Proc. natn. Acad. Sci. U.S.A.*, **54**, 752–756.

TOTH, B. (1963). *Proc. Soc. exp. Biol. Med.*, **112**, 873–875.

TOTH, B., and SHUBIK, P. (1966). *Natn. Cancer Inst. Monogr.*, **22**, 313–328.

TRAININ, N., PRECERUTTI, A., and LAW, L. L. (1964). *Nature, Lond.*, **202**, 305–306.

WALPOLE, A. (1958). *Ann. N.Y. Acad. Sci.*, **68**, 750–761.

WHEELOCK, E. F. (1966). *J. Bact.*, **92**, 1415–1421.

YANG, N. C., CASTRO, A. J., LEWIS, M., and WONG, T. W. (1961). *Science*, **134**, 386–387.

DISCUSSION

Mécs: Do the carcinogenic and non-carcinogenic compounds you used have different toxicities?

De Maeyer: The concentrations of carcinogenic aromatic hydrocarbons used to inhibit interferon synthesis were 10 to 100 times lower than those required to obtain a direct cytotoxic effect. Furthermore, growth of cultures of either mouse or rat embryo fibroblasts was not appreciably affected by concentrations of hydrocarbons that very markedly reduced interferon synthesis.

Chany: Were the X-irradiation experiments repeated *in vitro* in tissue culture? I am very impressed by the relatively small amount of energy needed to get these results.

De Maeyer: We did not study the effects of X-irradiation in tissue culture. My interpretation is that X-irradiation inhibits interferon synthesis in the animal by eliminating the interferon-producing cells, since we can restore this function by injecting bone marrow cells.

Gresser: Did you try urethane in tissue culture?

De Maeyer: In tissue culture urethane has no effect whatsoever on interferon synthesis. The explanation for this may be that urethane, in order to be carcinogenic, has to be hydroxylated (Boyland, E., and Nery, R. [1965]. *Biochem. J.*, **94**, 198–208). We are now going to try the hydroxylated compound in tissue culture.

Rotem: Further to Dr. Mécs' remark about possible toxicity, I would like to point out that we were able (Rotem, Z., Berwald, Y., and Sachs, L. [1964]. *Virology*, **24**, 483–486) to show that in hamster cells transformed *in vitro* with carcinogenic hydrocarbons the interferon yield was reduced. There was no residual material in the cells, as the assays were carried with cell lines that were passaged for three to five months after the original carcinogen treatment.

Pereira: Do the X-ray doses that are effective on the virus produce other effects, such as leukaemia?

De Maeyer: X-irradiation certainly has other effects. In mice exposed to 125 r. the lymphocytes disintegrate and disappear. The effect on granulocytes is not very pronounced, but at 250 r. they gradually diminish in the circulation. This is not because they are directly destroyed by the X-irradiation, but because the X-irradiation inhibits some stem cells in the bone marrow.

Finter: What is the LD_{50} in mice for this irradiation?

De Maeyer: It is somewhere between 500 and 1,000 r. but I do not know the exact figure.

Ho: I was impressed by the rapidity and the transient nature of the effect of urethane in mice. While it is nice to be able to correlate carcinogenic effect and inhibition of interferon production, would it not be more pertinent to study some of the more immediate metabolic effects of urethane—for example, whether it has effects similar to actinomycin which would explain some of these results?

De Maeyer: Dr. A. Kaye of the Weizmann Institute, who knows a lot about urethane, once said to me: "Don't ever study the mechanism of action of urethane, because it is a biochemical nightmare!"

Stoker: The same might be said of interferon!

De Maeyer: To come back to Dr. Ho's question, we are faced here with two different problems. We were interested in the effect of carcinogens on interferon and think we have explained part of their enhancing activity on virus replication in animals. But the second question is the mechanism by which carcinogens inhibit interferon.

Levy: We could examine the latter point in tissue culture a little more readily with some of the steroid-type agents. They affect RNA and protein synthesis in general.

Burke: And do they affect actinomycin-sensitive viruses?

De Maeyer: Yes, they do. We studied the effect of dimethylbenzanthracene and of 3,4-benzpyrene on vaccinia and herpes viruses and found an inhibition (De Maeyer, E., and De Maeyer-Guignard, J. [1964]. *Science*, **146**, 650–651). We also studied their effect on Semliki Forest virus and Sindbis virus and found no effect.

Burke: There is a suggestion of a correlation.

Rotem: Dr. A. Isaacs, Dr. F. Himmelweit and I carried out experiments along the same lines as Dr. De Maeyer (unpublished results). We did not study the age difference, but we used mice, about three to four weeks old, which are less susceptible to carcinogens than his. The idea was to study the reduction in interferon production after pretreatment with urethane, administered intraperitoneally 24 hours before irradiated or live Newcastle disease virus was administered intravenously. A reduction was seen in all animals, as compared to controls. NDV-induced interferon was harvested after four, six and eight hours. Although in the NDV-mouse system there is no question of replication of virus, we had to overrule the inhibitory effect of N-hydroxyurethane on virus growth as was shown by C. P. de Sousa, E. Boyland, and R. Nery (1965. *Nature, Lond.*, **206**, 688–689). They suggested that urethane, which is carcinogenic and has been used in the treatment of leukaemia and some forms of cancer, is metabolized by mammals to N-hydroxyurethane. This inhibited Shope fibroma virus, at least in cell cultures. That is why we used irradiated virus. We compared this with interferon induced by statolon. Youngner suggested that the interferon peak in the mouse serum is attained at about eight hours after intravenous administration. Our results fit very well with Dr. De Maeyer's results. There was a mean fivefold reduction of interferon in urethane-pretreated mice when live NDV was used as the inducer and the serum was harvested four hours after induction; the reduction was to eightfold after six hours, and was something of the same order with irradiated NDV. When statolon was used to induce interferon the reduction was never more than 1 to 3-fold. This suggests, though we have no direct evidence, that in NDV-induced interferon we are dealing with interferon synthesis, and in statolon-induced interferon with interferon release. However, the appearance of statolon-induced interferon is quite late so at the moment we have to ignore this suggestion. Dr. De Maeyer's results show that this effect of reduction in the interferon yield disappears after 72 hours. We did some experiments at different time intervals between injection of urethane and NDV. When the urethane was given simultaneously with NDV, the reduction noted was a small one. When the urethane was given one day before NDV the reduction in interferon yield was about sevenfold. This fits with Dr. De Maeyer's results. The effect still lasted when the inducer was given 14 days after the urethane administration. We have no data on interferon yields between these two periods. This might suggest that transformation of cells occurs in the animal, and it may account for the late effect of urethane on interferon yield *in vivo*.

De Maeyer: We have only done complete kinetic studies in two-month-old animals. As you say, the younger the animal the more susceptible it is to the interferon-inhibiting action of urethane. Maybe if we did complete kinetics in the young animal we would find the same.

Rotem: There was only a small difference between the two groups, but it does persist as long as 14 days.

Finter: Dr. De Maeyer may have explained one point that has long puzzled me, namely, the very different times at which peak levels of interferon have been found to occur after injections of NDV in different laboratories. Stinebring and Youngner (1964. *Nature, Lond.,* **204,** 712) found that the peak was 12 hours after injection, while other workers, including ourselves, find it at about six hours. Perhaps this could be due to the use of mice of different ages in the different laboratories. We have used relatively young mice.

De Maeyer: This is possible. In the literature the ages are often not given, but weights are given. Usually there is a certain correlation between the maximum peak, which appears at 12 hours in heavy mice, and at six hours in light mice.

Baron: The differences in time of maximum serum interferon are also connected with differences in the virus strain.

Fantes: When you use benzenoid analogues, before the actual carcinogens, what quantities of the analogues, on a molar basis, do you have to use? Do you use much more of them than of the actual carcinogens, and do you wash them off the cells first?

De Maeyer: The carcinogen is left on for 24 hours and then washed off. We have to add between 10 and 100 times more of the analogue to get the inhibition of the carcinogen and we have to leave it on the cells for 48 instead of 24 hours. Dr. Allison (Allison and Mallucci, 1964, *loc. cit.*) has studied the uptake of these polybenzenoid compounds quite extensively, and he says that the non-carcinogenic analogues also get into the cell, but less efficiently.

Andrewes: Does it have to be an analogue? Is the effect seen with any carcinogen?

De Maeyer: I have not studied it very extensively up to now, but 1,2-benzpyrene, which is non-carcinogenic, protects against 3,4-benzpyrene and 3-methylcholanthrene, whereas it does not seem to protect against the alkylating agent triethylenemelamine, for instance, nor against 4-nitroquinoline-N-oxide.

Andrewes: Have you any idea how it works?

De Maeyer: Not really.

Rotem: We also tried to reverse the effect of urethane by pretreating mice with different dosages of interferon, later giving urethane and an inducer. I would not say that we have been able to show any significant reversal.

Baron: Are there any examples of these carcinogens transforming cells in a system where there is apparently no virus, which would suggest that transformation can occur solely through the carcinogen? If this is the case, one would have to say that there are two actions of the carcinogen. Is that what you are proposing, that there are two actions?

De Maeyer: No, this has been misinterpreted. I do not believe at the present time that one can say that carcinogens act by way of viruses all the time. I think they can act directly on the cell.

Stoker: What is the evidence that they act directly on the cell?

De Maeyer: There is no more firm evidence for that than there is for saying that they always act by way of a virus.

Stoker: I was very glad to hear your results with irradiation, because it may explain a phenomenon we have observed, namely, that a sublethal dose of X-rays given to cells in culture increased the sensitivity to polyoma transformation.

Ho: Could the effect of the low dose of irradiation be partially due to another mechanism? We know that most of the rapidly proliferating cells and tissues in the body are susceptible to X-irradiation. One of the most susceptible is probably the intestinal epithelium. If such cells were affected, one might expect absorption of intestinal bacterial products such as endotoxin. This would produce a state of tolerance and thereby decrease the interferon levels produced after injection of virus. The difference in response to irradiation between NDV and Sindbis virus you showed may be explained by our finding that it is easier to make animals tolerant to NDV than to Sindbis.

De Maeyer: I do not think it is a very likely explanation. We find that at 125 or 250 r. there is no effect on Sindbis. I do not quite see why it should act only on the NDV-induced interferon. I think the best explanation—admittedly it is hypothetical—is on a cellular basis.

THE EFFECT OF INTERFERON PREPARATIONS ON FRIEND LEUKAEMIA IN MICE

I. Gresser[*], J. Coppey[*], D. Fontaine-Brouty-Boye[*], E. Falcoff[†], R. Falcoff[*], F. Zajdela[‡], C. Bourali[*], M. T. Thomas[*]

*Laboratories of Viral Oncology and Pathophysiology, Institut de Recherches Scientifiques sur le Cancer, Villejuif; †Groupe de Recherches sur les virus, Institut National de la Santé et de la Recherche Médicale, Hôpital Saint-Vincent du Paul, Paris; and ‡Unité de Physiologie Cellulaire, Institut du Radium, Orsay (Essonne)

INTERFERON (Isaacs and Lindenmann, 1957) has been shown to inhibit the multiplication of some oncogenic viruses and the cellular transformation induced by these viruses (Atanasiu and Chany, 1960; Allison, 1961; Strandström, Sandelin and Oker-Blöm, 1962; Bader, 1962; Lampson et al., 1963; Todaro and Baron, 1965; Kishida, Kato and Nagano, 1965; Oxman and Black, 1966). Little is known, however, concerning the effect of interferon on the murine leukaemia viruses.

There is some indirect evidence which suggests that Friend and Rauscher viruses may be sensitive to interferon. Wheelock (1966, 1967a) reported that inoculation of DBA/2 mice with certain doses of Sendai virus inhibited replication of Friend virus and retarded the evolution of Friend disease. Various polyanions which induce the production of interferon (Kleinschmidt and Murphy, 1965) have also been reported to inhibit the development of splenomegaly in Friend disease (Regelson, 1967; Regelson and Merigan, 1967; Wheelock, 1967b). However, two groups of workers reported that treatment of mice with interferon did not affect the evolution of Friend and Rauscher diseases (Wheelock, 1967b; Vandeputte et al., 1967).

In contrast to these results, concentrated preparations of interferon were shown to inhibit the development of splenomegaly induced by Friend virus in both Swiss and DBA/2 mice (Gresser et al., 1966, 1967a). This report reviews these findings and presents some recent data on the effects of interferon preparations on the evolution of Friend disease (Gresser et al., 1967b, d).

METHODS

Briefly the techniques employed were as follows. Swiss mice four to six weeks old were inoculated intraperitoneally with a 10 to 15 per cent extract of leukaemic spleen and killed three to five weeks later. Spleen weights provided a reliable criterion of infection and of extent of the disease (Rowe and Brodsky, 1959). Interferon was extracted from the brains of mice infected with West Nile virus (Finter, 1964a, 1965) or from sera and spleens of mice inoculated with Newcastle disease virus (NDV) (Baron and Buckler, 1963). Interferon preparations were assayed by standard plaque-reduction techniques utilizing monolayer cultures of mouse embryo fibroblasts or L cells inoculated with 50 to 100 plaque-forming units (p.f.u.) of vesicular stomatitis virus (VSV) (Wagner, 1961).

EXPERIMENTAL

Effect of interferon administered before inoculation of Friend virus

Intraperitoneal route. In Friend disease infectious virus can be consistently recovered from various tissues at varying intervals after viral inoculation (Friend, 1957). It seemed plausible that successive cycles of viral multiplication were responsible for successive cycles of cellular transformation. For this reason interferon was administered throughout the experimental period. In the experiments summarized below mice were inoculated intraperitoneally with interferon or normal mouse brain extract (as controls) 24 and three hours before viral inoculation and twice daily thereafter until the mice were killed.

Preliminary experiments suggested that daily intraperitoneal inoculations of 0·2 to 0·4 ml. of crude mouse brain interferon (usual titre 1:3,200) inhibited the development of splenomegaly in mice inoculated with Friend virus. Experiments utilizing tenfold concentrated preparations of interferon (titres: 1:14,000 to 1:67,000) were undertaken (Gresser *et al.*, 1966, 1967a, c) and the results may be summarized as follows:

(1) Concentrated mouse brain interferon preparations were more effective in inhibiting the development of splenomegaly than unconcentrated preparations.

(2) Concentrated interferon preparations were effective only when administered daily throughout the duration of the experiment. Administration of concentrated interferon for only three days was ineffective even though treatment *preceded* inoculation of Friend virus.

(3) Crude interferon preparations derived from sera and spleens of mice inoculated with NDV also inhibited the development of splenomegaly in mice infected with Friend virus.

(4) Interferon preparations were effective when administered to DBA/2 mice as well as to Swiss mice.

(5) The intraperitoneal route of inoculation of interferon was effective, whereas the intravenous route proved ineffective (this may have been related to a difference in the kinetics of diffusion of interferon and to the duration of serum interferon levels) (Gresser *et al.*, 1967*c*).

(6) Daily inoculation of control preparations of "normal" mouse brain or "normal" mouse serum-spleen mixtures neither inhibited nor enhanced the splenomegalic response to Friend virus.

(7) Repeated daily inoculation of concentrated interferon for four to six weeks did not induce the formation of neutralizing antibodies to interferon.

(8) Repeated intraperitoneal inoculation of interferon was well tolerated, although towards the third week a number of mice developed ascites.

Subcutaneous route. The development of ascites in mice inoculated intraperitoneally with concentrated interferon preparations made it desirable to inoculate interferon by another route. Furthermore it was considered of interest to inject interferon at a site other than the site of viral inoculation. Accordingly, a concentrated interferon preparation was inoculated subcutaneously 24 and three hours before viral inoculation and then twice daily throughout the four weeks the experiment lasted.

The results of this experiment demonstrated that subcutaneous administration of interferon was as effective in inhibiting the development of splenomegaly as the intraperitoneal route of inoculation (Gresser *et al.*, 1967*d*). Thus the mean spleen weight of infected mice treated with normal mouse brain extract was 1,208 mg., and of infected mice treated with interferon 257 mg. The mean spleen weight of uninoculated control mice in this experiment was 178 mg.

At the termination of the experiment, the titre of infectious Friend virus per unit weight of spleen was determined for each of several representative spleens from each group. One hundredfold less infectious virus was recovered from the spleens of mice treated with interferon than from the spleens of mice treated with normal mouse brain extract. Thus, treatment with interferon preparations inhibited not only the growth of the spleen but also viral multiplication (Gresser *et al.*, 1967*d*).

Administration of interferon after inoculation of Friend virus

Intraperitoneal route. The finding that interferon was effective when administered throughout the test period and ineffective when administered for only three days, even though it was given before viral inoculation, emphasized the importance of a long-term treatment in delaying the evolution of Friend disease. These results suggested, moreover, the possibility that interferon might be effective even if treatment were initiated after viral infection.

Mice in one group were treated intraperitoneally with interferon before viral inoculation, and in another group treatment was initiated 48 hours after viral inoculation. In both groups interferon treatment was continued throughout the experiment. Significant inhibition of splenomegaly was observed in both groups of mice treated with interferon (mean spleen weight of mice treated before viral inoculation: 322 mg.; of mice treated 48 hours after viral inoculation: 391 mg.) as compared to two viral control groups (mean spleen weight: 975 and 871 mg.) (Gresser *et al.*, 1967*b*).

Subcutaneous route. Since the subcutaneous route of inoculation proved successful when interferon was administered prophylactically, it was considered of interest to determine whether interferon administered by this route was also effective after inoculation of virus.

One group of mice was injected with concentrated interferon subcutaneously 24 hours after viral inoculation, and twice daily throughout the four weeks of the experiment. In a second group interferon treatment was stopped after the first week and the mice were kept without treatment for the remainder of the experiment. In a third group interferon treatment was initiated *one week after* viral inoculation and treatment was continued for the remaining three weeks of the experiment.

When the mice were killed four weeks after viral infection, it was apparent that interferon treatment initiated either one or seven days after viral inoculation was equally effective in retarding splenomegaly, provided that treatment had been continued daily thereafter. On the other hand interferon treatment for the first week, although appearing to diminish the size of the spleen initially, as judged by abdominal palpation, did not alter the ultimate splenomegalic response when the animals were left untreated for the ensuing three weeks. Experiments are in progress to determine whether there is a given period during which interferon treatment is most efficacious or whether the therapeutic effects observed depended on the duration of treatment and the total amount of interferon administered (Gresser *et al.*, 1967*d*).

Histology of the spleens of mice infected with Friend virus and treated with mouse brain interferon

The spleens of virus-infected mice inoculated with interferon were not only smaller than those of infected mice inoculated with control brain extract but histological differences were also noted (Gresser *et al.*, 1967*b*). Most of the leukaemic mice not receiving interferon had large spleens and the normal red pulp was extensively replaced by "Friend cells" (Friend, 1957; Zajdela, 1962). A considerable number of interferon-treated mice had small spleens containing only scattered foci of "Friend cells" and these could not be distinguished histologically from the occasional small spleen in untreated leukaemic mice. However, in the larger spleens of interferon-treated mice not only was the extent of Friend cell involvement less marked than that observed in the spleens (of similar size) of untreated leukaemic mice, but there appeared to be numerous foci of cellular maturation. This erythroid maturation was far less evident in the spleens of untreated leukaemic mice.

It is not clear how interferon preparations contribute to this erythroid maturation. It is possible that interferon acts at the level of individual virus-infected cells, thereby altering in some manner the virus-cell association. Perhaps a more likely possibility is that by reducing viral multiplication and therefore reducing the number of virus-infected cells the equilibrium between various splenic cell types is altered in such a manner as to favour cellular differentiation. A similar phenomenon has previously been observed in Friend-virus-infected mice treated with erythropoietin (Zajdela, 1962, unpublished observations)—namely inhibition of splenomegaly accompanied by histological evidence of erythroid maturation.

Effect of interferon preparations on survival of mice infected with Rauscher virus

In order to determine whether treatment with concentrated preparations of interferon prolonged the survival of virus-infected mice, experiments were undertaken (in collaboration with Dr. Leonard Berman and Dr. Guy de Thé) with BALB/c mice inoculated with Rauscher virus. Preliminary experiments have demonstrated that administration of concentrated interferon preparations by either the intraperitoneal or subcutaneous routes inhibits the development of splenomegaly in these mice and prolongs their life significantly.

Are the inhibitory effects observed in Friend disease attributable to interferon?

Since various biological effects observed with crude interferon preparations have not been observed with relatively purified preparations of interferon the question arises whether the inhibitory effects were due to interferon. It is possible that inhibition was mediated by mechanisms as yet undetermined or by another factor or factors present in the crude interferon preparations. Several observations, however, suggested that interferon was responsible for the inhibition observed.

(1) The preparations of interferon (as assayed *in vitro*) fulfilled various biochemical and biological criteria for classification as interferon.

(2) There was a direct correlation between the inhibitory effects in Friend disease and the interferon titre as assayed *in vitro* (VSV) or *in vivo* (EMC).

(3) Interferon preparations derived from different tissues and induced by different viruses were inhibitory.

(4) Interferon preparations inhibited the multiplication of Friend virus *in vivo*.

(5) Control tissue extracts were not inhibitory.

(6) There was no evidence that interferon preparations administered subcutaneously were toxic for mice as judged by total animal weights and weights of various viscera, nor did they appear to have any direct action on the haematopoietic system, as determined by reticulocyte counts, haematocrit and pathological examination of the spleen (Gresser *et al.*, 1967*d*).

Experiments in progress employing highly purified preparations of interferon may provide more direct evidence that the inhibitory effects *in vivo* are in fact attributable to interferon.★

DISCUSSSION

Many investigations have emphasized that interferon is effective when administered before viral infection and virtually ineffective when administered after viral infection (Isaacs and Lindenmann, 1957; Isaacs, 1963). Although these findings have cast some doubt on the therapeutic value of interferon (Hilleman, 1963, 1965; Ho and Postic, 1967), they may possibly reflect the choice of the experimental systems employed. Thus in acute viral diseases susceptible animal hosts were inoculated with virulent viruses and interferon was effective prophylactically, but afforded only negligible protection when given after viral inoculation (Finter, 1964*b*, 1966; Baron *et al.*, 1966).

The system we have chosen may be considered an example of a subacute infectious process. Multiplication of Friend virus occurs throughout the course of the disease and for this reason administration of interferon was continued daily throughout the test period. In contrast to the results obtained by others utilizing virulent viruses, it was not necessary to pretreat mice with interferon in order to retard the evolution of Friend disease. It was necessary, however, to continue interferon treatment after viral

★ These experiments when completed subsequently demonstrated that *highly purified* interferon proved as effective in inhibiting the development of splenomegaly as a crude interferon preparation of comparable titre (Gresser *et al.*, 1967*d*).

inoculation. Thus administration of interferon proved ineffective (as judged at autopsy four weeks later) if treatment initiated before viral inoculation was suspended several days later. Conversely, it was possible to retard the disease process when interferon treatment was initiated even one week *after* inoculation of virus, provided that interferon was subsequently administered over a long enough period and in sufficient quantity. These findings seem to us of some importance, since they suggest that other viral diseases of man and animals characterized by a long latent period or a subacute or chronic course may also be attenuated by adequate interferon treatment even after infection has been established in the animal host.

Friend disease may also be considered as a malignant process as well as a subacute disease (Friend, 1957; Metcalf, Furth and Buffett, 1959). In several other oncogenic virus-animal host systems, cellular transformation although related to the initial viral dose does not seem to depend on continued multiplication of infectious virus (Dulbecco, 1964). Our results suggest that in this respect Friend disease may differ from these systems. The finding that continued treatment with interferon reduced the level of infectious virus in the spleen and at the same time inhibited splenomegaly (manifested histologically as a reduction in the size and number of foci of Friend cells) suggested that successive cycles of viral multiplication throughout the course of the disease may have been in part responsible for progressive cellular transformation. It is not unexpected, therefore, that only continued interferon administration proved effective. Interferon administered for *only* a few days was ultimately without effect, since after an initial period of inhibition, viral multiplication may have ensued unchecked in the absence of interferon. Although it seems likely to us that interferon acted by repressing viral multiplication and thus cellular transformation, it should be emphasized that a direct action of interferon on virus-infected transformed cells has not been excluded. Whatever the mode of action, these observations suggest that even some virus-induced malignant processes may be attenuated or retarded by continued interferon therapy after viral infection.

SUMMARY

Concentrated preparations of mouse brain interferon administered either intraperitoneally or subcutaneously inhibited the development of splenomegaly induced by Friend virus in Swiss and DBA/2 mice. Interferon was effective when treatment was continued daily throughout most of the test period. Administration of interferon for several days proved ineffective even though treatment preceded viral inoculation. Interferon treatment initiated even one week after inoculation of virus was effective, provided that it was continued daily thereafter. One hundredfold less infectious virus per unit weight of spleen was recovered from the spleens of mice treated with interferon than from the spleens of untreated virus-infected mice. It seemed probable that continued repression of viral multiplication by interferon was related to the reduction in the size and number of foci of Friend cells observed in the spleens of mice treated with interferon. The relevance of these findings to the therapy of viral diseases and those malignant processes whose evolution depends on continued viral multiplication was discussed.

Acknowledgements

We are indebted to Mr. Philippe Lazar and Mrs. Suzanne Guéguen for analysing our experimental results, and to Drs. Charles Chany and Samuel S. Epstein for their critical review of the manuscript. We gratefully acknowledge the technical aid of Mlles Brigitte Galliot, Nicole Vanhaesebroucke, Sylvie Thomas, MM. Sylvain Gilly and Jean Michel Reymond, and the assistance of Mlle Madeleine Breuilh in preparing the manuscript for publication.

We should also like to express our gratitude to Dr. Sidney Farber for his constant encouragement and interest in the course of these investigations.

REFERENCES

ALLISON, A. C. (1961). *Virology*, **15**, 47.
ATANASIU, P., and CHANY, C. (1960). *C. r. hebd. Séanc. Acad. Sci., Paris*, **251**, 1687.
BADER, J. P. (1962). *Virology*, **16**, 436.
BARON, S., and BUCKLER, C. E. (1963). *Science*, **141**, 1061.
BARON, S., BUCKLER, C. E., FRIEDMAN, R. M., and McCLOSKEY, R. V. (1966). *J. Immun.*, **96**, 17.
DULBECCO, R. (1964). *J. Am. med. Ass.*, **190**, 721.
FINTER, N. B. (1964*a*). *Nature, Lond.*, **204**, 1114.
FINTER, N. B. (1964*b*). *Br. med. J.*, **2**, 981.
FINTER, N. B. (1965). *Nature, Lond.*, **206**, 597.
FINTER, N. B. (1966). *Br. J. exp. Path.*, **47**, 361.
FRIEND, C. (1957). *J. exp. Med.*, **105**, 307.
GRESSER, I., COPPEY, J., FALCOFF, E., and FONTAINE, D. (1966). *C. r. hebd. Séanc. Acad. Sci., Paris*, **263**, 586.
GRESSER, I., COPPEY, J., FALCOFF, E., and FONTAINE, D. (1967*a*). *Proc. Soc. exp. Biol. Med.*, **124**, 84.
GRESSER, I., COPPEY, J., FONTAINE-BROUTY-BOYE, D., FALCOFF, R., FALCOFF, E., and ZAJDELA, F. (1967*b*). *Nature, Lond.*, **215**, 174.
GRESSER, I., FONTAINE, D., COPPEY, J., FALCOFF, R., and FALCOFF, E. (1967*c*). *Proc. Soc. exp. Biol. Med.*, **124**, 91.
GRESSER, I., FONTAINE-BROUTY-BOYE, D., FALCOFF, E., COPPEY, J., FALCOFF, R., and ZAJDELA, F. (1967*d*). In preparation.
HILLEMAN, M. R. (1963). *J. cell. comp. Physiol.*, **62**, 337.
HILLEMAN, M. R. (1965). *Am. J. Med.*, **38**, 751.

Ho, M., and Postic, B. (1967). In *First International Conference on Vaccines against Viral and Rickettsial Diseases of Man*, pp. 632–649. Washington, D.C.: PAHO/WHO Scientific Publication 147.

Isaacs, A. (1963). *Adv. Virus Res.*, **10**, 1.

Isaacs, A., and Lindenmann, J. (1957). *Proc. R. Soc. B*, **147**, 258.

Kishida, T., Kato, S., and Nagano, Y. (1965). *C. r. Séanc. Soc. Biol.*, **159**, 782.

Kleinschmidt, W. J., and Murphy, E. B. (1965). *Virology*, **27**, 484.

Lampson, G. P., Tytell, A. A., Nemes, M. M., and Hilleman, M. R. (1963). *Proc. Soc. exp. Biol. Med.*, **112**, 468.

Metcalf, D., Furth, J., and Buffett, R. F. (1959). *Cancer Res.*, **19**, 52.

Oxman, M. N., and Black, P. H. (1966). *Proc. natn. Acad. Sci. U.S.A.*, **55**, 1133.

Regelson, W. (1967). In *Atherosclerosis and the Reticuloendothelial System*, in press.

Regelson, W., and Merigan, T. (1967). *Am. Ass. Cancer Res.* **8**, 56.

Rowe, W. P., and Brodsky, I. (1959). *J. natn. Cancer Inst.*, **23**, 1239.

Strandström, H., Sandelin, K., and Oker-Blöm, N. (1962). *Virology*, **16**, 384.

Todaro, G. J., and Baron, S. (1965). *Proc. natn. Acad. Sci. U.S.A.*, **54**, 752.

Vandeputte, M., De Lafonteyne, J., Billiau, A., and De Somer, P. (1967). *Arch. ges. Virusforsch.*, **20**, 235.

Wagner, R. R. (1961). *Virology*, **13**, 323.

Wheelock, E. F. (1966). *Proc. natn. Acad. Sic. U.S.A.*, **55**, 774.

Wheelock, E. F. (1967a). *J. natn. Cancer Inst.*, **38**, 771.

Wheelock, E. F. (1967b). *Proc. Soc. exp. Biol. Med.*, **124**, 855.

Zajdela, F. (1962). *Bull. Ass. fr. Étude Cancer*, **49**, 351.

DISCUSSION

Merigan: Some preliminary results that we have obtained with Dr. Henry Kaplan and Miriam Lieberman in general support your findings, Dr. Gresser. Passive intraperitoneal administration of interferon to mice that had received X-irradiated lymphoma virus apparently also prolonged survival from that disease.

Levy: Some years ago we showed that a characteristic of Friend virus disease is that, many days before the enlarged spleens are seen, an increased uptake of phosphorus into the cell is detectable, that is at about a day and a half after administration of the virus. This increasing uptake of phosphorus was very rapidly altered by chemotherapeutic drugs. It might be possible to use this technique instead of the spleen weight for assessing the effect of interferon after a short time.

Gresser: We have undertaken some experiments with ^{59}Fe (Mirand, E. A., Prentice, T. C., Hoffman, J. G., and Grace, J. T. [1961]. *Proc. Soc. exp. Biol. Med.*, **106**, 423), with inconclusive results; we have not tried phosphorus. As to chemotherapeutic drugs, we have done some preliminary experiments with 6-mercaptopurine and mitomycin C in mice, but we soon ran into problems of toxicity. Experiments on Friend leukaemia utilizing toxic substances are difficult to interpret (Sidwell, R. W., Dixon, G. L., Sellers, S. M., Maxwell, C. F., and Schabel, F. M. [1965]. *Proc. Soc. exp. Biol. Med.*, **119**, 1141). Is one acting directly on the disease process or indirectly through a toxic action?

Stoker: The two possibilities you mentioned were inhibiting multiple cycles and a direct action on the transformed cells. If the interferon action applies generally to RNA viruses, then if there is a direct action on the cells, it would be possible, perhaps, to untransform Rous cells or mouse sarcoma cells in culture.

Gresser: We are doing those experiments now, in association with Dr. L. Berman, but we have no results at present. We are maintaining transformed mouse cells from the Harvey strain of murine sarcoma virus under concentrated mouse interferon. As to the other point, I am not sure that the interferon inhibitory effects I mentioned are applicable to all RNA viruses. Two exceptions come to mind. One stems from the work of Lampson and his co-workers (1963, *loc. cit.*), who showed that the administration of large amounts of interferon, even six hours after inoculation with the Rous virus, did not alter the subsequent appearance of tumours. The second example comes from some experiments we did with Dr. Chany (unpublished observations) in which the rhabdomyosarcoma virus of Moloney was inoculated into mice intramuscularly. Concentrated interferon was inoculated at the same site before viral inoculation and daily thereafter without any observable inhibitory effect. This suggests that it is not sufficient to refer to RNA viruses—there may be numerous reasons why some viruses may be susceptible to this sort of continued interferon treatment and why other viruses may not be susceptible or may even counteract the action of interferon.

Finter: Can you test the relative sensitivity to interferon *in vitro* of Friend virus and, say, Semliki or other viruses?

Gresser: Yes, we have done some experiments along these lines. The problem is that this virus multiplies at very low levels *in vitro*, and it is an extremely difficult system to work with. For example in Friend-virus-infected mouse embryo cell cultures we recovered after several weeks approximately 5 SD_{50} (median spleen-dose) when the virus was titred back into the mouse. In the virus-infected and interferon-treated cultures we were unable to detect any virus. Thus Friend virus seemed to be sensitive to interferon *in vitro*, but I cannot compare its sensitivity to that of Semliki Forest virus because of the difficulties inherent in the *in vitro* techniques with Friend virus.

Finter: Is it strictly necessary to give interferon daily after infection with Friend virus? If so, this seems to imply that the effect of the interferon is wearing off rather rapidly, so that perhaps you are working with a dose which is only just effective. This might explain your failure to get any significant effect with interferon given prophylactically. Again the question of the sensitivity of the virus to interferon comes in. In our experiments with Semliki Forest virus in mice, we found that 100 units were needed to protect if given 24 hours before virus infection, but 5,000 units if given six days before infection. So the protective effect of the interferon fell off with time, but not at an extremely rapid rate.

Gresser: We have not examined this aspect and have only given interferon daily or twice daily.

Ho: J. Armstrong (doctoral thesis, Graduate School of Public Health, University of Pittsburgh, 1967) in our department has worked with DNA viruses. He showed that interferon inhibited *in vitro* transformation of hamster embryonic cells by adenovirus 12. However, using adeno 12, SV40 and SV 7, he was unable to inhibit oncogenesis in the hamster host. This, of course, may be explained by dosage effects and so on, but it is also possible that one should not extrapolate from *in vitro* transformation to *in vivo* oncogenesis.

Chany: The fact that we inject these mice with interferon every day, or even twice a day, is perhaps related to Dr. Baron's observation that in order to maintain the antiviral state, a constant interferon level is needed in the organism. I think this really explains the necessity for the continuous injection of large amounts of interferon.

Finter: Perhaps the position is that if one gives a sufficiently large dose of interferon, it will still protect even after some time, during which there may nevertheless be a considerable decay in its antiviral effect. With a dose on the verge of the minimum effective one, the effect may fall after a slight decay to below the level at which virus multiplication is resumed, in accordance with Dr. Baron's findings.

Baron: Perhaps the question boils down to this: is the same total amount of interferon more effective if it is spread out or if it is given in one dose?

Merigan: In mice with X-irradiated lymphoma virus we have been observing prolongation of life with interferon injection three times weekly, although I think obviously this is conditioned by the intrinsic interferon-sensitivity of the virus and the relative doses of the interferon. I do not think we can interpolate easily between them, but I certainly think one might stop other types of mouse leukaemia with constant but less frequent dosages than you use, Dr. Gresser.

Baron: Do the mice infected with these various leukaemia viruses actually produce interferon, Dr. Gresser? Obviously the virus is sensitive to interferon during infection because of the effectiveness of passive administration of interferon. If the infected mice do not produce a large amount of interferon, are these mice capable of responding to another inducer of interferon while they are infected?

Gresser: In answer to your first question on the induction of interferon by Friend virus: as a positive control we inoculated NDV and measured serum and spleen interferon at five, 12 and 24 hours. The peak level was 1:5,000 at five hours. When we inoculated a 10 per cent Friend spleen extract intravenously, interferon was not detected in the serum at five hours but at 24 hours small amounts of interferon were detected (1:20 to 1:40) (Gresser *et al.*, 1967c, *loc. cit.*). No interferon was detected after inoculation of normal spleen extract. The problem of interpreting these findings, as illustrated from your own work (Baron and Buckler, 1963, *loc. cit.*), is related to the actual amount of virus inoculated. The *in vivo* assay techniques of Friend virus are imprecise and it is difficult to know how much virus is present in a given preparation. For example our preparations usually titre $10^3 SD_{50}$/ml. but in terms of physical particles there is clearly a much greater number. This low interferon response therefore means little. We have also assayed serum and spleen seven, 14, 21, 28, 35, 37, and 45 days after inoculation of Friend virus and have not detected interferon in mice with the disease (Gresser *et al.*, 1967c, *loc. cit.*).

As to your second question: we infected mice with Friend virus, and three and six weeks thereafter inoculated NDV as an interferon inducer. These Friend-virus-infected mice produced almost as much serum and spleen interferon (the difference was of questionable significance) as the uninfected mice inoculated with NDV (Gresser *et al.*, 1967c, *loc. cit.*). We did not test the capacity of these mice to produce interferon shortly after infection with Friend virus. Wheelock reported (Wheelock, E. F. [1966]. *Proc. natn. Acad. Sci. U.S.A.*, **55**, 774) a decrease in the interferon response of Friend-virus-infected mice during the period after viral infection, but by two to three weeks I believe their "interferon response" was similar to that of control mice, as in our experiments.

Andrewes: I believe that Metcalf and others (Metcalf, D., Furth, J., and Buffett, R. F. [1959]. *Cancer Res.*, **19**, 52) have suggested that the Friend disease has a sort of double pathology—I think Metcalf called it a reticulosis plus an erythroblastosis, or something like that—and there has been a suggestion that one might occur without the other. Do you believe in this, and does it complicate the issue at all?

Gresser: The disease described by Friend (Friend, C. [1957]. *J. exp. Med.*, **105**, 307) and subsequently by Metcalf, Furth and Buffett, was considered a reticulosarcoma. I think it is agreed now that the "Friend" cells are in fact pro-erythroblasts (Zajdela, 1962, *loc. cit.*). In the one or two-month period that concerned us the disease process is one of the erythroid series and not a reticulosarcoma. Several months later there may be a myeloid phase.

GROUP DISCUSSION

Stoker: In this final session I shall ask for any further comments or afterthoughts on the main groups of topics we have discussed, in the order we have talked about them, and then for comments on any points which have not been tackled at all.

INDUCING AGENTS

Stoker: Is it possible that Alick Isaacs was right when he suggested that nucleic acid is essential to induce interferon? From what we have heard, the inducers used in intact animals are very difficult to interpret, because a stimulation of latent virus infection, or something like that, is not ruled out. So it is perhaps best to narrow the field to the inducers which work in tissue culture, and this, I understand, brings it down to viruses and statolon. No evidence given here proves that statolon is free of nucleic acid.

Joklik: Has anyone any information on how many nucleic acid molecules, or how many virus particles, are needed to cause stimulation of interferon production? Obviously the implications are different if it turns out that only one is needed rather than 1,000, for instance. But it is not enough to know how much virus one has to add; one must know how many of these particles enter the cell.

Chany: It is almost impossible to answer the question. Infectious and non-infectious viruses can produce interferon, but we do not know whether non-infectious virus contains incomplete viral genome or whether it contains active genome at all.

Joklik: Leaving aside the question of whether it is complete or incomplete, one wants to get away from any multiplication or amplification effect inside the cell. By using purified labelled virus, it ought to be possible to find out whether one virus particle is sufficient to cause interferon production.

Andrewes: One of my difficulties in writing the obituary of Alick for the Royal Society is that we know that all the fundamental work that he did at the beginning was very sound and valuable, but some of his ideas, particularly some of his later work, apparently have not stood up. Opinions as to which parts of his work are perfectly all right and which are not would be very useful. I gather that his enthusiasm for the idea that the main stimulus to interferon was foreign nucleic acid is not generally accepted now. Is that so?

Finter: When these findings were first published, we made several attempts to repeat them, but without success. I know that Dr. Fantes had the same experience. The method used for assay may be relevant to the results which Alick obtained, and Dr. Rotem may be able to help us here. Could some factor other than interferon, perhaps residual amounts of the nucleic acids added to the cultures, have been responsible for the inhibition of the challenge virus which was observed? If I recall the published protocols correctly, it is not clearly stated whether the assay plates were washed thoroughly before the challenge virus was added.

Rotem: The difficulty was applying the RNA to the cells and not all experiments were reproducible. It is true to say that only high molecular weight RNA worked, but not a low molecular weight RNA, or a degraded one. The titres were very low, about $1:8$, but the properties of the material were perfectly all right; we could identify it as interferon. Also there were slight differences between the interferons that were produced in chick and in mouse cells, especially in their heat sensitivity. Virus-induced chick and mouse interferons also differ in this property. This was the evidence that we got at the time for considering RNA as an interferon inducer.

Baron: One of Alick's last papers reassesses the role of nucleic acid as the inducer; in it he wrote that he was doubtful that nucleic acids were in fact proven to be the inducer (Isaacs, A. [1965]. *Aust. J. exp. Biol. med. Sci.*, **43**, 405).

Gresser: I would like to suggest the following experiment: it has been shown that titres of interferon are often higher *in vivo* than *in vitro* after inoculation of viruses or other substances. The inoculation of polio RNA into the allantois of the embryonated egg—which apparently has very little RNase (Denys, P., and Prinzie, A. [1962]. *Virology*, **17**, 216), and in which only a single cycle of multiplication occurs—might induce the production of interferon.

Crick: Is there an animal virus for which the protein part alone stimulates interferon production?

Burke: We tried using empty capsids of Semliki Forest virus to induce interferon formation and it failed for technical reasons.

Pereira: Many people must have added purified virus proteins to cells in culture, but I do not know of any report that they induced interferon formation.

Chany: We have found that purified measles haemagglutinin does not induce interferon or interference. Of course, it is possible that the envelope is responsible for the derepression of interferon, not the haemagglutinin itself.

Crick: Possibly the haemagglutinin does not get into the cell.

Stoker: Have any experiments been done to see whether the nucleic acids that are used do get in?

Chany: Our experiments with nucleic acids were also negative. We don't know whether they get in.

Rotem: Treatment of nucleic acids with RNase destroyed their ability to induce interferon. RNA, which was ineffective as an interferon inducer in cells of the same species as that from which it was prepared, became capable of inducing interferon in such cells after treatment with nitrous acid.

Baron: The Pfizer group originally claimed to have substantiated the finding that nucleic acids stimulate the interferon system, but they have now partly withdrawn that claim. They still get an antiviral effect of nucleic acids but it is specific for certain viruses (Takano, K., Warren, J., Jensen, K. E., and Neal, A. L. [1965]. *J. Bact.,* **90,** 1542).

Kleinschmidt: Whether the nucleic acids are found to be inducers of interferon or not, the paper by Rotem, Cox, and Isaacs (Rotem, Z., Cox, R. A., and Isaacs, A. [1963]. *Nature, Lond.,* **197,** 564–566) was certainly the inducer that made us bring statolon out of the refrigerator.

Crick: Does heat shock to cells produce interferon?

Wagner: We have not tried that, but we did add a lot of materials of a particulate nature, thinking that some sort of membrane interaction might produce pinocytosis, possibly membrane fragments breaking off which would enter the cell and induce interferon. We tried plastic particles, Thorotrast, and things like that, in a number of cells, and never got any interferon. Again, we have no idea whether these substances were getting on or into the cells.

Burke: We tried things which might disturb cellular DNA in some way—very low doses of u.v. light, and of mitomycin—but we got no interferon.

Finter: The cell treated with interferon can distinguish between cellular messenger RNA and viral messenger RNA, so we know that these two types of RNA must differ. Could there perhaps be a specific mechanism in the cell for the recognition of viral nucleic acid, which triggers off the formation of interferon?

Crick: The difficulty is to establish whether it is the viral RNA that does it. This is why one wonders whether there is any less specific thing which, in cell culture, will produce interferon.

Levy: But even if you establish that viral RNA itself will induce interferon formation, this does not really mean that it is an exclusive property of nucleic acid. Viral RNA might be just one of the insults that will stimulate interferon.

Mécs: M. A. Gharpure (1965. *Virology*, **27**, 308–319) in Professor Stoker's laboratory found that pretreatment of host cells by heat prevents growth of DNA but not RNA viruses, probably through inhibition of DNA-dependent RNA synthesis. Therefore we can suppose that this pretreatment makes interferon production impossible by DNA viruses, assuming that this is preceded by viral messenger-RNA synthesis.

Merigan: The trachoma agents are interesting in their ability to produce interferon in tissue culture (Hanna, L., Merigan, T. C., and Jawetz, E. [1957]. *Am. J. Opthal.*, **63**, 1151). Strains which readily infect in tissue culture are good interferon inducers *in vitro*. Some of these agents do not invade, say, mouse cells in tissue culture, but they can be forced in by centrifugation, after which one gets a yield of interferon. On the other hand, if the agent is first heat-inactivated by exposure to 60°c one can still make the particles enter the cell, but they do not produce interferon.

Chany: What happens if the agent is u.v.-irradiated?

Merigan: That hasn't been done yet. As I mentioned earlier, these agents offer an interesting chance to look at the intracellular events that might be correlated with the stimulus to interferon production.

Fantes: Borecký and co-workers (Borecký, L., Lackovič, V., Blaškovič, D., Masler, L., and Šikl, D. [1967]. *Acta virol.*, *Prague*, (Engl. ed.) **11**, 264) reported that mannan was capable of inducing interferon. If so, that would not only take away the virus part of the inducer, but also the polyanionic part.

Burke: The product was not very well characterized. There were no titres in the paper, and one of the physical properties was odd: I think it was labile at pH 2, which one would not expect it to be.

Levy: Since a number of the RNA viruses can induce interferon, and since these RNA viruses presumably have no connexion with the nucleus, the means of induction of interferon would have to be at least partially indirect. If interferon represents a derepression, which is a nuclear phenomenon, then either something other than the virus gets into the nucleus, or there is a very transient connexion of the input virus with the nucleus.

Ho: Phytohaemagglutinin is another non-viral, non-nucleic-acid substance that has been reported to induce interferon (Wheelock, E. F. [1965]. *Science*, **149**, 310). One of the original merits of Dr. Isaacs' nucleic acid theory, as I understand it, is that not only is foreign nucleic acid an inducer of interferon, but it is also the target against which the interferon acts. In this respect, there is a generalization one can make in the whole field of interferon induction and action, namely, that those viral agents which induce interferon best are also agents against which interferon acts best. This interesting phenomenon requires some explanation, and so far Dr. Isaacs' is the only one postulated. It should be kept in mind in many of our discussions.

Baron: One other inducer of interferon in tissue culture—aside from phyto-haemagglutinin, which may perhaps be special because it acts only in white cells—is rickettsia infection. Hopps and co-workers found that rickettsia infection of chick embryo tissue culture was an excellent inducer of interferon. The rickett-siae are not sensitive to the action of interferon, whereas the TRIC agents are. Rickettsia is a larger organism, presumably more independent of the host, and in tissue culture it can induce interferon but is not sensitive to its action. This work has not been published except in abstract form, but I have seen the evidence and it is very convincing (Hopps, H. E., Kohno, S., Kohno, M., and Smadel, J. E. [1964]. *Bact. Proc.*, 155).

HETEROGENEITY OF INTERFERONS

Stoker: Dr. Gresser, you had a point about over-purifying.

Gresser: Many of the properties of interferon described several years ago were subsequently found, when interferon was purified, to be due to impurities. It is apparent, therefore, that viruses induce the liberation of a whole variety of factors. I think it is a mistake to ignore these, Furthermore it is possible that interferon may act synergistically with some of these factors. When the specific activity of purified preparations of interferon is investigated we may be introducing another artifact, an experimental one, since *in vivo* interferon may be acting entirely differently.

Tyrrell: These other factors would include not only things that might work synergistically, but also things like blocker, or stimulon.

Chany: We find that some viruses resistant to interferon, such as the Moloney sarcoma, are not blocked by interferon *in vivo*. The same preparations block Moloney or Friend leukaemia viruses. The Moloney sarcoma virus reverses interferon action just as adenovirus 12 does. It seems possible that some of these viruses resistant to interferon are resistant because they produce stimulons. If we really want to use interferon as a therapeutic agent, we might have to get rid of such antagonists.

Baron: Dr. Merigan has had some experience which supports Dr. Gresser's point of view on the question of whether interferon disappears from fluids around cells. He used pure versus impure interferon, and the pure interferon disappeared from the tissue culture fluid much more rapidly than the impure interferon. Yet the antiviral activity was equal in both cultures, the implication being that per-haps there were stabilizers in the impure material, which prevented non-specific inactivation of interferon (Merigan, T. C., Winget, C. A., and Dixon, C. B. [1965]. *J. molec. Biol.*, **13**, 670).

Ho: Interferon may consist of more than one substance or type of molecule. This could be one of the reasons why purification is difficult.

Stoker: Yes, that is possible. This brings us back to the awful problem of defini-tion. Obviously there are classes of substance of widely different molecular weight which have similar biological effects. Whether they all work through exactly the same mechanism does not seem to be clear. The work showing that interferons of different molecular weights all act through induction of an inhibitory protein was not fully clear to me.

Wagner: We have not compared the mechanisms of action of the different interferons.

Stoker: The high molecular weight substance might, therefore, work through some entirely different mechanism.

Levy: Along these lines, it might be useful to evolve a definition of "interferon" which includes a mechanism of action. It may not be practical at this time to define each substance that we isolate by its mechanism of action, but one should be prepared to reject a substance as interferon if it turns out to be working by a mechanism totally different from the way viral-induced interferon works.

Kleinschmidt: M. Boxaca and K. Paucker have claimed (1967. *Fedn Proc. Fedn Am. Socs exp. Biol.*, **26**, 363) that the antibody to the low molecular weight mouse interferon also neutralizes the higher molecular weight interferon. Since antibodies are very specific, this would indicate that at least a portion of the larger molecular weight interferon must be similar to the low molecular weight material.

Andrewes: Dr. Isaacs at first thought that interferon was non-antigenic, but it has turned out that at least in certain circumstances it is antigenic. Is it ever antigenic in the same species of animal?

Chany: With Dr. Falcoff and his colleagues we have done experiments in humans. We injected them intravenously with WBC interferon, and interferon prepared in the amniotic membrane. As stated earlier, these interferons have different molecular weights. In leukaemia patients, injected intravenously with a total amount of more than 3 litres of a preparation of WBC interferon, we observed no trace of antibody production which would block the action of interferon.

Burke: We tried to prepare an antibody in rabbits to chick interferon, and we obtained one which would precipitate and neutralize the activity of crude interferon preparations. We came to the conclusion that a reaction was occurring which was carrying down interferon, but that it was not a true interferon antiserum. Most people would agree that interferon is very weakly antigenic in heterologous species. Proof that it is non-antigenic or antigenic in a homologous species is therefore much more difficult to discover.

Fantes: Interferon probably appears to be poorly antigenic because only very small amounts, by weight, have so far been injected.

De Maeyer: Is it a smaller amount of antigen than the amount present in a dose of inactivated polio vaccine, for instance?

Fantes: Many times smaller.

Gresser: Interferon may be inducing the formation of precipitin-type antibodies. We would *not* detect these since we test interferon by biological assay.

There are some enzymes, I believe, which induce precipitins but not antibodies which block their action.

Pereira: The sensitivity of the antigenicity test is impressive: minute amounts of certain proteins are required to stimulate a very good antibody response under appropriate conditions. Obviously, different proteins vary in their capacity to stimulate antibody production, but if we have to arrange these in some order, I would put interferon at the lower end of the scale.

Merigan: We have tried to detect antibody to interferon in heterologous species by an approach which doesn't seem to have been reported before. We incubated interferon preparations with serum from animals that had been given large amounts of interferon, and then subjected these preparations to molecular sieve chromatography. Even if interferon were to be active in the antigen-antibody complex, then we would still be able to pick up the presence of specific antibody because it should have a displacement in its emergence volume on Sephadex G100. This did not occur, even in animals that had been injected with good amounts of interferon for one year. From the literature it is clear that any anti-serum which has been produced is quite weak; it will only neutralize a small number of units of interferon.

ACTION OF ANTIVIRAL PROTEIN

Stoker: We are just getting to the point that Dr. Levy raised on antiviral proteins and the mechanism of action. We should be quite clear as to the differences between the three systems which have been studied, Dr. Joklik's, Dr. Marcus's, and Dr. Levy's.

Levy: Dr. Joklik is working with the messenger RNA of a DNA virus in infected mouse cells, Marcus is working with an RNA virus in a cell-free system derived from chick cells, and we are working with an RNA virus, both in infected mouse cells and in a cell-free system.

Marcus incubates ribosomes from control and interferon-treated chick cells with labelled or unlabelled Sindbis virus RNA. He finds that control ribosomes bind and translate the viral RNA. Ribosomes from interferon-treated cells bind the viral RNA to a lesser extent and do not translate it: Marcus attributes this to the fact that these ribosomes contain a protein which inhibits translation. He reports the formation of detectable amounts of a large polysome in the cell-free system. With interferon-type ribosomes, he gets a decreased amount of polysome with Sindbis RNA, and no translation. Joklik and I both agree that binding of the viral RNA in the *in vivo* system is inhibited in interferon-treated cells. Joklik has suggested that the viral RNA may have been altered, but I am more inclined to think it is the ribosome that has been changed. I feel that the effect is primarily an alteration of a ribosomal subunit. We do find the formation of a polysome, or a polysome-like structure, in interferon-treated cells, but it is non-functional or only poorly functional. In this regard our results bear some resemblances to Marcus's cell-free system. But our cell-free system results are different from his in that we don't see binding, and I think this is why we do not get translation. We do not get binding in the interferon-treated cells at the 40 S subunit level.

Sonnabend: Dr. Friedman, working on a similar problem with Semliki Forest virus in chick cells, had results which differed from yours. Friedman has clearly shown that SFV RNA associated with a 65 S cytoplasmic particle when he infected chick cells with labelled virus, and that this association was not altered by pretreatment of the cells with interferon.

Levy: The differences are that Marcus sees the formation of a polysome *in vitro*; we see the formation of a defective polysome *in vivo*. I am not sure the differences are really major ones.

Joklik: Then what differences are the major ones?

Levy: It may be possible to explain, when we know more about it, why we do not get the *in vitro* binding in the way Marcus does. Even with control ribosomes, we get nothing like the big polysomes he sees. This is really one of the critical differences.

Martin: I think there are quite large differences as far as binding is concerned between your work and Marcus and Salb's. If I recall correctly, Marcus saw about 60 per cent of binding of the viral RNA to the ribosomes from interferon-treated cells as compared with control ribosomes, whereas you essentially get no binding.

Levy: *In vivo*, we do see some binding, which bears marked resemblances to Marcus's *in vitro* work.

Joklik: At the moment one would like to think that there is just one mechanism rather than two, but it is the combination of messenger RNA with ribosomes or translation in formed polyribosomes that is inhibited. You have the best of both worlds, Dr. Levy: you find non-translation of some polyribosomes, and non-formation of others!

Levy: I can go either way, I suppose!

Ho: How do you explain your *in vitro* results?

Levy: With the interferon-treated cells *in vivo* we never see an association of the input labelled viral RNA with a ribosomal subunit. We also do not get a functioning polysome. I tentatively conclude from this that passage through a 40 S ribosomal subunit is a necessary step for the formation of a functional polysome. We can get a polysome-like structure in the absence of association with a ribosomal subunit, but it just does not function. And this may be the kind of polysome that Marcus sees, which is formed but does not function.

Stoker: I am interested in recognition of viral messenger. If it is true that animal virus RNA is recognized in this respect, but that host cell RNA, polyuridylic acid and probably TMV RNA, are not recognized, this would then indicate that the RNA from the sensitive animal viruses must have a positive recognition sign rather than a negative one, so to speak. Something must be present which is different to other sorts of RNA.

Levy: I have no idea what this recognition is, but there could be a whole gradation of recognition or non-recognition ranges, even within animal viruses. I am not sure that the TMV RNA should be put into a totally different class. Maybe we should consider it in the same way as an animal virus RNA not recognized by the interferon ribosome.

Kleinschmidt: Is there any evidence at all on structural differences between viral and host cell nucleic acids? Is there any evidence that viral nucleic acid, say, gets methylated, or something of this sort, when it gets into the cell?

Joklik: There is no evidence at all.

Crick: It is possible that in the mammalian cells there are no polycistronic messages, and in mammalian viruses there are.

Joklik: In vaccinia the messages must be monocistronic.

Crick: They are small, but do you know for sure that there are not two cistrons there?

Joklik: The S value is similar to that of the host cell RNA.

Crick: But there could still be two genes there. I agree that it does not look like that.

Joklik: Small vaccinia virus messenger RNA molecules seem to be as small as 8 S. 10 S is about the median sedimentation coefficient, but there is quite a bit of stuff smaller than 10 S.

Burke: Above and beyond this, we have to explain the variation in binding to explain the different sensitivity of various viruses.

Crick: As I understand it, we have not established the differences in binding in all the cases of viruses of different sensitivity. The most promising thing would be to pursue this binding *in vitro*, because there you have a clear-cut assay.

Joklik: Dr. De Maeyer, did the bone marrow experiments you described suggest that most of the interferon in the animal was made in bone marrow?

De Maeyer: No, certainly not. We give a fairly heavy irradiation dose, 1,000 r., which knocks out the bone marrow completely; it is a lethal dose: the animal develops leucopenia and dies after about a week. Immediately after irradiation, we inject isologous bone marrow, 10^7 cells to one series, and 10^5 to the other. Then at various intervals we follow the restoration of interferon production after injection of virus.

The picture of restoration of interferon production is quite similar to that of the restoration of circulating leucocytes. So it is not the bone marrow itself; it is the cells that are derived from the stem cells in the transfused bone marrow that are probably responsible for the restoration of interferon production.

Burke: Could the differences with the various benzpyrenes be explained by an alternative hypothesis, Dr. De Maeyer? That is, one could say that the nuclear membrane is permeable to the benzpyrenes that are carcinogenic, and impermeable to the ones that are non-carcinogenic; in the ones where the nuclear membrane is permeable, damage occurs to nuclear RNA and a nuclear property such as the production of interferon cannot then be expressed. The production of interferon and the carcinogenesis do not have to be tied together.

De Maeyer: No, I was not trying to tie them together. This explanation is quite possible. However, nobody has ever really proved that these compounds get into the nucleus.

Burke: Is there any effect on RNA synthesis with these compounds?

De Maeyer: They might inhibit DNA-dependent RNA synthesis, but this has not been demonstrated directly, as far as I know.

Burke: The ability to produce interferon is a property of the cell nucleus, and clearly it is rather easily disturbed. When we washed our cells halfway through interferon production, interferon-producing ability was damaged much more easily than the ability to produce virus. Various types of slightly traumatic treatment of the nucleus might just disturb it.

De Maeyer: Yes, we know that u.v.-irradiation of cell cultures will inhibit interferon synthesis (De Maeyer-Guignard, J., and De Maeyer, E. [1965]. *Nature, Lond.*, **205**, 985–987).

Levy: But you inhibit RNA synthesis. Could this not explain the inhibition of interferon production?

Burke: With the fowl plague–NDV system, one would predict, if this is true, that fowl plague would be sensitive to the carcinogens and that NDV would be insensitive to the carcinogens.

De Maeyer: Yes, because fowl plague is inhibited by actinomycin and NDV is not.

Levy: But more precisely cell growth should be affected, should it not?

De Maeyer: It is not affected appreciably at concentrations of hydrocarbon that inhibit interferon production almost completely.

INFORMATION EXCHANGE GROUP

Stoker: Many of you are concerned about reaching some decision on what we ought to call "interferon". It was suggested that we should discuss this, but I do not think it would be very fruitful at this stage. If you feel that it would be wise to publish suggestions about definitions for the future, it probably should not come from this symposium, but perhaps it could come from the Information Exchange Group which already exists. Dr. Baron, could you say a bit about what is going to happen to the IEG, which is now presumably finishing?

Baron: As you know, seven information exchange groups were originally set up. Ours was No. 6 and had a maximum of 250 members, which is the membership now. The largest of the others was the Nucleic Acid Protein Chemistry Group, which had well over 1,000 members and which perhaps deluged its membership with preprints. The editors of the biochemical journals declared that these preprints were in effect publications, and that they would not publish anything in the future which had first gone through an IEG. The IEG system was considered by the National Institutes of Health to be an experiment in communication, so the NIH decided that in face of this journal opposition they should terminate the present operation of the IEGs and turn them free of the NIH. In doing so, the NIH indicated that they believed that the idea was worth while and could evolve to an acceptable status. Shortly thereafter, the journal editors who had condemned the IEG functions wrote a letter to *Science* saying they were sorry that the IEGs were being disbanded, and that what they really meant was that the IEGs should have been modified, but continued. To date ours is the only group that has made an attempt to continue our communication system.

A committee was elected, which has negotiated with the American Institute for Biological Sciences, to operate an information exchange programme which would disseminate abstracts of work being prepared for publication, plus the tables and figures. In other words, the meat of the work would be sent, but not a full article, which is in agreement with what the biochemical journal editors will accept in the way of communication. The name of the Group has been changed to the "Interferon Scientific Memorandum". The idea was that each communication would be limited to eight pages, which would be photographed and reduced 50 per cent to reduce costs. The American Institute of Biological Sciences, a nonprofit making organization, has submitted a contract proposal to the NIH on these lines and hopefully expects this will be approved. We have had informal approval but we must go through all the fiscal people. The amount of the contract will be very small, no more than $12,000 (hopefully less) per year, which is considered to be cheap for the prevention of unnecessary duplication of research, which is expensive.

We have had many suggestions and have tried to incorporate almost all of these into the system. Incidentally, the vote to continue the IEG was overwhelming: 93 per cent of those replying voted to continue because they felt it was valuable, and something like 80 per cent of the membership replied, which I think is even more of a vote of confidence.

Stoker: Well, I am afraid our time is now up, and this anyway seems a good point on which to close. I am sure Alick Isaacs would have approved of our meeting and the spirit in which you have all participated. I hope that you have enjoyed yourselves as much as I have.

INDEX OF AUTHORS*

Numbers in bold type indicate a contribution in the form of a paper;
numbers in plain type refer to contributions to the discussions

* Indexes compiled by Mr William Hill.

INDEX OF SUBJECTS

Printed in England by Spottiswoode, Ballantyne & Co. Ltd., London and Colchester